CRASH COURSE

Infectious Diseases

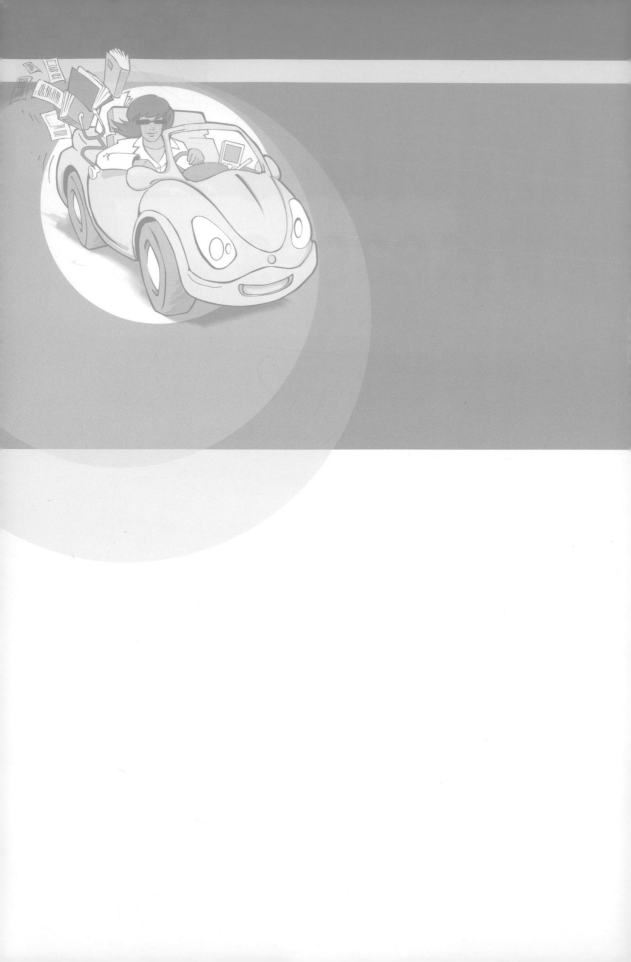

CRASH COURSE

Infectious Diseases

Series editor
Daniel Horton-Szar
BSC (Hons) MBBS (Hons) MRCGP
Northgate Medical Practice,
Canterbury

Faculty advisor
Christopher P. Conlon
MA MD FRCP
University Reader in Infectious
Diseases and Tropical Medicine,
University of Oxford,
Consultant Physician,
John Radcliffe Hospital,
Oxford

Emma Nickerson
MRCP
Senior House Officer on medical rotation,
Oxford Radcliffe Hospitals NHS Trust,
Oxford

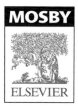

MOSBY

ELSEVIER

Edinburgh • London • New York • Oxford • Philadelphia • St Louis • Sydney • Toronto 2007

MOSBY
ELSEVIER

An imprint of Elsevier Limited

Commissioning Editor:	Fiona Conn/Alison Taylor
Development Editor:	Hannah Kenner
Project Manager:	Emma Riley
Designer:	Sarah Russell
Cover Designer:	Stewart Larking
Icon Illustrations:	Geo Parkin
Illustration Manager:	Gillian Richards
Illustrator:	Hardlines Studio

First published 2007

ISBN-13: 978-0-7234-3387-3

British Library Cataloguing in Publication Data
A catalogue record for this book is available from the British Library

Library of Congress Cataloging in Publication Data
A catalog record for this book is available from the Library of Congress

Notice
Knowledge and best practice in this field are constantly changing. As new research and experience broaden our knowledge, changes in practice, treatment and drug therapy may become necessary or appropriate. Readers are advised to check the most current information provided (i) on procedures featured or (ii) by the manufacturer of each product to be administered, to verify the recommended dose or formula, the method and duration of administration, and contraindications. It is the responsibility of the practitioner, relying on their own experience and knowledge of the patient, to make diagnoses, to determine dosages and the best treatment for each individual patient, and to take all appropriate safety precautions. To the fullest extent of the law, neither the Publisher nor the Authors assume any liability for any injury and/or damage to persons or property arising out or related to any use of the material contained in this book.

Printed in China

Preface

It can be a daunting prospect to learn about infectious diseases as a medical student and junior doctor – there is just so much to know! Too often there is that looming nightmare of rapidly approaching exams or the start of a new attachment when you realize you don't have the information you want at your fingertips. This book is written with that in mind: with its key points highlighted in tables, diagnostic algorithms and Hints and Tips boxes for quick and easy access; and multiple self-assessment questions to ensure you have grasped the essentials, in the varying formats you are likely to encounter.

I hope the very practical approach proves helpful, especially in the 'patient presents' section (Part 1) and Part 3 on taking a history, examining and investigating the patient with an infectious disease.

This is the book I wanted to have as I was attempting finals and my subsequent MRCP examinations so I hope you feel the same. Good luck!

Emma Nickerson

More than a decade has now passed since work began on the first titles of the Crash Course series, but medicine never stands still and the work of keeping this series relevant for today's students is an ongoing process. This title builds upon the success of the preceding books, keeping the series up to date with the latest medical research and developments in pharmacology and current best practice.

As always, we listen to feedback from the thousands of students who use Crash Course and have made further improvements to the layout and structure of the books. Each chapter now starts with a set of learning objectives, and the self-assessment sections have been enhanced and brought up to date with modern exam formats. We have also worked to integrate points of clinical relevance into the basic medical science material, which will not only add to the interest of the text but will reinforce the principles being described.

Despite fully revising the books, we hold fast to the principles on which we first developed the series: Crash Course will always bring you all the information you need to revise in compact, manageable volumes that integrate basic medical science and clinical practice. The books still maintain the balance between clarity and conciseness, and providing sufficient depth for those aiming at distinction. The authors are medical students and junior doctors who have recent experience of the exams you are now facing, and the accuracy of the material is checked by senior faculty members from across the UK.

I wish you all the best for your future careers!

Dr Dan Horton-Szar
Series Editor

Dedication

To my loving family.

Contents

Contents

Contents

THE PATIENT PRESENTS WITH

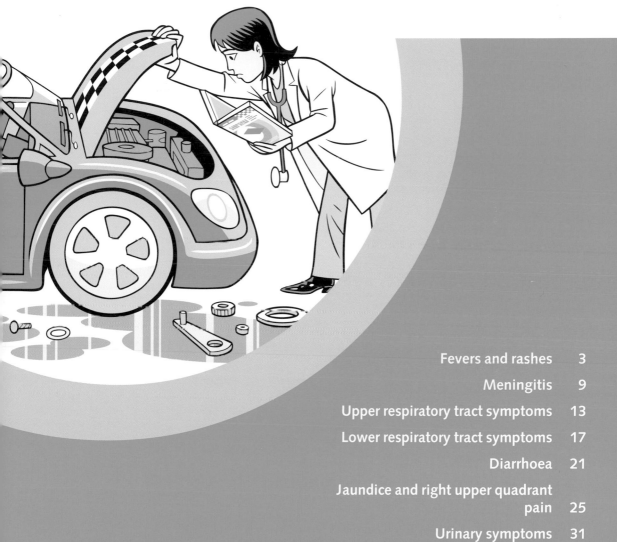

Fevers and rashes

Objectives

In this chapter you will learn:

- To recognize the childhood exanthemas
- Which childhood exanthemas can be immunized against
- What to look for when examining a rash
- Which infections may require radiographs as part of their investigation
- How to distinguish between measles and rubella.

The conditions covered in this chapter are the childhood exanthemas (see Fig. 1.1), as well as other infectious causes of a rash, where a fever can be part of the clinical picture (see Fig. 1.2).

Mumps cannot be included as a childhood exanthema because it does not involve a rash.

Drug reactions can produce a variety of skin rashes (see Fig. 1.3).

Almost all patients with infectious mononucleosis who are given ampicillin will develop a maculopapular rash as a result.

A *rash* is defined as an eruption on the skin, which is temporary. The appearance of a rash and its distribution is usually sufficient for diagnosis. If you do not recognize the rash then there is usually time to seek advice, the crucial exception is with purpura when in the case of meningococcal septicaemia a matter of minutes to hours delay can be life-threatening.

A *fever* is a body temperature greater than 37.2°C, with 36.9°C being the normal body temperature. It is important to record the actual temperature measured as not all illnesses can produce a high fever, e.g. greater than 39°C.

HISTORY

If someone presents with a rash you need to ask about the rash itself:

- Is there one single lesion or are there multiple ones?
- What areas of the body are involved? If more than one, what was the order of progression?
- Is the rash itchy?
- Does the rash involve mucosal surfaces such as the mouth or the conjunctiva?
- Has this ever occurred before?

In children the index of suspicion for a rash being one of the childhood exanthemas would be high, as these are common. Further questions to help elucidate the causative agent for a childhood exanthema would be:

- How old is the patient?
- Has the patient completed all the childhood immunizations, or what childhood illnesses has the patient already had? (See Fig. 1.5.)
- Have any of the patient's siblings/relatives or school friends/colleagues been complaining of similar symptoms?
- Does the patient have a sore throat, cough or sore red eyes?
- Does the patient have any associated joint pains?
- Does the patient feel miserable or have a fever?
- Does the patient work in a high-risk area, e.g. in a microbiology or research laboratory?

The MMR vaccination was only introduced in 1988; prior to that, girls received rubella aged 12 years.

In adults particularly, other considerations need to be borne in mind such as:

- Recent travel history
- Awareness of insect bites
- Other past medical history
- Changes in any medications including non-prescription items
- Associated symptoms, e.g. sore throat, cough, diarrhoea, meningitis, abdominal pain, weight loss, night sweats, chest pain, arthralgia, confusion.

EXAMINATION

When looking at someone's rash you need to be asking yourself:

- Is there one single lesion or are there multiple ones?
- What areas of the body are involved?

Fig. 1.1 Childhood exanthemas

Chickenpox
Measles
Rubella
Scarlet fever
Rheumatic fever
Erythema infectiosum

Fig. 1.2 Other infectious causes of a rash

Lyme disease	
Typhus	
Erythema multiforme	
with fever	Stevens–Johnson
without fever	Herpes
	Mycoplasma
	Orf
Erythema nodosum with fever	
(commonly)	Streptococcus
	Mycobacteria, e.g. leprosy, tuberculosis
(less commonly)	Leptospirosis
	Yersinia
	Viral infections
	Fungal infections
Purpura with fever	Meningococcal septicaemia
	Differential with haematological malignancies and possible neutropenic sepsis

- Are the affected areas in sun-exposed sites?
- What is the nature of the rash, e.g. macular/papular/vesicular/crusting/blistering? (See Fig. 1.6.)

Fig. 1.3 Examples of rashes caused by drugs

Rash	Causative drugs
Contact dermatitis (erythema around site of application)	Topical antibiotics, e.g. chloramphenicol, sulphonamides
Diffuse erythema	Penicillins
Erythema multiforme	Barbiturates, sulphonamides, penicillins
Erythema nodosum	Sulphonamides, oral contraceptive pill
Fixed drug reaction (patch of erythema recurs whenever drug given)	Tetracyclines, paracetamol
Blistering eruption	Barbiturates, sulphonamides, salicylates
Photosensitivity rash (rash in exposed areas)	Tetracyclines, sulphonamides, amiodarone
Stevens–Johnson syndrome (erythema multiforme with vesicles involving the mucosae, e.g. mouth, conjunctivae)	Sulphonamides, penicillins
Anaphylaxis	Penicillins
Erythroderma (whole body erythema)	Sulphonamides, gold
Toxic epidermal necrolysis (erythema, blistering and loss of epidermis) (see Fig. 1.4)	Penicillins, sulphonamides, barbiturates

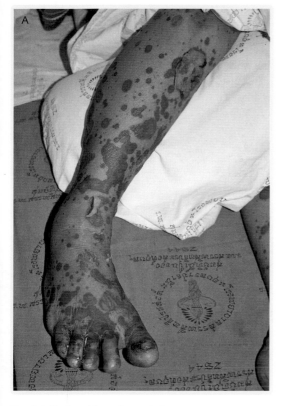 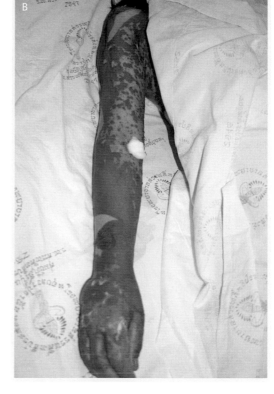

Fig. 1.4 Toxic epidermal necrolysis.

Fig. 1.5 Childhood vaccination programme	
2, 3 and 4 months	Diphtheria, tetanus, pertussis (DTP) Polio *Haemophilus influenzae* type b (Hib) Meningococcal group C (Men C)* Pneumococcal (PCV)**
12–15 months	Measles, mumps, rubella (MMR) *Haemophilus influenzae* type b (Hib) Meningococcal group C (Men C) Pneumococcal (PCV)
3–5 years (pre-school)	Diphtheria, tetanus, pertussis (DTP) Polio Measles, mumps, rubella (MMR)
13–18 years (school leavers)	Diphtheria, tetanus Polio

Meningococcal group C given in months 3 and 4
**Pneumococcal given in months 2 and 4*

- Is there a clear demarcation of the lesions or is the border indistinct?
- Do the lesions vary in size?
- Is there normal skin between the lesions?
- Is the rash itchy, e.g. can you see scratch marks?

- Is there mucosal or conjunctival involvement?
- Is there any skin loss?

There may also be additional signs on examination that are associated with rashes and fevers, as shown in Figure 1.7.

INVESTIGATIONS

Many of the childhood exanthemas do not require diagnostic tests; they are identified clinically. In certain cases it may be important to confirm the clinical diagnosis with:

- Serology
- Viral culture or PCR (polymerase chain reaction) of vesicular fluid.

In some cases there may be a concern about the underlying cause for the infection, or the causative agent is not immediately apparent and blood tests are necessary:

- Full blood count – check for neutropenia as a predisposition to infection. Viral infections give

Fig. 1.6 Terms used to describe rashes with their meanings and examples

Terms	Description	Examples
Macular	Erythema, not raised	Rubella, scarlet fever
Maculopapular	Erythema, raised	Measles, erythema infectiosum, drug reaction
Vesicular	Small fluid-filled blisters	Chickenpox
Purpura	Dark, purplish, non-blanching	Meningococcus, thrombocytopenia
Eschar	Single, black, crusted ulcer	Typhus
Target lesions	Ring of erythema with central erythema spot but clear area between the two	Erythema multiforme
Erythema nodosum	Raised red lesions on shins	Erythema nodosum
'Slapped cheeks'	Erythema across cheeks	Erythema infectiosum
Erythema chronicum migrans	Red area around bite with definite margin	Lyme disease
Erythema marginatum	Pink coalescent rings	Rheumatic fever
Bullae	Tense blisters	Drug reaction
Koplik spots	Grains of salt on red background in the mouth	Measles
Pruritus	Itchy lesions	Chickenpox, erythema infectiosum
Dermatomal	Rash in distribution of dermatome	Shingles

rise to a leucocytosis, usually lymphocytosis, whereas bacterial infections produce a neutrophilia. Thrombocytopenia can be detected which may have given rise to purpura.

- Blood film – may identify a haematological malignancy which led to impaired immunity or thrombocytopenia.
- Blood cultures – to isolate the infective cause of sepsis.
- Cerebrospinal fluid (CSF) examination – to detect *Neisseria meningitidis* or meningitis complicating Lyme disease or mumps. For the interpretation of results see Chapter 2.
- Throat swab for culture of *Streptococcus pyogenes*.

Imaging may be required in particular infections to check for complications, such as:

- Chest radiograph for pneumonitis in chickenpox infection
- Joint radiographs in rheumatic fever.

Cardiac investigations are necessary when Lyme disease and rheumatic fever have been diagnosed:

- Electrocardiogram (ECG) – to check the PR interval and to identify complete heart block in Lyme disease as both first- and third-degree heart block are complications.
- Echocardiogram (Echo) – to look for pericardial and myocardial involvement in rheumatic fever.

A summary algorithm demonstrating how to approach diagnosing the cause of a rash is shown in Figure 1.8.

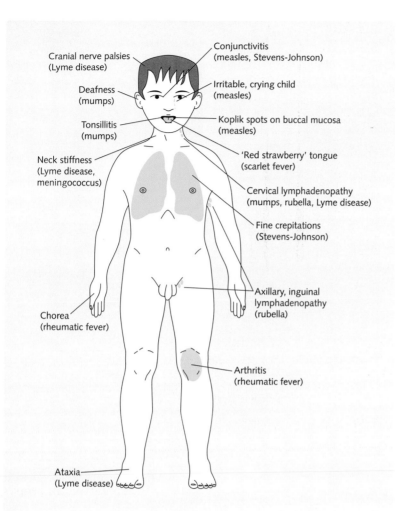

Cranial nerve palsies
(Lyme disease)

Conjunctivitis
(measles, Stevens-Johnson)

Deafness
(mumps)

Irritable, crying child
(measles)

Tonsillitis
(mumps)

Koplik spots on buccal mucosa
(measles)

Neck stiffness
(Lyme disease,
meningococcus)

'Red strawberry' tongue
(scarlet fever)

Cervical lymphadenopathy
(mumps, rubella, Lyme disease)

Fine crepitations
(Stevens-Johnson)

Chorea
(rheumatic fever)

Axillary, inguinal
lymphadenopathy
(rubella)

Arthritis
(rheumatic fever)

Ataxia
(Lyme disease)

Fig. 1.7 Examination findings associated with fevers and rashes (shown on body map).

Fig. 1.8 Diagnostic algorithm for rashes. * Sick, irritable child.

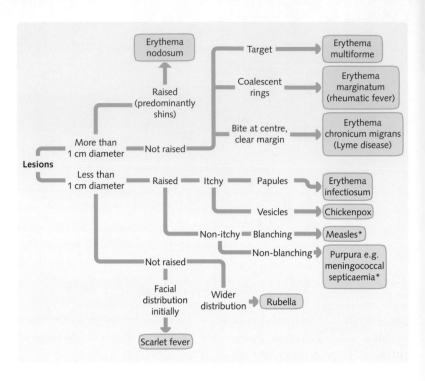

In this chapter you will learn:

- The triad of symptoms that indicates meningitis
- How to differentiate between meningitis and encephalitis at the bedside
- How to calculate the Glasgow Coma Score (GCS), e.g. for a patient who opens their eyes, withdraws their limbs and grunts when a painful stimulus is applied
- The CSF findings in bacterial meningitis
- The investigations that would be appropriate for a patient with a purpuric rash and meningitis.

Meningitis is a symptom triad of headache, neck stiffness and photophobia. It indicates that there is inflammation of the meninges, the triple layer of membranes overlying the brain and extending down the spinal cord. The causes of meningitis can be:

- Bacterial, e.g. pneumococcus, meningococcus, *Haemophilus influenzae* type b, tuberculosis
- Viral, e.g. enteroviruses, herpes simplex virus, mumps
- Fungal, e.g. cryptococcus, candida.

The most important infective differential diagnosis is encephalitis, usually caused by herpes simplex virus (HSV). The distinguishing factor clinically is that encephalitis usually results in an altered level of consciousness and focal neurological signs whereas meningitis does not, although the two can coexist.

HISTORY

The aim of the history is twofold: first to confirm that the triad of meningitis is present and secondly to ascertain the most likely causative agent. If the symptoms were rapid in onset and are more severe, a bacterial cause is more likely, whereas a more insidious onset with a flu-like illness initially and less severe symptoms makes a viral aetiology more likely. The age of the patient is significant, as neonates, children and adults have a different causative profile (see Ch. 15). Immunocompromised patients and pregnant women may have more unusual organisms causing meningitis, e.g. *Listeria monocytogenes*. A

contact history is very useful to obtain as this may identify an outbreak of meningitis cases.

You must ask specifically about a rash associated with the meningitis and whether this blanches or not, as purpura occurs with meningococcal meningitis. If a patient has a purpuric rash without neck stiffness then this may represent meningococcal septicaemia. Both cases warrant immediate treatment with antibiotics.

It is important to assess the neurological status, in particular asking if there has been any cognitive impairment, mood changes, drowsiness, fitting or focal signs, such as limb weakness or speech involvement, as these features would make encephalitis a more likely diagnosis.

EXAMINATION

An overall assessment of the patient needs to be made rapidly, checking for a purpuric rash; signs of shock, e.g. tachycardia, hypotension; and the Glasgow Coma Score (GCS; see Fig. 2.1). If these are present or there is a depressed GCS then urgent medical therapy is required and senior team involvement.

To assess if there is neck stiffness ask the patient to touch their chest with their chin; if the patient is unable to do this then attempt to perform this movement passively. Kernig's sign should be tested also, looking for meningitis (see Fig. 2.2).

Fig. 2.1 Glasgow Coma Score

Score	Eye opening	Best verbal response	Best motor response
1	No response	No response	No response
2	Open to pain	Non-verbal sounds	Extensor posture to pain
3	Open to command	Inappropriate words	Flexor response to pain
4	Open spontaneously	Confused speech	Withdraws to pain
5		Orientated	Localizes to pain
6			Obeys command

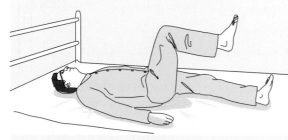

1. Patient lies on bed with one hip and knee flexed.

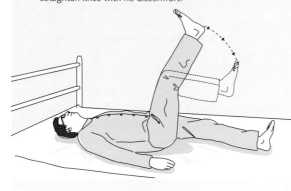

2. Examiner helps patient to straighten knee while the hip is kept flexed. Positive result if pain in neck results from straightening knee. Negative result if patient able to straighten knee with no discomfort.

Fig. 2.2 How to test for Kernig's sign.

A central and peripheral neurological examination must be performed to check for focal neurological signs.

INVESTIGATIONS

The mainstay of diagnosing meningitis and its causative organism is a lumbar puncture for cerebrospinal fluid (CSF) examination (see Fig. 2.3).

A lumbar puncture is contraindicated when:

- There are signs of raised intracranial pressure, e.g. papilloedema, focal neurological signs, reduced consciousness, falling pulse and rising BP
- There is a serious coagulation defect
- There is an infection at the site of needle insertion.

In viral encephalitis the CSF results are similar to those of viral meningitis. During microscopy of the CSF, the identification of the causative organism with Gram staining may be possible. Fungal hyphae can be seen in fungal cases. The CSF will also be cultured so

Fig. 2.3 CSF results distinguishing normal, bacterial, TB, viral and fungal causes of meningitis

	Normal	Bacterial	Tuberculosis	Viral	Fungal
Appearance	Clear colourless	Turbid	Viscous, turbid	Clear	Viscous, clear
WCC (per mm³)	0–5	500–10 000 polymorphs	< 500 lymphocytes/ polymorphs	< 1000 lymphocytes	< 500 lymphocytes/ polymorphs
Glucose	> 2/3 blood glucose	Very low	Low	Normal	Low
Protein (g/l)	0.15–0.4	High	Very high	Raised	Very high

that the organism can be confirmed and antibiotic sensitivities checked. PCR (polymerase chain reaction) may be performed to check for *Neisseria meningitidis, Streptococcus pneumoniae* or herpes simplex virus.

The other tests performed for meningitis are:

- Blood cultures – to identify bacterial causes
- Serology – to identify viral causes
- Throat swab for *Neisseria meningitidis, Streptococcus pneumoniae*
- PCR on blood for *Neisseria meningitidis*.

Other tests for encephalitis are:

- CSF and blood serology
- CT or MRI scan – shows diffuse oedema, especially in the temporal lobes, and may be used to exclude other causes of focal neurological changes
- Electroencephalogram (EEG) – to show slow wave changes typical of encephalitis.

A summary algorithm demonstrating how to approach a patient with suspected meningitis is shown in Figure 2.4.

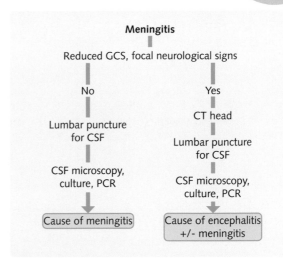

Fig. 2.4 Diagnostic algorithm for meningitis.

Upper respiratory tract symptoms

In this chapter you will learn:

- What bacteria can cause an upper respiratory tract infection
- Which infections give rise to a tonsillar exudate
- The symptoms that suggest the development of otitis media
- Where the 'cervical' lymph nodes are to be found
- How to distinguish between glandular fever and streptococcal pharyngitis.

The upper respiratory tract extends from the point of entry at either the nostrils or the oral cavity down to the trachea. Predominantly viral and bacterial infections affect this tract, ranging from minor infections such as the common cold (viral) and non-specific upper respiratory tract viral illnesses in children to more serious infections:

- Viral:
  - Croup (viral laryngotracheobronchiolitis)
  - Influenza (influenza A and B viruses)
  - Glandular fever (Epstein–Barr virus)
- Bacterial:
  - Epiglottitis (*Haemophilus influenzae* type b)
  - Whooping cough (*Bordetella pertussis*)
  - Streptococcal pharyngitis (*Streptococcus pyogenes*)
  - Diphtheria (*Corynebacterium diphtheriae*).

Upper respiratory tract infections can progress to cause otitis media if the Eustachian tube becomes blocked, or sinusitis should one or more of the sinus cavities be unable to drain.

HISTORY

Upper respiratory tract infections typically commence with coryza, i.e. a running nose and sneezing. The other features are shown in Figure 3.1:

If you suspect epiglottitis then keep the child calm, and only someone able to intubate should examine the child, because airway obstruction may occur.

Symptoms suggestive of otitis media should be specifically enquired about:

- Earache
- Impaired hearing
- Difficulty equalizing pressure in the ears

and those implying there is sinusitis:

- Feeling of pressure, fullness or pain over the sinus areas.

EXAMINATION

The examination involves:

- Tonsils – look for enlargement, exudate and a false membrane.
- Sinuses – press over the sinus areas to assess for tenderness (see Fig. 3.2).
- Ears – view the outer ear and then using an otoscope note the appearance of the eardrum, specifically looking for a fluid level behind the drum and drum perforation.
- Cervical lymphadenopathy – examine for enlarged lymph nodes (see Fig. 3.3) and if present comment on their size, mobility and texture.

INVESTIGATIONS

- Haematology – a raised white cell count is a non-specific finding in any infection: neutrophilia with bacterial infections and lymphocytosis in viral infections. Atypical lymphocytes suggest

Fig. 3.1 Symptoms associated with upper respiratory tract infections

	Common cold	Childhood viral URTI	Croup	Influenza	Glandular fever	Epiglottitis	Whooping cough	Strep. pharyngitis	Diphtheria
Fever	–	+	+	+	+	+	±	+	–
Malaise	+	+	–	+	+	–	+	+	–
Sore throat	–	–	+	+	+	+	+	+	+
Tonsillar enlargement ± exudate	–	–	–	–	+ Exudate	–	–	+ Exudate	+ Exudate
Cervical LN	–	–	–	–	+	–	–	+	+
Respiratory distress ± stridor	–	–	+ Stridor	–	–	+ Stridor	+ Stridor	–	–
Cough	–	+	Bovine	+	–	–	Whoop	–	–
Rash (viral exanthema)	–	±	–	–	–	–	–	–	–

+ present; – absent; LN, lymphadenopathy

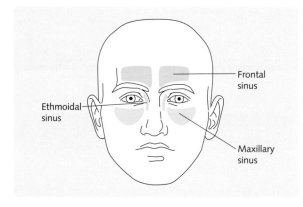

Fig. 3.2 Sinus locations.

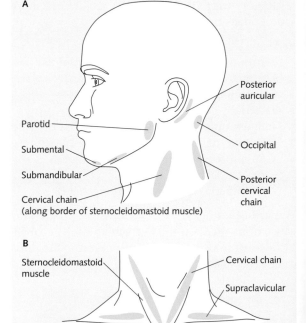

Fig. 3.3 Location of lymph nodes.

glandular fever. A monospot or Paul–Bunnell test detects glandular fever.

- Biochemistry – raised CRP (C-reactive protein) occurs in infection. Deranged liver function tests with a hepatitic pattern, i.e. AST (aspartate transaminase) and ALT (alanine transaminase) raised most prominently, are seen in glandular fever.
- Microbiology – throat swabs for *Haemophilus influenzae* type b, *Streptococcus pyogenes* and *Corynebacterium diphtheriae*, and nasopharyngeal swabs for *Bordetella pertussis* should be taken. Blood cultures may isolate *Haemophilus influenzae* type b and *Streptococcus pyogenes*, and cultures of discharging fluid from the ear can be taken for otitis media. Although it is possible to test serology to identify the viral cause of the common cold, croup or influenza, the cost of this cannot usually be justified as it does not affect the management of the condition.

- Imaging – by means of plain radiographs or an MRI scan of the sinuses, may be useful in sinusitis as it demonstrates the fluid-filled cavities.

A summary algorithm demonstrating how to approach the diagnosis of the cause of an upper respiratory tract infection is shown in Figure 3.4.

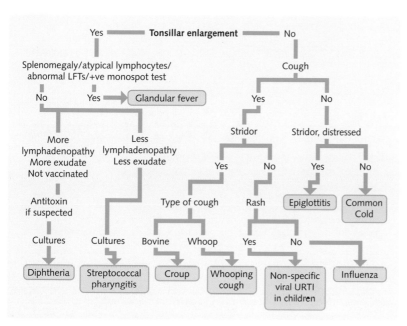

Fig. 3.4 Diagnostic algorithm for upper respiratory tract symptoms. LN, lymphadenopathy.

Lower respiratory tract symptoms

Objectives

In this chapter you will learn:

- Which are the atypical pneumonias
- What defines a hospital-acquired infection
- The symptoms that are associated with pneumonia
- The signs you can pick up from examining the chest in someone with lobar pneumonia
- How the severity of a pneumonia is assessed.

The lower respiratory tract is distal to the trachea, involving bronchi, bronchioles and alveolar air spaces. The majority of infections that present to the hospital setting are bacterial. The organism responsible varies depending whether the infection was acquired in the community or in hospital.

Community-acquired bacterial infections:

- *Streptococcus pneumoniae*
- *Haemophilus influenzae* } typical pneumonia
- *Klebsiella pneumoniae*
- *Staphylococcus aureus* (rare)
- *Mycoplasma pneumoniae*
- *Legionella pneumophila*
- *Chlamydia pneumoniae* } atypical pneumonias
- *Chlamydia psittaci*
- *Coxiella burnetii*

- *Mycobacterium tuberculosis*.

Community-acquired viral infections:

- Influenza viruses.

Hospital-acquired infections:

- *Haemophilus influenzae*
- *Escherichia coli*
- *Klebsiella pneumoniae*
- *Serratia* species
- *Pseudomonas aeruginosa*
- *Staphylococcus aureus*.

For lower respiratory tract infections in immuno-compromised patients, see Chapter 25.

HISTORY

The symptoms suggestive of a lower respiratory tract infection need to be clarified:

- Fever, rigors
- Productive cough and the colour and volume of the sputum
- Haemoptysis (coughing up blood)
- Pleuritic chest pain
- Night sweats, malaise
- Confusion in the elderly.

Beware that bleeding gums can blood-stain the saliva and when patients spit out phlegm and saliva together they consider that they are coughing up blood.

The history should also attempt to elucidate the most likely culprit organisms for the infection. A significant differentiating factor is where the infection was acquired, either in the community or in hospital, which is defined as 2 or more days after admission. The patient's place of work may be relevant, e.g. air conditioning in an office for legionella infection, coal mining leads to an increased risk of COPD (chronic obstructive pulmonary disease), farm workers for coxiella infections. People who keep birds, especially parrots, are at an increased risk of contracting a pneumonia due to *Chlamydia psittaci* and so one should enquire about pets and hobbies. A recent travel history is important as different antibiotic resistance patterns are seen, e.g. penicillin-resistant pneumococcus in Spain, and air-conditioning is more commonplace in humid countries. Any contact with tuberculosis either abroad or at home ought to be noted and infection excluded.

Patients will be susceptible to respiratory tract infections if they have an underlying respiratory condition such as asthma, cystic fibrosis, COPD or a reduced ability to expand the chest, e.g. severe kyphoscoliosis or myasthenia gravis. Other groups will be more prone to aspiration pneumonia, e.g. following a stroke when the gag reflex is impaired or in alcoholics who induce a reduced level of consciousness.

EXAMINATION

On approaching the patient there may be a number of clues around the bedside, e.g. inhalers or a peak expiratory flow meter indicating asthma or COPD. From taking the history it may be apparent that the patient is confused and an Abbreviated Mental Test Score (see Fig. 4.1) can give a rough quantification of this, which is useful to monitor.

On inspection, note if the patient is tachypnoeic (increased rate of breathing), dyspnoeic (distressed or difficulty breathing) or using accessory muscles of respiration and whether the patient appears cachectic. Also look for nicotine-stained fingers, clubbing and peripheral (fingers) and central (lips and under tongue) cyanosis. Check the shins for erythema nodosum.

Fig. 4.1 Abbreviated Mental Test Score

1. How old are you?
2. What is your date of birth?
3. What time of day is it (to nearest hour)?
4. What is the year?
5. Name the hospital you are in.
6. Can you recognize two people nearby, e.g. doctor, nurse?
   Please remember the following address: 42 West Street (check immediate recall).
7. Count backwards from 20 to 1.
8. What was the address I asked you to remember?
9. Who is the current Prime Minister?
10. When did the First World War start?

Scoring:
1 point for each question to give score out of 10
A score ≤ 8 indicates confusion

On respiratory examination, check for lymphadenopathy, the position of the trachea and any scars over the chest wall indicating surgery or chest drain placement (usually mid-axillary line). Observe if there is any asymmetry of chest wall movement on expansion, percuss for dullness and listen for crepitations, bronchial breathing, pleural rub, reduced or absent breath sounds. To complete the examination, look at the temperature chart to see the height and pattern of the temperature and check the sputum pot.

INVESTIGATIONS

- Peak flow (if asthmatic) – to give a guide as to the severity of the exacerbation: < 50% of normal/predicted PEFR (peak expiratory flow rate) is severe and < 25% of normal/predicted PEFR is life-threatening.
- Arterial blood gas (ABG) – to guide oxygen therapy, aiming to maintain the P_aO_2 > 10 kPa. A P_aO_2 ≤ 8 kPa is one of the markers of severity for a community-acquired pneumonia. The P_aCO_2 reflects the rate of breathing (rapid respirations blow off CO_2) and is especially important in treating patients with either asthma or COPD.
- Chest radiograph – look for lobar/patchy consolidation, cavities, hyperexpanded lung fields, hilar lymphadenopathy, raised or flattened hemidiaphragms. Those features seen in patients with an infective exacerbation of COPD are shown in Figure 4.2.
- Haematology – raised white cell count (WCC), WCC differential showing neutrophilia in a bacterial infection.
- Blood film – red blood cell agglutination suggests *Mycoplasma pneumoniae* infection.

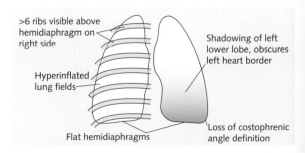

Fig. 4.2 Infective exacerbation of COPD, on a chest radiograph diagram.

- Biochemistry – raised CRP (C-reactive protein) indicating infection; raised urea and low albumin are severity markers; low sodium and abnormal liver function tests (LFTs) suggest an atypical pneumonia.
- Sputum microscopy and cultures – to identify the organism responsible.
- Bronchoalveolar lavage/gastric lavage specimens for microscopy and culture – to attempt to isolate *Mycobacterium tuberculosis*.
- Blood cultures – to identify the organism responsible, as sputum cultures have a poor detection rate.
- Urinary legionella antigen – rapid way of diagnosing legionella infection.
- Serology – acute and convalescent titres to identify the atypical pneumonias.
- Skin testing for tuberculosis – Mantoux testing (see Ch. 26).

Capillary blood gas testing, e.g. from pinprick to ear lobe, can be used to monitor oxygen therapy in patients with COPD, which reduces the requirement for multiple, more painful arterial stabs.

SEVERITY SCORING

The British Thoracic Society have devised a 5-point score to identify those patients at an increased risk of death or requiring an intensive care unit (ITU) admission (see Fig. 4.3).

Fig. 4.3 CURB-65 severity scoring

The **CURB-65** is determined as follows:
- **C**onfusion (assessed by Abbreviated Mental Test Score)
- **U**rea > 7 mmol/l
- **R**espiratory rate ≥ 30 breaths/minute
- **B**P with systolic < 90 mmHg and/or diastolic < 60 mmHg
- Age ≥ **65** years

A score of:
≤1 indicates low risk, possibly suitable for home treatment
 2 indicates increased risk, requiring in-hospital care
≥3 is severe pneumonia, with increased risk, e.g. score 3 gives 17% risk of death/ITU and score 5 is a 57% risk of death/ITU

There are other markers of severity in community-acquired pneumonia which may influence decisions made on the management of lower CURB-65 scoring cases, for instance someone who scored 1 but possessed a number of the other severity markers would be less suitable for treatment at home. These are:

- Clinical:
  - Underlying disease
  - Atrial fibrillation
  - Multilobar involvement
- Laboratory:
  - Serum albumin < 35 g/l
  - Hypoxia $P_aO_2 \leq 8$ kPa
  - Leucopenia < 4×10^9/l
  - Leucocytosis > 20×10^9/l.

A summary algorithm demonstrating how to approach managing a patient with a lower respiratory tract infection is shown in Figure 4.4.

Fig. 4.4 Diagnostic algorithm for lower respiratory tract symptoms.

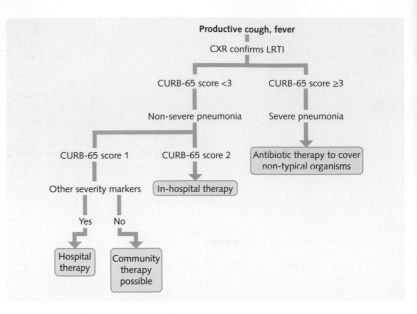

Objectives

In this chapter you will learn:

- The differential diagnosis of acute diarrhoea
- The factors from the history that would raise the suspicion of an infective aetiology for an episode of diarrhoea
- What biochemical abnormalities occur with severe diarrhoea
- The differential diagnosis for a dilated colon.

Diarrhoea is an increased frequency and volume of stool passed. It is defined as > 300 g of loose stool passed in 24 hours. Diarrhoea is extremely common and most people will experience it during their lifetime. The nature of the diarrhoea reflects the origin of the problem: watery diarrhoea comes from the small bowel, whereas bloody diarrhoea results from an inflamed large bowel.

Food poisoning relates to diarrhoea and/or vomiting resulting from the ingestion of infected foodstuffs. This may be toxin-related, e.g. *Staphylococcus aureus*, *Escherichia coli* (enterotoxigenic; ETEC), or due to bacteria, e.g. *Bacillus cereus*, *Salmonella enteritidis*.

The differential diagnoses for acute and chronic diarrhoea are shown in Figures 5.1 and 5.2 respectively.

HISTORY

Pointers in the history that suggest an infective cause of diarrhoea are:

- Sudden onset
- Suspicious or different food eaten
- Other people affected and whether they ate the same food (i.e. an outbreak)
- Associated with or preceded by vomiting
- Recent travel history.

In order to work out the most likely organism causing the diarrhoea, it is important to clarify the following information:

- Whether the diarrhoea is watery or bloody in nature

- How long the patient has had diarrhoea
- If there were any preceding symptoms
- If there is associated abdominal pain or vomiting
- Whether the patient has received broad-spectrum antibiotic treatment recently.

The causes of food poisoning are outlined in Figure 5.3.

EXAMINATION

On inspection, does the patient look dehydrated: in particular note the skin turgor and mucous membranes; and if more severe, whether the patient is tachycardic or hypotensive.

Young people compensate for shock well, only manifesting hypotension when there has been profound fluid loss. A more sensitive sign is postural hypotension.

Make a note of any scars on the abdomen from previous surgery which may have resulted in blind loops of bowel where bacterial overgrowth could occur. On abdominal examination, palpate for masses and abdominal tenderness; frank peritonism reflects colitis progressing to toxic dilatation of the colon, which is rare.

On digital rectal examination, check for faecal impaction leading to overflow diarrhoea, for any masses and observe the colour of any stool on the glove and whether blood or mucus is present. To finish, look at the temperature chart for fevers.

Fig. 5.1 Acute diarrhoea

Watery	Bloody
Change in diet	Shigella (late disease)
Food poisoning, e.g. *Staph.*	Salmonella
aureus, ETEC, *Bacillus*	Campylobacter
cereus, shigella (early	*Escherichia coli* (EHEC, EIEC)
disease), *Clostridium*	*Entamoeba histolytica*
perfringens, *Yersinia*	
enterocolitica	
Cholera	
Rotavirus	
Other viruses, e.g. astro-	
viruses, small round viruses	

Toxic megacolon usually occurs in ulcerative colitis and Crohn's disease but can be seen in infective colitis, e.g. with salmonella or campylobacter.

Any masses felt should be investigated further as there may be pathology underlying the diarrhoea, e.g. colonic carcinoma, or the infective diarrhoeal illness was merely coincidental.

Fig. 5.2 Chronic diarrhoea

Watery	Steatorrhoea	Bloody
Parasites, e.g. *Cryptosporidium*	Giardia	Pseudomembranous colitis
parvum, *Isospora belli*	Tropical sprue	(from *Clostridium difficile*)
Clostridium difficile	Coeliac disease	Inflammatory bowel disease
Inflammatory bowel disease	Cystic fibrosis	Colonic carcinoma
Colonic carcinoma	Crohn's disease	Radiation colitis
Thyrotoxicosis	Chronic pancreatitis	
Laxative abuse	Pancreatic	
Pancreatic carcinomas, e.g.	carcinoma	
gastrinoma, VIPoma		
VIP, vasoactive intestinal peptide		

Fig. 5.3 Causes of food poisoning

Organism	Source	Incubation period	Associated symptoms	Recovery
Staphylococcus aureus	Enterotoxins in canned food, processed meats, milk, cheese	2–6 hours	Vomiting and abdominal discomfort	12–24 hours
E. coli 0157:H7	Undercooked beef, raw cow's milk	12–48 hours	Haemorrhagic colitis	10–12 days
Bacillus cereus	Spores in food esp. rice	1–6 hours	Vomiting	Rapid
Clostridium perfringens	Spores in food survive boiling	8–22 hours	Cramping pain	2–3 days
Clostridium botulinum	Spores survive cooking, need anaerobic conditions, e.g. canned/bottled food	18–36 hours	Paralysis from neuromuscular blockade	10–14 days
Salmonella species	Undercooked meat esp. chicken	12–24 hours	Vomiting, fever	2–5 days
Campylobacter jejuni	Undercooked meat esp. chicken; milk	48–96 hours	Fever, malaise, abdominal pain	3–5 days
Shigella species	Contaminated food, some strains have spores	28 hours	Fever, malaise, abdominal pain, tenesmus	Few days

Source: Kumar P, Clark M. Clinical Medicine, 4th edn. Edinburgh: Saunders; 1998: Table 1.21

INVESTIGATIONS

- Haematology – raised WCC (white cell count) with infection; lowered haemoglobin if marked blood loss in diarrhoea.
- Biochemistry – raised CRP (C-reactive protein) with infection; low potassium, sodium and chloride if severe diarrhoea, and raised urea if dehydrated.

- Stool microscopy and culture – to identify causative agent.
- Blood cultures – to identify the causative bacteria.
- Plain abdominal radiograph – check for dilated colon.

A summary algorithm demonstrating how to approach diagnosing the infectious causes of diarrhoea is shown in Figure 5.4.

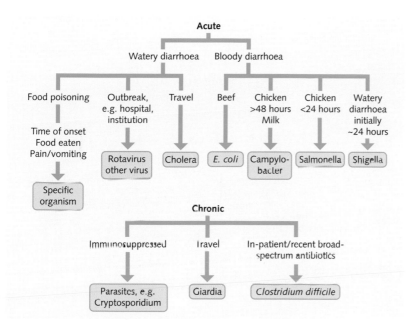

Fig. 5.4 Diagnostic algorithm for infective diarrhoea.

Jaundice and right upper quadrant pain

Objectives

In this chapter you will learn:

- Which infections can result in jaundice
- The risk factors for hepatitis C infection
- What the presence of HBsAg, anti-HBc IgG and HBeAg indicate
- Which investigations give a more accurate assessment of liver damage
- Which infections of the liver can give rise to right upper quadrant pain
- What signs there are at the bedside in acute cholecystitis.

JAUNDICE

Jaundice describes the yellow colouring of the skin and sclerae due to an elevated bilirubin level in the blood. To be clinically detectable the bilirubin needs to exceed 35 µmol/l. Jaundice can be prehepatic, hepatic or posthepatic in origin (see Fig. 6.1).

The infections to consider in a jaundiced patient include:

- Viral hepatitis: A, B, C, D and E
- Epstein–Barr virus (EBV)
- Cytomegalovirus (CMV)
- Leptospirosis
- Toxoplasmosis
- Hydatid disease

Fig. 6.1 Causes of jaundice

Prehepatic	Haemolysis
	Abnormal erythropoiesis
	Gilbert's syndrome (conjugation enzyme defect)
Hepatic	Drugs, e.g. rifampicin, erythromycin
	Alcohol
	Infections, e.g. viral hepatitis, Epstein–Barr virus, cytomegalovirus
	Cirrhosis, e.g. from Wilson's disease
	Chronic liver disease, e.g. chronic hepatitis C virus infection
Posthepatic	Intrahepatic obstruction, e.g. primary biliary cirrhosis, primary sclerosing cholangitis
	Extrahepatic obstruction, e.g. cancer of pancreatic head, gallstones

- Tropical infections, e.g. malaria, typhoid, dengue fever and yellow fever (see Ch. 24).

History

The aspects of the history which point towards an infective cause for jaundice are:

- An acute onset of symptoms
- Associated diarrhoea and vomiting, e.g. with hepatitis A and E
- Associated fever and lymphadenopathy, e.g. with EBV, CMV, toxoplasmosis
- Associated myositis and conjunctivitis, e.g. with leptospirosis
- Associated rash, e.g. with toxoplasmosis, leptospirosis.

A broad range of questions need to be asked, particularly covering lifestyle issues to differentiate between the potential infective causes of jaundice, as shown in Figure 6.2.

HIV can be contracted via the same risk factors as for hepatitis B and C, i.e. sexually, vertically and via blood products, so those identified as at risk should be encouraged to undergo HIV testing in addition.

A number of drugs used to treat infections can in themselves cause jaundice:

- Antituberculous agents: rifampicin, isoniazid, pyrazinamide

- Antibacterial agents: flucloxacillin, co-amoxiclav, erythromycin, cephalosporins
- Antifungal agents: fluconazole, itraconazole.

Examination

Inspection of the patient is a large part of the examination for jaundice. Beyond looking for a yellow discoloration of the skin and sclerae, check for the peripheral stigmata of chronic liver disease, i.e. gynaecomastia, scratch marks, purpura, spider naevi in the drainage area of the superior vena cava (> 5 is significant); palmar erythema, Dupuytren's contracture, clubbing and leuconychia on the hands. The presence of these signs indicates that the liver is cirrhotic, which from the viewpoint of infection could only result from chronic hepatitis B or C.

A maculopapular rash can be seen with CMV or EBV (if a sore throat is treated with ampicillin before a diagnosis is made). Conjunctivitis would raise the suspicion of leptospirosis. Cervical lymphadenopathy is found in EBV, CMV and toxoplasmosis infections.

On abdominal examination palpate all four quadrants for tenderness and masses, then moving from the right iliac fossa feel superiorly for hepatomegaly and diagonally to the left upper quadrant for splenomegaly. Testing for shifting dullness and a fluid thrill would elicit ascites, which may reflect a cirrhotic liver.

If there is a suspicion of toxoplasmosis then check for neurological signs, and if considering CMV infection then check for retinitis with a fundoscope.

Investigations

- The hepatitis viruses can be detected with serology:
  - Hepatitis A: IgM anti-HAV
  - Hepatitis B (see Fig. 6.3 and Fig. 19.2)
  - Hepatitis C: anti-HCV, viral RNA PCR
  - Hepatitis D: anti-HDV, HDV Ag
  - Hepatitis E: anti-HEV.
- Serology can also be checked for EBV, CMV, *Toxoplasma gondii*, *Leptospira interrogans* and *Echinococcus granulosus*.
- Full blood count – eosinophilia is typically seen in hydatid disease.
- Blood film – looking for the atypical lymphocytes of EBV infection.
- Monospot test – specifically for EBV.
- Blood cultures – to isolate *Leptospira interrogans*.

Fig. 6.2 Risk factors for infective causes of jaundice

Risk factor	Infection
Seafood consumption	Hepatitis A and E
Outbreak (e.g. food poisoning)	Hepatitis A and E, toxoplasmosis
Travel history	Hepatitis A and E, malaria, yellow fever, typhoid, dengue fever
Job/hobby/travel involving water contact	Leptospirosis
Intravenous drug abuse (previous or current)	Hepatitis B and C
Sexual history	Hepatitis B and C, cytomegalovirus
Prolonged symptoms over months	Hepatitis B and C
Kissing contact, especially as young adult	Epstein–Barr virus
Recipient of blood products pre-1990	Hepatitis C
Transplant recipient/ immunosuppression	Cytomegalovirus
Animal contact	Hydatid disease

Fig. 6.3 Hepatitis B serology results

	HBsAg	Anti-HBs	Anti-HBc IgM	Anti-HBc IgG	HBeAg	Anti-HBe	HBV DNA
Acute infection (early)	+	−	+	−	+	−	+
Acute infection (later)	+	±	+	+	±	+	+
Post-infection	−	+	−	+	−	−	−
Chronic infection (low infectivity)	+	−	−	+	−	+	±
Chronic infection (high infectivity)	+	−	−	+	+	−	+
HBV vaccination	−	+	−	−	−	−	−

HBsAg, hepatitis B surface antigen; HBc, hepatitis B core protein; HBeAg, hepatitis B e antigen

- Urine cultures – to isolate *Leptospira interrogans*.
- Liver function tests, conjugated and unconjugated bilirubin – to confirm a hepatitic cause for the jaundice and exclude other non-infectious differential diagnoses.
- Liver synthetic function, i.e. albumin, prothrombin time (PT) – these tests give a more accurate assessment of the insult to the liver than transaminase levels.
- Renal function – creatinine levels in combination with the PT are used in the King's criteria for assessing patients requiring liver transplantation in acute liver failure. Also in cases of leptospirosis it is important to check for renal failure, which can occur in Weil's disease.
- Imaging: ultrasound scan or CT scan of the abdomen – to identify the cystic lesions of hydatid disease (see Fig. 6.4) or if the infectious diagnosis was in doubt. A chest radiograph and CT scan of the head are necessary in hydatid disease to look for further cysts.
- Liver biopsy – can be taken for both histology and culture.
- Aspiration of cystic fluid for culture in cases of hydatid disease.

A summary algorithm demonstrating how to approach diagnosing the infectious causes of jaundice is shown in Figure 6.6.

RIGHT UPPER QUADRANT PAIN

The differential diagnosis for right upper quadrant pain is shown in Figure 6.5.

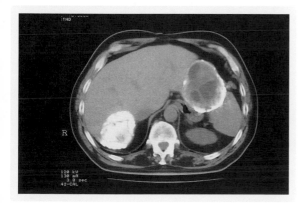

Fig. 6.4 CT scan showing liver cysts.
Source: Conlon CP, Snydman DR. Mosby's Colour Atlas and Text of Infectious Diseases. Edinburgh: Mosby; 2000: Fig. 9.47.

History

As with any history of pain, the exact nature of the right upper quadrant pain needs to be detailed. A useful mnemonic is *SOCRATES*.

Site	right upper quadrant
Onset	sudden/gradual
Character	sharp/dull/colicky
Radiation	to shoulder tip
Alleviating factors	position
Timing	constant/intermittent/ length of intervals between pain
Exacerbating factors	fatty foods/position
ASsociated features	vomiting/seizures.

There may have been symptoms preceding the onset of the pain, e.g. jaundice, dark urine and pale stools from obstructing gallstones. Jaundice in association with right upper quadrant pain also occurs in cholangitis and hydatid disease, although the latter more commonly presents with right upper quadrant pain alone than with jaundice. A high fever and rigors suggest cholecystitis or cholangitis. Classically abscesses give a fever pattern of daily spikes. Vomiting occurs with acute cholecystitis.

The infection may be precipitated by surgery or instrumentation (e.g. ERCP – endoscopic retrograde cholangiopancreatography) to the biliary tree or abdominal cavity. A past medical history of gallstones, where the gall bladder has not been removed, would increase the suspicion of a biliary tract infection. Recent foreign travel to the tropics places an amoebic abscess in the differential diagnosis. Close work with sheep and dogs is a risk factor for hydatid disease.

Examination

The first aspect to note is how unwell and distressed the patient appears. Infections of the biliary tract and bacterial liver abscesses cause the patient to be more symptomatic. The patient may be jaundiced, suggesting cholangitis, acute cholecystitis with gallstones obstructing the common bile duct, or rarely hydatid disease.

On abdominal examination palpate the abdomen gently initially, as there may be guarding and rebound tenderness in the right upper quadrant indicative of

Fig. 6.5 Causes of right upper quadrant pain

Liver infections	Others
Bacterial liver abscess	Duodenal ulcer
Amoebic liver abscess	Congestive hepatomegaly
Viral hepatitis	Pyelonephritis
Cholangitis	Appendicitis
Cholecystitis	Right-sided lower lobe pneumonia
Hydatid disease	

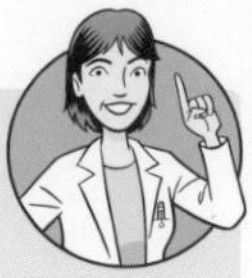

Murphy's sign is elicited by placing two fingers gently into the right upper quadrant and then asking the patient to take a deep breath in. When an inflamed gallbladder moves downwards with inspiration and hits the examiner's fingers the patient usually takes in a sharp gasp of air with the pain, and this is a positive result. NB: the result is only significant if no similar response is elicited when done with the fingers placed on the left upper quadrant.

peritonism with acute cholecystitis. Care also needs to be taken when feeling for hepatomegaly, as this can be tender in all the infective differential diagnoses. Murphy's sign is positive in acute cholecystitis.

Investigations

- Full blood count – raised WCC (white cell count) with infection; eosinophilia seen in hydatid disease.
- Liver function tests – show a raised bilirubin and an obstructive picture, i.e. alkaline phosphatase and gamma-glutamyl transpeptidase (GGT) more markedly raised than the transaminases with biliary tract infections and less often with hydatid disease.
- Blood cultures – to identify the causative organism.
- Aspirated contents of abscess for culture – to identify the causative organism.
- Serology for *Entamoeba histolytica* and *Echinococcus granulosus*.
- Imaging – an ultrasound scan can demonstrate a dilated biliary tree, gallstones and abscesses and cysts in the liver. A CT scan of the abdomen is better for identifying the source of sepsis for a bacterial liver abscess.

A summary algorithm demonstrating how to approach diagnosing the infectious causes of right upper quadrant pain is shown in Figure 6.7.

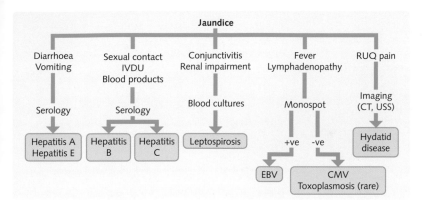

Fig. 6.6 Diagnostic algorithm for jaundice.

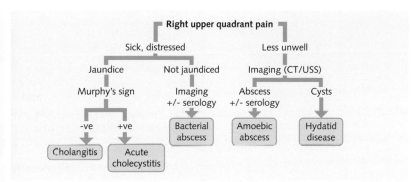

Fig. 6.7 Diagnostic algorithm for right upper quadrant pain.

Urinary symptoms

Objectives

In this chapter you will learn:

- To recognize the symptoms that suggest the patient has pyelonephritis rather than just a UTI
- Who is at risk of developing a UTI
- What the urine dipstick shows with a UTI
- Who should have an ultrasound scan of the renal tract.

Urinary tract infections can involve the urethra and bladder, which would constitute a urinary tract infection (UTI), or ascend to affect the kidney when it becomes pyelonephritis.

HISTORY

The symptoms that specify there is a urinary tract infection are:

- Dysuria – pain or burning sensation on passing urine
- Frequency – increased number of times in the day that the desire to urinate is felt
- Nocturia – need to get up at night to pass urine
- Haematuria – blood seen in the urine.

In the elderly the only manifestation of a UTI may be confusion. Older patients should have their mental state assessed (see Ch. 4).

The suspicion that a UTI may have progressed to pyelonephritis is raised by finding the following symptoms:

- Abdominal pain that classically radiates from loin to groin
- Fevers, usually more pronounced in pyelonephritis
- Rigors, as these imply bacteraemia.

In cases of urinary tract tuberculosis there will be the additional constitutional symptoms typically associated with TB, namely weight loss, malaise and night sweats.

The other important aspect of the history is to explore any predisposing factors:

- Female sex (as the urethra is shorter)
- Diabetes mellitus
- Congenital urinary tract abnormalities
- Neuropathic bladder, e.g. from spinal cord compression, multiple sclerosis
- Outflow obstruction such as in prostatic hypertrophy
- Urinary catheter in situ
- Predisposition to stones, e.g. hypercalciuria, gout
- Past medical history of tuberculosis elsewhere in the body.

The location of the patient when the infection manifested affects the likelihood of the causative organism: 95% of infections from the community are due to *Escherichia coli*, whereas nosocomial (hospital-acquired, i.e. > 2 days after admission) infections cover a broader range of organisms and the resistance to antibiotics is liable to be higher.

EXAMINATION

Looking around the bedside can often reveal clues as to the underlying cause of an infection, such as blood glucose monitoring equipment, or a catheter bag strapped to the edge of the bed frame. The patient's demeanour can distinguish between a simpler UTI and pyelonephritis: patients with pyelonephritis are restless since they cannot get comfortable with the abdominal pain and they usually look more unwell, sweaty and feverish. Dehydration is assessed from the skin turgor, mucous membranes, jugular venous pressure (JVP), pulse and blood pressure (lying and standing for a postural BP).

On abdominal examination, palpate all areas including the loins to elicit both suprapubic tenderness and loin or back pain. Palpate the kidneys to check their presence and gauge for size. In men a digital rectal examination to assess prostate size and regularity may be appropriate. Any neurological symptoms obtained from the history should prompt a neurological examination, with particular attention paid to any sensory deficits. The examination is completed by checking the temperature chart for the fever pattern.

INVESTIGATIONS

- Urine dipstick – this simple bedside test is highly useful. An infection gives positive results for nitrites, leucocytes, sometimes blood and less often protein. A diabetic patient may have glucose detected in the urine and ketones if they are type 1, although the latter are present in the fasted state.
- Urine microscopy – gives a quantification of the RBC (red blood cells) and WBC (white blood cells) in the urine; any bacteria present can be Gram stained to assist with identification. The technique can distinguish sterile pyuria, which is a feature of urinary tuberculosis.
- Urine cultures – to identify the organism and then antibiotic sensitivity patterns can be tested, which is particularly important with infections partially treated prior to admission or in nosocomial infections when resistance is more likely.
- Blood cultures – to identify the organism, especially in cases where there have been rigors as these indicate bacteraemia.
- Imaging – an ultrasound scan of the renal tract may be indicated to exclude hydronephrosis, obstruction and renal calculi. If the history suggests calculi (loin pain and haematuria) then a plain radiograph known as a KUB (kidneys, ureters and bladder) followed by intravenous contrast to perform an intravenous urogram (IVU) are carried out to find the number, location and size of any calculi (Fig. 7.1).

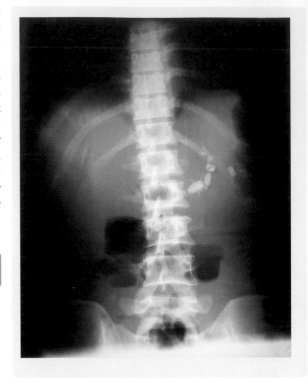

Fig. 7.1 KUB showing multiple renal calculi.

Many catheterized patients will permanently have positive results for an infection on dipstick testing. In these cases treatment has to be aimed at symptoms and proven cultured infections.

All males presenting with their first urinary tract infection should have an ultrasound scan of the renal tract before discharge, as also should females who suffer with recurrent infections. Males are less prone to UTIs so an anatomical abnormality as a cause is more likely.

A summary algorithm demonstrating how to approach diagnosing the cause of urinary symptoms is shown in Figure 7.2.

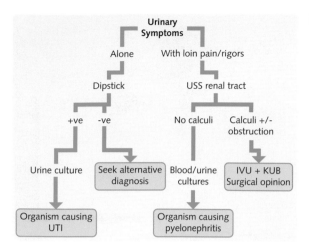

Fig. 7.2 Diagnostic algorithm for urinary symptoms.

Genital symptoms

8

Objectives

In this chapter you will learn:

- The differential diagnosis of urethral discharge
- The risk factors for candidiasis
- The signs and symptoms that are associated with gonorrhoea
- Which infections give rise to oral ulcers, in addition to genital ones
- How the causes of genital ulceration are differentiated.

Symptoms arising from the genital region are, in the vast majority of cases, due to sexually transmitted infections (STIs). These include:

- Syphilis
- Gonorrhoea
- Non-gonococcal urethritis
- Chlamydia
- Candidiasis
- Trichomoniasis
- Genital warts
- Genital herpes (herpes simplex virus 1 and 2) (HSV-1 and -2)
- Chancroid
- Lymphogranuloma venereum
- Granuloma inguinale
- HIV (see Ch. 25).

The differential diagnosis of oral and genital ulceration includes the small vessel vasculitis Behçet's disease and lichen planus. The other features of Behçet's disease are uveitis, arthritis, erythema nodosum, abdominal pain, meningoencephalitis and pathergy reaction (pustule formation at site of skin injury, e.g. venepuncture site). Lichen planus produces a white lacy pattern on the oral mucosa more commonly than ulceration. In other areas of the skin, especially the wrists and ankles, it manifests as raised purplish plaques with a network of white lines across known as Wickham's striae.

HISTORY

The description of the symptoms suffered begins the process of delineating which organism is responsible.

- Urethral discharge and urethritis suggest gonorrhoea, non-gonococcal urethritis, chlamydia, candidiasis and trichomoniasis.
- Warty lesions on the external genitalia could be due to human papillomavirus or the condylomata lata of secondary syphilis.
- Genital ulcers can occur in genital herpes, syphilis, chancroid, lymphogranuloma venereum and granuloma inguinale.
- Oral ulcers, with or without genital ulceration, are seen in HSV and syphilis.

Further questioning should be directed to risk behaviour and other associated symptoms.

As regards risk behaviour:

- Sexual history including the number of sexual partners, whether casual or regular partners, any contact with sex workers, sexual orientation and practices, date of last intercourse
- Usage of barrier contraception, e.g. condoms, diaphragms and any spermicidal lubricants, and whether condom failure was suspected
- Any known symptoms in partners or their sexual history
- Antibiotic use, steroid therapy, oral contraceptive pill and pregnancy can all predispose to candidiasis.

The associated symptoms of sexually acquired infections are:

35

- Fever, malaise and lymphadenopathy suggesting secondary syphilis
- Fever, headache and myalgia accompanying HSV infection
- Pharyngitis occurring in gonococcal infections and secondary syphilis
- Rashes: maculopapular in secondary syphilis, pustular in gonorrhoea
- Arthritis complicating gonorrhoea and non-gonococcal urethritis if part of Reiter's syndrome
- Conjunctivitis completing the triad for Reiter's syndrome, with urethritis and arthritis
- Pelvic pain and infertility indicating progression to pelvic inflammatory disease (PID).

EXAMINATION

Given that the examination required is more intimate than for most complaints, patients need to be put at their ease by having a private room, ideally one that someone cannot burst into, and a chaperone present to prevent any allegations of non-professional conduct.

Initially inspect the external genitalia for visible discharge, erythema, ulceration (Fig. 8.1) and wart lesions. Palpate for lymphadenopathy in the inguinal region, in particular noting if this is tender, and in males examine the testes. In female patients, a bimanual vaginal examination is warranted to check for cervical and adnexal tenderness and discharge not visible externally.

A more general examination is necessary to look for the related features of sexually transmitted infections.

- General inspection – to assess if the patient looks unwell, as gonorrhoea can result in septicaemia.
- Mouth – ulcers on the lips occur in HSV and 'snail track' ulcers in the oropharynx in syphilis.
- Eyes – conjunctivitis is part of the triad for Reiter's syndrome.
- Skin – pustular skin lesions local to the genitalia and thighs are seen in gonorrhoea, and a generalized maculopapular rash suggests secondary syphilis.
- Abdomen – pelvic tenderness occurs with PID secondary to gonorrhoea and chlamydia. A digital rectal examination may elicit tenderness in proctitis due to gonorrhoea and chlamydia.
- Swollen joints – can arise from a septic arthritis in gonococcal infections or as part of Reiter's syndrome.

INVESTIGATIONS

- Swabs – for microscopy and culture should be taken from any discharge visible, ulcers, suppurating lymph nodes, urethral meatus in males and high vaginal and cervical swabs in women.
- Dark-ground microscopy of exudate from chancres – for syphilis.
- Viral PCR from vesicles or ulcers – for HSV.
- Blood cultures – in suspected gonococcal infections.
- Joint aspiration – microscopy and culture for causative organism.

Fig. 8.1 Causes of genital ulceration

Condition	Organism	Genital ulcers	Inguinal lymphadenopathy	Oral ulcers
Genital herpes	HSV-2, less often HSV-1	Painful, shallow ulcers	Tender lymph nodes	Yes, with HSV-1 usually
Syphilis	*Treponema pallidum*	Painless ulcer (chancre) in primary syphilis (Fig. 8.2)	Painless lymph nodes	Yes, in secondary syphilis
Chancroid	*Haemophilus ducreyii*	Painful, deep necrotic ulcers (Fig. 8.3)	Tender lymph nodes	No
Lymphogranuloma venereum	*Chlamydia trachomatis* (serotypes L1–L3)	Painless, small ulcers	Tender lymph nodes which discharge	No
Granuloma inguinale	*Calymmatobacterium granulomatis*	Painless, velvety ulcers	No lymph nodes	No

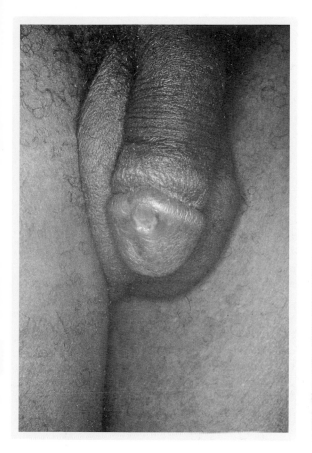

Fig. 8.2 Syphilitic chancre.
Source: Conlon CP, Snydman DR. Mosby's Colour Atlas and Text of Infectious Diseases. Edinburgh: Mosby; 2000: Fig. 10.30b.

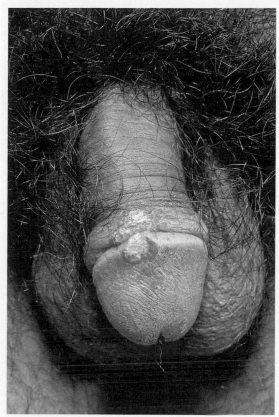

Fig. 8.3 Chancroid ulcer.
Source: Conlon & Snydman, 2000: Fig. 10.43.

Summary algorithms demonstrating how to approach diagnosing the cause of genital ulcers and discharge are shown in Figure 8.4.

Fig. 8.4 Diagnostic algorithms for genital symptoms.

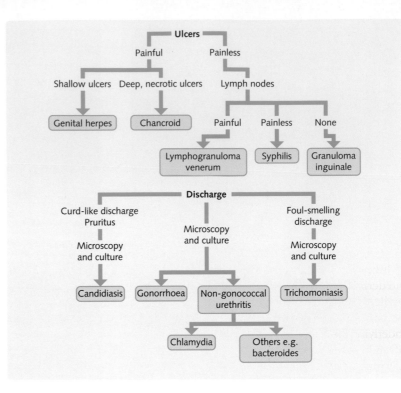

Objectives

In this chapter you will learn:

- The risk factors for cellulitis
- The clinical findings that would suggest there may be osteomyelitis
- What investigations are required if the erythema extends over a joint
- The management of extreme pain associated with erythema.

Cellulitis is an infection of the subcutaneous tissues and dermis. Clinically it appears as an area of warm, swollen erythema; if this extends over a joint then the concern is that there may be a septic arthritis underlying the skin infection. Osteomyelitis describes infection of the bone, rather than the joint cavity, and may present as cellulitis.

HISTORY

The history needs to cover a number of areas:

- Port of entry for bacteria – the commonest is probably athlete's foot, the fungal infection that produces cracks in the skin between the toes, resulting in lower leg cellulitis. Intravenous drug users are liable to infections around their sites of venepuncture. Any break in the skin due to trauma, ulcers or a bite may result in infection.
- Susceptibility – the risk of cellulitis is increased in diabetes mellitus due to hyperglycaemia; in peripheral neuropathy from the inability to feel trauma to the extremities; in peripheral vascular disease due to the poor blood supply impairing healing and a tendency to ulceration; in obesity from pressure areas and immobility.
- Systemic features – fevers, sweats and rigors may indicate bacteraemia, rather than just a localized infection.
- Risk of MRSA (methicillin-resistant *Staphylococcus aureus*) – any recent hospital admissions and the length of stay; whether MRSA screening has previously been performed and the results.
- Treatment pre-admission – patients may have received a course of antibiotics from their GP

prior to admission, and it is useful to know what antibiotics and the dose, to judge if it was inadequate dosing or possible antibiotic resistance that precipitated admission.

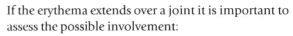

If there is a history of trauma with skin penetration, the patient's tetanus immune status must be confirmed and immunization considered.

If the erythema extends over a joint it is important to assess the possible involvement:

- Range of movement of the joint – in septic arthritis, joint movement is extremely restricted due to pain. In acute osteomyelitis of the lower limb, weight-bearing is likely to be reduced.
- Time course – whether the erythema started over the joint and spread outwards or started at a distant point and extended towards the joint.
- Prosthetic material – whether the joint has been replaced leaving metalwork in situ or there has been recent instrumentation, such as an arthroscopy.

EXAMINATION

The examination is almost entirely careful inspection. Note the distribution and extent of the erythema and then by drawing around the edge any expansion or resolution can be judged from the time of admission (Fig. 9.1).

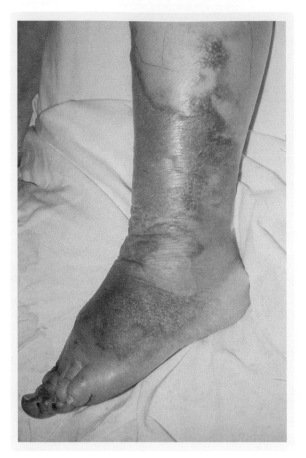

Fig. 9.1 Cellulitis.
Source: Conlon CP, Snydman DR. Mosby's Colour Atlas and Text of Infectious Diseases. Edinburgh: Mosby; 2000: Fig. 11.6.

Specifically look for any broken skin, particularly cracks between the toes, and if there are any ulcerated areas whether bone is visible at the base. It is important to describe the ulcer base with reference to slough, exudate, necrotic tissue, margins and depth. In intravenous drug users particularly, there may be abscesses at the sites of venepuncture.

A life-threatening complication not to miss is necrotizing fasciitis. This presents with an unwell patient in excruciating pain, with vesicles and a dusky colour to the skin of the affected area. On a plain radiograph gas may be visible within the tissues. Necrotizing fasciitis requires urgent surgical debridement.

Check for any temperature difference compared with an unaffected area with the back of the hand (more sensitive test). Using a tape measure, record the circumference of an infected limb compared to the unaffected one to quantify any swelling. Palpate for local lymphadenopathy. Using a metal probe, press into an ulcer to see whether it is possible to probe down to bone to assess likely bony involvement.

An erythematous, warm, swollen lower limb has the differential diagnosis of cellulitis and a deep vein thrombosis (DVT). NB: they can coexist, for example in an elderly immobile woman who has venous ulcers that become infected.

If the area of erythema includes a joint, additionally palpate for bony tenderness, feel for an effusion and assess both the passive and active range of movement of the joint.

Septic arthritis can destroy a joint in a matter of hours, so making the diagnosis rapidly and urgently referring for a surgical washout is critical.

INVESTIGATIONS

- Haematology – a raised WCC (white cell count), usually neutrophilia in a bacterial infection.
- Biochemistry – a raised CRP (C-reactive protein) indicates an infection.
- Blood cultures – to identify causative organism, and check for antibiotic sensitivities.
- Abscess aspiration/incision and drainage specimens for culture – to find bacterial cause; higher detection rate than blood cultures.
- Joint fluid aspiration – microscopy and culture to ascertain if septic arthritis present and, if so, isolate the organism responsible.
- Deep bone biopsies (from debridement procedure) – for culture if osteomyelitis suspected.
- Imaging – plain radiographs and/or MRI to look for joint destruction in septic arthritis and changes suggestive of osteomyelitis.

- Blood glucose level – in diabetic patients to check for hyperglycaemia while infected and whether a sliding scale of insulin is required to improve glycaemic control, and in patients not known to be diabetic a fasting glucose is warranted to ensure the infection is not a presentation of diabetes mellitus.

A summary algorithm demonstrating how to approach managing cellulitis is shown in Figure 9.2.

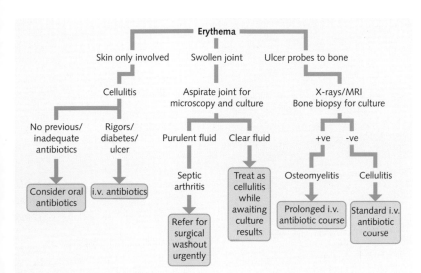

Fig. 9.2 Diagnostic algorithm of cellulitis.

Complications from intravenous drug use

Objectives

In this chapter you will learn:

- What information it is important to elicit from a drug history
- How cellulitis and a DVT can be differentiated
- What investigations are indicated in a breathless intravenous drug user (IVDU)
- The symptoms and signs that would suggest endocarditis.

A number of problems are particularly experienced by those who inject themselves with illicit drugs, namely:

- Cellulitis and abscesses
- Endocarditis, especially tricuspid valve involvement
- Septic emboli, e.g. to lungs
- Blood-borne viruses, e.g. HIV, hepatitis C and B
- Thrombosis, i.e. deep vein thrombosis (DVT) and pulmonary embolus (PE).

When you are the doctor who will be prescribing the methadone it is prudent to confirm the dose with the GP before giving methadone, to establish it is correct. The patient may just want to receive more or may have been selling it and is therefore not able to tolerate the high dose quoted.

HISTORY

In this setting a detailed drug history is required:

- How long have intravenous drugs been used?
- What drugs are used?
- How much is spent on a daily basis?
- How is the habit funded?
- What sites are used for injection?
- Have any courses of rehabilitation been undertaken, and have any been successful?
- Is the general practitioner (GP) prepared to prescribe methadone?
- Does the patient know his hepatitis C/B or HIV status?
- Have needles ever been shared with other users? Is their infectious status known?

Given the variety of complications that can arise from intravenous drug use, the symptoms suffered cover all systems:

- Skin: pain, erythema, swelling and warmth around injection sites with enlarged local lymphadenopathy occur with cellulitis, abscesses and DVTs.

- Respiratory: breathlessness and a productive cough imply a lower respiratory tract infection possibly due to septic emboli, whereas breathlessness, haemoptysis and pleuritic chest pain are more indicative of a pulmonary embolus. The upper respiratory tract symptoms of a sore throat, local lymphadenopathy and a flu-like illness may herald HIV seroconversion.
- Cardiovascular: swelling of the ankles suggests heart failure in endocarditis.
- Abdominal: jaundice with mild right upper quadrant pain hints at acute hepatitis C or B infection.
- Systemic: fevers, rigors and malaise are non-specific but in this setting could be present with cellulitis, endocarditis, septic emboli or HIV.

EXAMINATION

More commonly than in other scenarios the patients may have multiple coexisting sequelae of their intravenous drug habit, so attention needs to be paid particularly to searching for all the potential complications.

Botulism (a descending flaccid paralysis) can complicate intravenous drug use as a result of anaerobic conditions at injection sites allowing growth of the *Clostridium botulinum* introduced by the needle. High-risk practices for contracting clostridial infections are needle-sharing, use of citric acid as a solvent and injecting into muscles or just under the skin ('skin-popping') rather than directly into the vein.

- Skin – looking for cellulitis and abscesses around injection marks with local lymphadenopathy, and the differential diagnosis of an erythematous, tender, swollen, warm lower limb being DVT; jaundice of the skin and sclerae suggesting acute hepatitis; a maculopapular rash raising the possibility of an HIV seroconversion.
- Hands – Osler's nodes (on fingertip pulps) and Janeway lesions (macules on palms) indicating infective endocarditis.
- Nails – splinter haemorrhages occurring with infective endocarditis, and mild clubbing in subacute cases of infective endocarditis.
- Eyes – jaundice of the sclerae suggesting hepatitis; pallor of the conjunctivae indicating anaemia and Roth spots on the retina both occurring in endocarditis.
- Respiratory – a generalized wheeze resulting from smoking heroin; a pleuritic rub more strongly suggesting pulmonary embolus than infective consolidation in the lung.
- Cardiovascular – a new murmur being infective endocarditis until proved otherwise.
- Abdominal – right upper quadrant tenderness and/or hepatomegaly hinting at hepatitis; splenomegaly suggesting endocarditis.

To finish the examination check the temperature chart for the pattern of the fevers.

INVESTIGATIONS

- Urine dipstick – to check for microscopic haematuria in endocarditis.
- Haematology – raised WCC (white cell count) seen in infection, with a neutrophilia in bacterial infections; anaemia occurs in infective endocarditis; atypical lymphocytes and leucopenia raise the suspicion of HIV.
- Biochemistry – raised CRP (C-reactive protein) in infection; abnormal liver function tests (LFTs) with transaminases AST and ALT most deranged in hepatitis; impaired renal function due to glomerulonephritis may occur in infective endocarditis.
- Blood cultures – to identify the bacteria causing the infection; multiple sets should be taken, ideally three separated in time or venepuncture site, especially in suspected endocarditis.
- HIV testing – patient needs to be properly counselled before the test (see Ch. 25).
- Hepatitis B and C screening – to check for current infection as well as carrier status.
- Arterial blood gas – to look for hypoxia, likely to be more severe with a PE than septic emboli to the lungs.
- Imaging – chest radiograph to look for septic emboli; a CT pulmonary angiogram or ventilation/perfusion ($\dot{V}/\dot{Q}$) scan (see Fig. 10.1) to detect a PE; an Echo (echocardiogram) to search for vegetations (see Fig. 23.4) and valvular regurgitation in endocarditis; an ultrasound and Doppler scan of the lower limb vasculature to diagnose a DVT; an abdominal ultrasound scan to assess for hepatomegaly and splenomegaly.

A summary algorithm demonstrating how to approach diagnosing the complications of intravenous drug use is shown in Figure 10.2.

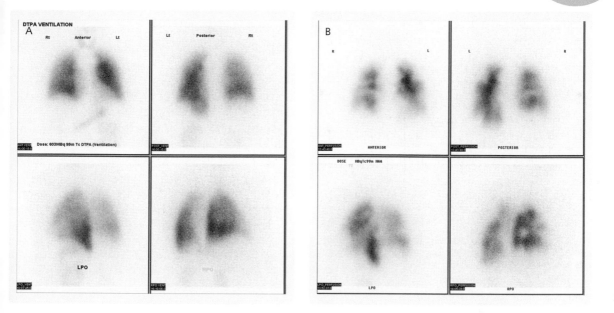

Fig. 10.1 V̇/Q̇ scan: (A) the V̇ (ventilation) scan shows defects which do not match with the defects on (B) the Q̇ (perfusion) scan, indicating a pulmonary embolus.

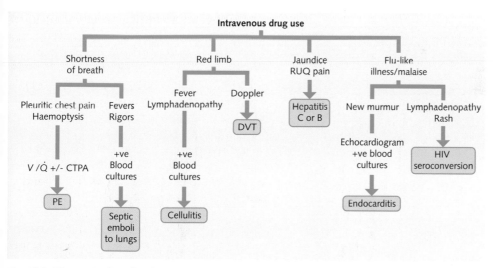

Fig. 10.2 Diagnostic algorithm for intravenous drug use complications. CTPA, computerized tomography pulmonary angiogram.

Unwell from abroad

Objectives

In this chapter you will learn:

- The most important infection to consider in any returned traveller with a fever, and how it is investigated
- The differential diagnosis of a traveller with diarrhoea
- What infections can give rise to respiratory symptoms
- The differential diagnosis of a pruritic rash.

It pays to remember that unwell returned travellers may not have an infection related to their travel. The most important infection to exclude in any returning traveller is malaria, as this can be rapidly fatal. The list of differential diagnoses should therefore be malaria, malaria, malaria, and then consideration of any of the following:

- Amoebiasis
- Brucellosis
- Dengue fever
- Giardia
- Japanese B encephalitis
- Leishmaniasis
- Leprosy
- Relapsing fever
- Schistosomiasis
- Trypanosomiasis
- Typhus
- Typhoid, paratyphoid
- Viral haemorrhagic fevers
- Worm infections
- Yellow fever.

The time elapsed since being overseas affects the likelihood of various infections being the culprit, as shown in Figure 11.1.

HISTORY

A travel history should involve enquiring about:

- Countries visited (including stopovers on journeys), the length of time overseas and amount of time since return

- Activities undertaken while overseas, e.g. backpacking in rural areas, water contact such as white water rafting, swimming in lakes
- Water supplies for drinking and washing (especially brushing teeth)
- Types of food eaten and the places eaten at
- Awareness of insect or other bites, use of insect repellent and nets over the bed at night
- Symptoms while abroad and if any other travellers were similarly affected
- Vaccinations prior to the trip and whether antimalarial prophylaxis was taken, including whether taken correctly.

The nature and duration of any symptoms suffered needs to be clarified:

- Insect bites: classically daytime bites are more likely to cause dengue fever and African trypanosomiasis, whereas evening bites make malaria, leishmaniasis and American trypanosomiasis (Chagas' disease) more likely.
- Diarrhoea can be due to gastroenteritis, cholera, giardia, amoebiasis, typhoid, paratyphoid, schistosomiasis, tapeworm infection and strongyloidiasis.
- Abdominal pain occurs in typhoid, paratyphoid, schistosomiasis, visceral leishmaniasis, trypanosomiasis, giardia, amoebiasis, tapeworm, roundworm and hookworm infections.
- Worms seen in the stool could result from threadworm, hookworm or tapeworm infection.
- Haematemesis and melaena suggest haemorrhagic dengue fever or any of the other viral haemorrhagic fevers.

Fig. 11.1 Infective causes of a fever in descending order of likelihood

<3 weeks since return	>3 weeks since return
Malaria	Malaria
African trypanosomiasis	Brucellosis
Dengue fever	Liver abscess
Typhoid, paratyphoid	Typhoid, paratyphoid
Tick typhus	Visceral leishmaniasis
Hepatitis A	Hepatitis B, C or E
Brucellosis	Tuberculosis
Viral haemorrhagic fevers	HIV seroconversion
	Filariasis

- Urinary symptoms: frequency, dysuria and haematuria may be due to schistosomiasis, rather than just a simple urinary tract infection.
- Rigors and high fevers are classic for malaria.
- Night sweats may be due to malaria, tuberculosis, brucellosis or visceral leishmaniasis.
- Cough can be a part of the symptoms for typhoid, paratyphoid, tuberculosis, schistosomiasis, visceral leishmaniasis and strongyloidiasis.
- Chest pain occurs in typhoid, paratyphoid and trypanosomiasis.

EXAMINATION

On inspection of the patient there may be many clues to the diagnosis:

- Anaemia (pallor of conjunctivae) could be due to haemolysis in malaria, typhoid, paratyphoid and typhus, or blood loss from hookworm infestation of the bowel.
- Jaundice (yellow discoloration of sclerae and skin) suggesting malaria or a viral hepatitis from a food poisoning outbreak, e.g. hepatitis A.
- 'Rose spots' (maculopapular rash) due to typhoid or paratyphoid.
- Morbilliform (measles-like) rash occurs with Chagas' disease, dengue fever and typhus.
- Petechiae would indicate haemorrhagic dengue fever.
- Subcutaneous nodules occur in cysticercosis.
- Crusted ulcers healing by scarring are the hallmark of cutaneous leishmaniasis.

- Hyperpigmentation of the face, hands, feet and abdomen occurs in visceral leishmaniasis, also known as kala-azar (meaning black sickness).
- Lymphangitis (erythematous, tender, palpable lymphatics) is seen in filariasis.
- Elephantiasis (gross leg lymphoedema) (see Fig. 24.19) and hypopigmentation appear in filariasis.
- Hypopigmentation in association with anaesthesia is classic for leprosy.
- Hyperaesthesia, particularly in the ulnar nerve distribution, arises in African trypanosomiasis.
- 'Cutaneous larva currens' (a rapidly migrating pruritic urticaria) over the lower limbs and trunk is seen in strongyloidiasis.
- 'Cutaneous larva migrans' (a slow moving erythematous snaking pattern which is intensely itchy) occurs with a non-human hookworm infection of the skin.
- Non-migrating pruritic urticaria in combination with lymphoedema occurs in *Loa loa* infections.

The other clinical features to look for are shown in Figure 11.2.

INVESTIGATIONS

- Full blood count – haemolytic anaemia is a complication of malaria, typhoid, paratyphoid and typhus. Eosinophilia occurs in worm infections.
- Renal function – can be impaired in malaria and typhus.
- Liver function tests – can be deranged in typhoid, paratyphoid, amoebic abscesses and schistosomiasis.
- Thick and thin blood films (three sets required, separated in time) – to detect malaria parasites and identify the species (Fig. 11.3). Evening (between 9 p.m. and 1 a.m.) thick and thin blood films for *Wuchereria bancrofti*.
- Commercial malarial antigen test kit (e.g. Optimal) – to identify *Plasmodium falciparum*, which can give rise to cerebral malaria.
- Blood cultures – to identify the organism responsible for infection.
- Blood glucose – to check for hypoglycaemia, critical in cases of falciparum malaria and since the required treatment, quinine, can cause hypoglycaemia as it releases insulin.

Fig. 11.2 Signs in returned travellers

Signs	Causes
Conjunctival suffusion	Dengue, viral haemorrhagic fevers, yellow fever, typhus, Japanese B encephalitis, trypanosomiasis, cysticercosis
Fever ≥40°C	Malaria
Lymphadenopathy	Typhoid, paratyphoid, dengue, brucellosis, visceral leishmaniasis, trypanosomiasis, filariasis
Relative bradycardia	Typhoid, paratyphoid, yellow fever
Pericardial rub	Typhoid, paratyphoid
Respiratory signs	Typhoid, paratyphoid, schistosomiasis, Chagas' disease
Hepatosplenomegaly	Malaria, schistosomiasis, typhoid, paratyphoid, trypanosomiasis, brucellosis
Splenomegaly	Visceral leishmaniasis, typhus
Focal neurology	Cysticercosis, cerebral malaria, Japanese B encephalitis, schistosomiasis, trypanosomiasis, leprosy
Cognitive impairment	Typhoid, paratyphoid, trypanosomiasis, cysticercosis, Japanese B encephalitis

- Urine dipstick – to detect haemoglobinuria in falciparum malaria.
- Urine specimens for microscopy and culture (including midday sample for schistosomiasis)
- Stool cultures including for ova, cysts and parasites – to detect schistosomiasis, giardia, typhoid, paratyphoid and worm infections.
- Bone marrow cultures – to detect brucella, typhoid, paratyphoid and leishmania.
- Skin lesion biopsies – a margin sample is needed to detect the leishmania protozoa. Skin smears for acid-fast bacilli and nerve biopsies can be helpful in diagnosing leprosy. Biopsies of subcutaneous nodules in cysticercosis can be diagnostic.
- Duodenal aspirates for culture – can detect typhoid, paratyphoid, strongyloidiasis and brucella infections.
- Lymph node aspirates for culture – can detect leishmaniasis and trypanosomiasis.
- Liver biopsy – to demonstrate the inflammatory response in schistosomiasis.
- Cerebrospinal fluid (CSF) examination – in suspected cases of trypanosomiasis.
- Serology – acute and convalescent results to detect the causative organism.
- PCR (polymerase chain reaction) – for *Mycobacterium leprae* detection.

Fig. 11.3 Blood film for falciparum malaria.

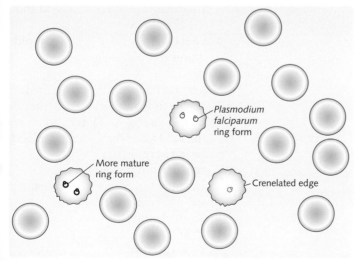

Plasmodium falciparum ring form

More mature ring form

Crenelated edge

- Electrocardiogram (ECG) – before treatment with quinine, since this can lengthen the QT interval.
- Imaging – CT of the head when focal neurology is found on examination, to detect the cause. Chest radiograph to investigate the respiratory signs found in typhoid, paratyphoid, schistosomiasis and Chagas' disease. An abdominal ultrasound scan to study the hepatosplenomegaly seen in a number of tropical infections or for biliary obstruction resulting from roundworms. A renal tract ultrasound scan to look for morbidity resulting from schistosomiasis infection. Barium studies can show up roundworms in the gastrointestinal tract.

Summary algorithms demonstrating how to approach diagnosing infections in returning travellers are shown in Figure 11.4.

> Many of the microscopy or culture samples require particular preparation, media or stains for optimal results, which are important to check before collection.

Fig. 11.4 Diagnostic algorithms for the returned traveller.

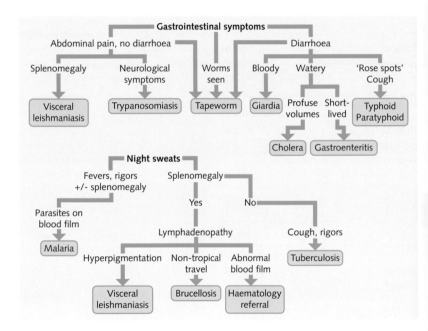

Fever when immunocompromised

Objectives

In this chapter you will learn:

- The potential sources of immunosuppression
- How the respiratory opportunistic infections are differentiated
- The bedside differences between the oral opportunistic infections
- What investigations should be performed on the CSF of an immunocompromised patient with neurological symptoms
- How the fungal skin rashes can be differentiated.

Patients who are immunocompromised for whatever reason are liable to contract opportunistic infections. The initial part of the history should cover details of the immunocompromised state, as in Figure 12.1.

Immunocompromised patients can have the same infections as immunocompetent people but in addition one needs to consider the infections in Figure 12.2.

RESPIRATORY INFECTIONS

History

Symptoms suggestive of a respiratory cause for feeling unwell would be:

- Dry or productive cough
- Purulent sputum with or without haemoptysis
- Breathlessness on exertion
- Night sweats, malaise and weight loss
- Previous lung disease which could lead to cavitation
- Skin rash prior to the onset of respiratory symptoms.

In HIV, opportunistic infections are more prevalent once the CD4 count is less than 200×10^6/ml. Once such an infection has been diagnosed, that is known as AIDS-defining. The full list of AIDS-defining infections is in Chapter 25.

Examination

On inspection of the patient a vesicular pruritic rash with widespread distribution should raise the suspicion of varicella pneumonia. A cachectic patient hints at tuberculosis. On auscultation of the chest there may be no additional sounds to hear or a variable distribution of crepitations. Apical crepitations are suggestive of tuberculosis. A dull percussion note, reduced breath sounds and reduced vocal fremitus may indicate an empyema occurring with nocardia infection. In addition, asking the patient to walk around with a saturation probe on a finger may elicit a decrease in saturations with exertion, as is seen in PCP and CMV pneumonia. The examination should be completed by looking in the sputum pot to check for the purulence of the sputum and for haemoptysis, which is seen with mycobacterial and nocardia infection.

Investigations

- Chest radiograph – may appear normal or show increased shadowing with an alveolar (e.g. PCP), apical (e.g. TB) or diffuse (e.g. VZV) distribution. A round lesion with a crescent of air above it describes an aspergilloma (fungal ball in previously formed lung cavity; Fig. 12.3).
- Sputum microscopy and culture – including for acid-fast bacilli (AFB), fungal hyphae and spores.
- Bronchoalveolar lavage (BAL) washings or lung tissue biopsy – microscopy for fungus of PCP.
- Serology – to identify CMV, VZV and *Aspergillus precipitans*.
- Blood cultures – for identification of MAI.

Fig. 12.1 Issues related to immunosuppression

Causes	Details to cover

Immunosuppressive drug regimen	Timetable and drugs involved in regimen
	Any prophylaxis given to prevent opportunistic infections
	Can regimen be reduced or stopped temporarily
	Examples of regimens:
	    to prevent rejection of transplanted organ
	    to treat malignancy
	    to prevent flare-ups in inflammatory disease such as rheumatoid arthritis, ulcerative colitis, vasculitis

HIV	Latest CD4 count and viral load Treatment and compliance Previous opportunistic infections and prophylaxis given Date of diagnosis and source of infection If acquired via blood-borne source, other viruses checked (hepatitis B, C) Who knows diagnosis? Who must not find out?
Congenital immunodeficiency	Problems encountered previously Treatment and prophylaxis given

Fig. 12.2 Infections occurring in immunosuppressed patients

Respiratory infections	*Pneumocystis carinii* pneumonia (PCP) Cytomegalovirus (CMV) pneumonitis – rare in HIV *Mycobacterium tuberculosis* *Mycobacterium avium-intracellulare* (MAI) – tends to be disseminated Varicella zoster virus (VZV) pneumonia Aspergillosis Nocardia
Oral infections	Candidiasis Epstein–Barr virus (EBV) – glandular fever Herpes simplex virus 1 (HSV-1) stomatitis
Gastrointestinal infections	Oesophageal or disseminated candidiasis CMV colitis *Cryptosporidium parvum* *Isospora belli* Microsporidia *Mycobacterium avium* complex Giardiasis
CNS infections	Toxoplasmosis Cryptococcal meningitis Tuberculous meningitis Encephalitis (HSV, VZV)
Eye infections	CMV retinitis Toxoplasmosis
Skin infections	Fungal, e.g. tinea, pityriasis versicolor VZV (chickenpox) Herpes zoster (shingles)

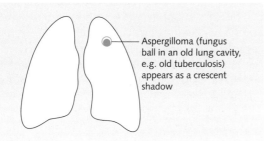

Fig. 12.3 Chest radiograph diagram showing the 'crescent' of an aspergilloma.

Aspergilloma (fungus ball in an old lung cavity, e.g. old tuberculosis) appears as a crescent shadow

A summary algorithm demonstrating how to approach diagnosing respiratory infections in immunocompromised patients is shown in Figure 12.4.

ORAL INFECTIONS

History

The complaints include:

- Lesions or plaque in the oral cavity or on the lips
- Sore throat.

Examination

Inspection of the mouth may demonstrate vesicles or ulcers on the lips with HSV or white clumps/plaque on the tongue and buccal mucosa with oral candidiasis.

A differential diagnosis of white plaque on the tongue is oral hairy leukoplakia, which is associated with EBV. This can be distinguished from oral candidiasis as it extends to cover the lateral borders of the tongue which candida does not.

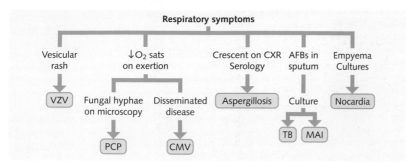

Fig. 12.4 Diagnostic algorithm for respiratory symptoms in an immunocompromised patient.

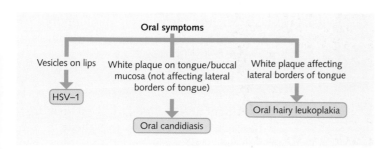

Fig. 12.5 Diagnostic algorithm for oral symptoms in an immunocompromised patient.

Investigations

Diagnosis is mostly clinically but the following may be performed:

- Microscopy and culture of oral plaque material
- Serology from vesicular fluid.

A summary algorithm demonstrating how to approach diagnosing oral symptoms in immuno-compromised patients is shown in Figure 12.5.

ABDOMINAL INFECTIONS

History

The symptoms suffered are:

- Dysphagia (difficulty swallowing) and odynophagia (pain on swallowing) indicating oesophageal candidiasis
- Diarrhoea, especially if it has occurred over a prolonged period or is explosive in nature – may be watery or bloody
- Abdominal pain associated with the diarrhoea
- Malabsorptive symptoms, e.g. steatorrhoea, bloating, flatulence and weight loss
- Weight loss associated with night sweats.

Examination

On inspection, look for evidence of recent weight loss and whether the patient appears dehydrated. Check in the mouth for candida. Palpate the abdomen for tenderness and hepatosplenomegaly.

Investigations

- Stool microscopy for bacteria, ova, cysts and spores.
- Stool culture – to identify the causative organism.
- Barium swallow – shows 'moth-eaten' appearance to oesophagus with oesophageal candidiasis (Fig. 12.6).
- Abdominal radiograph – loops of dilated bowel are seen in CMV colitis.
- Serology – to check for CMV.
- Blood cultures – to identify MAI.
- Oesophagogastroduodenoscopy (OGD) – shows ulceration and white plaques of oesophageal candidiasis.
- Rectal tissue biopsy – for inclusion bodies indicating CMV colitis.

A summary algorithm demonstrating how to approach diagnosing gastrointestinal infections

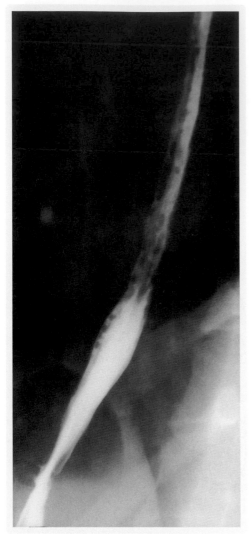

Fig. 12.6 Barium swallow showing ulceration due to candida.
Source: Conlon CP, Snydman DR. Mosby's Colour Atlas and Text of Infectious Diseases. Edinburgh: Mosby; 2000: Fig. 9.2.

in immunocompromised patients is shown in Figure 12.7.

CENTRAL NERVOUS SYSTEM INFECTIONS

History

A number of the following symptoms may be present:

- Triad of meningitis: headache, photophobia and neck stiffness

- Cognitive impairment
- Seizures
- Focal deficits, e.g. limb weakness, visual impairment.

Examination

The Glasgow Coma Score should be calculated to assess consciousness (see Ch. 2). If possible, a rudimentary evaluation of mental function using the Abbreviated Mental Test is useful (see Ch. 4). Both peripheral and central nervous system examinations are required to elicit any potential focal signs, e.g. hemiparesis or ophthalmoplegia, and note should be taken of whether there is any photophobia. The patient should have the neck checked for stiffness and Kernig's sign tested (see Ch. 2).

Investigations

- CT or MRI of the head (Fig. 12.8) – if there are any focal neurological signs, to evaluate them and to check it is safe to perform a lumbar puncture.
- Lumbar puncture (LP) – to obtain cerebrospinal fluid (CSF) for microscopy and culture.
- Serology – to identify toxoplasmosis, HSV and VZV.
- PCR (polymerase chain reaction) on CSF for HSV.
- Electroencephalogram (EEG) – to show the slow wave changes typical of encephalitis.

A summary algorithm demonstrating how to approach diagnosing CNS infections in immunocompromised patients is shown in Figure 12.9.

EYE INFECTIONS

History

The patient reports visual disturbances either related to decreased acuity or due to 'floaters' across the visual field.

Examination

An ophthalmoscope is required as there is usually nothing abnormal to see externally. On fundoscopy an appearance of 'pizza pie' or 'cheese and ketchup' (i.e. ischaemic areas and haemorrhages) indicates CMV retinitis, whereas in toxoplasmosis there tends to be chorioretinal scarring with ischaemia.

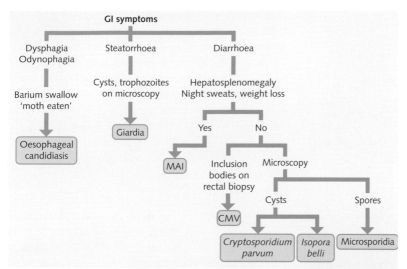

Fig. 12.7 Diagnostic algorithm for gastrointestinal symptoms in an immunocompromised patient.

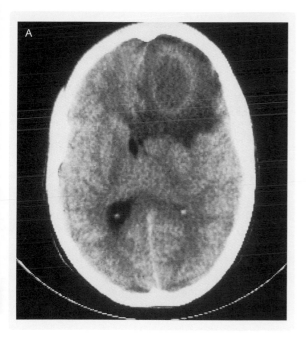

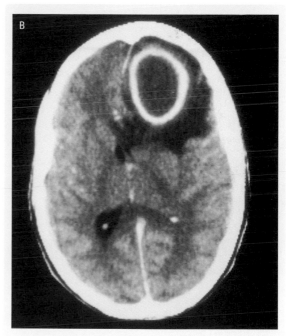

Fig. 12.8 CT scan of the brain with contrast showing brain abscess:

(A) pre-contrast;
(B) post-contrast.

Source: Conlon & Snydman, 2000: Fig. 7.11.

HSV-1 and -2 can cause retinitis in conjunction with encephalitis but the patient is usually so unwell that this aspect is not highlighted and the intravenous aciclovir used, treats all complications.

Investigations

The diagnosis is usually clinical, but serology can be used to confirm the clinical suspicion.

A summary algorithm demonstrating how to approach diagnosing ocular infections in immunocompromised patients is shown in Figure 12.10.

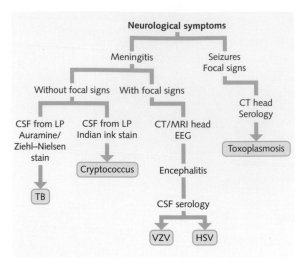

Fig. 12.9 Diagnostic algorithm for neurological symptoms in an immunocompromised patient.

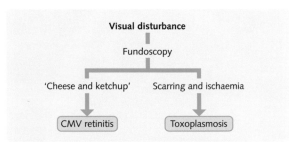

Fig. 12.10 Diagnostic algorithm for eye symptoms in an immunocompromised patient.

SKIN INFECTIONS

History

The patient will be suffering with a rash, the details of which need to be clarified.

- Are there itchy vesicles?
- Is the distribution widespread or only at specific sites?
- Are the lesions large or small?
- Are the lesions 'ring'-shaped?
- Are lesions itchy?
- Are there pigmentation changes to the skin?
- Is there nail involvement?

Examination

Large, slightly itchy ring-shaped lesions with a red scaly outer region and a clear central area occur in ringworm. The fungus can also infect the scalp leading to patches of hair loss, moist skin folds (erythema and not a ring shape) and nails where it tends to cause discoloration and onycholysis (lifting of nail from nail bed). A brown scaly rash in white-skinned patients or a loss of pigment in tanned or black-skinned patients is indicative of pityrosporum infection. Vesicles in a single or two neighbouring dermatomes with an abrupt stop at the midline define shingles, whereas a widespread distribution occurs in chickenpox. The lesions are painful in shingles but merely itchy in chickenpox.

In immunocompetent patients shingles affects a single dermatome but in immunocompromised patients more than one consecutive dermatome may be involved and it can disseminate to cover the whole body.

Investigations

Often the diagnosis can be made clinically but the following tests may be useful to confirm:

- Skin scrapings for fungus identification on potassium hydroxide examination and fungal culture
- Viral PCR of vesicle fluid
- VZV serology.

A summary algorithm demonstrating how to approach diagnosing skin infections in immuno-compromised patients is shown in Figure 12.11.

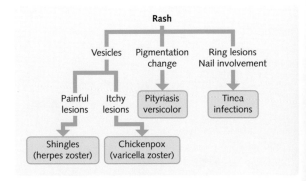

Fig. 12.11 Diagnostic algorithm for a rash in an immunocompromised patient.

Serology tends to be a less helpful investigation in immunocompromised patients as they have an impaired immune response, and tissue samples for culture are much better. A more aggressive approach to acquiring tissue is required, such as using endoscopy and bronchoscopy to obtain biopsies. The effect of being able to make a diagnosis and treat the appropriate infection can be more marked than with immunocompetent patients.

Pyrexia of unknown origin

Objectives

In this chapter you will learn:

- Which rheumatological conditions need to be considered when investigating a pyrexia of unknown origin (PUO)
- Which tumours can produce a fever
- The classical fever patterns
- How the investigations of a PUO should be approached.

Pyrexia of unknown origin (PUO) is defined as an illness of > 3 weeks' duration with a temperature > 38 °C documented on several occasions without any diagnosis after 1 week of evaluation in hospital.

A series of studies undertaken in the 1990s looking at the causes of PUO found the results in Figure 13.1. The causes in each of the categories are shown in Figure 13.2.

The pattern of the fever is classically supposed to help in the diagnosis but sadly this tends not to be very useful in practice. Some examples are shown in Figure 13.3.

HISTORY

The history cannot be too detailed! All aspects of the patient's life need to be covered, however trivial something may initially seem. For the definition of a PUO to be fulfilled the diagnosis is clearly not straightforward, so all potential diagnoses need to be entertained.

- Rigors – would be uncommon in a tumour-related fever.
- Weight loss – if unintentional should ring alarm bells for tumours and tuberculosis.
- Known heart valve problems or valve replacement are particular risk factors for endocarditis.
- Past medical history – especially problems that were never fully explained in the past. Any psychiatric problems in the past or courses of counselling undertaken. Any blood products received prior to 1990 when hepatitis C screening was introduced or in the early 1980s before HIV was fully described.

- Past surgical history – any operations and if any prosthetic material left in situ.
- Drugs – any changes to regular medications in the last few months. All substances taken including over-the-counter preparations, alternative therapies and illicit drugs need to be asked about.
- Family history.
- Tuberculosis contacts – amongst close family and friends, while in the UK and abroad.
- Travel – the countries and timing of any visit abroad. Any problems suffered by the patient or any travelling companions while away. The types of activities undertaken and style of travelling. Malaria prophylaxis taken if required for places visited.
- Immunizations – childhood vaccination programme received, any adult boosters and vaccines for foreign travel. Any problems encountered.
- Work – jobs done, whether any of these involved occupational exposures and the protective measures taken.
- Hobbies – particularly those involving water contact, animals or time in forests.
- Pets, insect and animal contact – intentional contact or otherwise (particularly bites and ill-health of animal).
- Alcohol – current weekly unit intake and whether consumption has been heavier in the past.
- Sexual history – sexual orientation, number of partners and whether regular or casual, whether 'safe sex' practiced. Any previous sexually transmitted infections, treatment taken and whether partner was screened also.

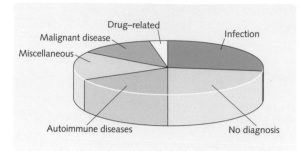

Fig. 13.1 Categories of possible causes of pyrexia of unknown origin.

Fig. 13.2 Causes of pyrexia of unknown origin by category

Category	Example causes
Infection	Bacterial: endocarditis, intra-abdominal, e.g. abscess, tuberculosis, complicated urinary tract infections, brucella Viral: cytomegalovirus (CMV), Epstein–Barr virus (EBV), HIV Amoebic: abscesses Arthropod-borne: leishmaniasis
Autoimmune diseases	Temporal arteritis, polymyalgia rheumatica Still's disease, rheumatoid arthritis Systemic lupus erythematosus, polyarteritis nodosa Rheumatic fever
Malignant disease	Lymphomas Renal carcinoma Carcinoma metastasizing to liver
Drug-related	e.g. cephalosporins, carbapenems
Miscellaneous	Alcoholic hepatitis Granulomatous diseases, e.g. sarcoidosis Self-induced, factitious

EXAMINATION

A thorough examination of all systems to ensure no subtle signs are missed is vital. Daily re-examination to detect progressive changes may also be invaluable.

General

Inspect patients to make an assessment of how unwell they appear; then run through a checklist in your head to look particularly for anaemia, jaundice, cyanosis, any skin rashes, lesions or swellings.

Hands

Look for clubbing, splinter haemorrhages (endocarditis), leuconychia (hypoalbuminaemia) and stigmata of chronic liver disease such as palmar erythema, Dupuytren's contracture and spider naevi. Joint swelling, pain and deformity would raise the suspicion of arthropathies such as rheumatoid arthritis or systemic lupus erythematosus (SLE).

Lymphadenopathy

Check all potential palpable sites, i.e. cervical, axillary and inguinal nodes. The size, texture and mobility of the nodes can help distinguish between fixed, craggy, firm malignant nodes and soft, rubbery, mobile nodes that result from an infection.

Fig. 13.3 Fever patterns

	Pattern	Examples
Intermittent fevers	Sporadic	Subacute bacterial endocarditis, tuberculosis, filarial fever, amyloidosis, brucella
Daily fever spikes	Daily	Abscess, malaria, schistosomiasis
Remitting	Diurnal variation but not dipping to normal	Amoebiasis, malaria, salmonella, Kawasaki disease, CMV
'Saddleback fever'	Fever for 7 days then no fever for 3 days	Borrelia, leptospirosis, dengue, ehrlichia
Pel–Ebstein fever	As above but longer periodicity	Hodgkin's lymphoma (very rare to see this classical pattern)

Cardiovascular

Any new regurgitant murmur in association with a fever should be considered as endocarditis until proven otherwise. A pericarditic rub may result from a viral pericarditis with or without myocarditis.

Respiratory

Upper lobe crepitations in particular raise the suspicion of tuberculosis. Fine crepitations in the mid-zones may represent sarcoidosis. An area of collapse or a pleural effusion could result from a carcinoma that may be metastasizing to the liver.

Abdominal

Any areas of tenderness or palpable masses should be investigated further to look for abscesses, peritoneal tuberculosis or cancer, e.g. renal carcinoma.

INVESTIGATIONS

The exact investigations chosen will depend on the potential diagnoses thrown up by the history and examination findings. Generally attention should be focused on any abnormalities found rather than blindly investigating, as this tends to be more fruitful.

Haematology

A raised haemoglobin could reflect inappropriately raised erythropoietin from a renal carcinoma. Neutrophilia indicates a bacterial infection whereas lymphocytosis tends to occur with viral infections. Eosinophilia can occur with parasite infections and drug-related fevers. Lymphopenia may suggest HIV. Atypical lymphocytes are seen with EBV, HIV and haematological malignancies. A high erythrocyte sedimentation rate (ESR) should lead to the suspicion of temporal arteritis, polymyalgia rheumatica (PMR) or tuberculosis.

Biochemistry

Impaired renal function could relate to a renal carcinoma, leptospirosis or the glomerulonephritis associated with SLE. Abnormal liver function tests (LFTs) occur in hepatitis but are a very late feature of liver metastases. A raised alkaline phosphatase may be the only abnormality resulting from a liver abscess.

Raised calcium and ACE (angiotensin-converting enzyme) levels suggest sarcoidosis. Tumour markers may be helpful, e.g. alpha-fetoprotein for hepatocellular carcinoma, CA 125 and CA 19-9 for both pancreatic and colonic carcinomas.

Urine dipstick test

Microscopic haematuria is one of the embolic phenomena resulting from endocarditis. Renal tuberculosis can give rise to nitrite and leucocyte positive results. Proteinuria may indicate impaired renal function resulting from a tumour.

Immunology

A positive rheumatoid factor is in fact not very specific for rheumatoid arthritis and can also be raised in other connective tissue diseases, e.g. SLE and systemic sclerosis. Hypergammaglobulinaemia may reflect a connective tissue disease or sarcoidosis.

Biopsies

Biopsies can be taken for both histology and cultures to try to elucidate a diagnosis. Any significantly enlarged lymph nodes should be biopsied, choosing the most accessible one(s) to biopsy. A bone marrow trephine and biopsy can be very informative. If temporal arteritis is suspected a temporal artery biopsy should be obtained, this can be up to 10 days after starting steroid treatment. Skin lesions, unidentified masses or peritoneal thickening seen on scanning should be biopsied to attempt to obtain a diagnosis.

Cultures

Cultures are necessary to identify the organism causing the fever. Multiple sets of blood cultures separated in time and space increase the chances of significant positive results; at least three sets are required to diagnose endocarditis. Some fastidious organisms may require prolonged culture in order to grow. Depending on the circumstances it may be appropriate to culture a variety of fluids including urine, aspirated pleural fluid, aspirated synovial fluid, aspirated pericardial fluid and CSF. In suspected tuberculosis the specimens, which can be collected for microscopy and culture to look for acid-fast bacilli, are sputum, early-morning urine, gastric lavage fluid, bronchoalveolar lavage washings and peritoneal fluid specimens.

Serology

Serology can be checked to ascertain the hepatitis B and C status in terms of infection and carriage; and to test for HIV and other infections, e.g. leptospirosis and CMV.

Echocardiography

Transthoracic imaging to look for vegetations and valvular destruction should be the first choice as it is non-invasive but if this appears normal then a transoesophageal echocardiogram (TOE) is required to exclude endocarditis.

Imaging

A chest radiograph can demonstrate bilateral hilar lymphadenopathy (sarcoidosis), pleural fluid, shadowing of the lung lobes, the scarring of old tuberculosis and the cavities of active tuberculosis. An ultrasound scan of the abdomen is an effective way to look for liver abscesses. Either a CT or MRI scan of the whole body (i.e. chest, abdomen and pelvis) can be carried out to look for lymphadenopathy, fluid, organ integrity, masses and abscesses.

It is important to consider the radiation exposure of the scan you are requesting, especially in younger patients, as excessive exposure can result in malignancies. As a result many young patients have an MRI scan in preference to search for the cause of their PUO.

A trial of stopping all medications

This is used to assess if a drug may be the cause of the fever. In cases where there are multiple potentially culprit drugs, each drug should be restarted if required in succession with 2–3 days between to tease out the offending drug.

In modern medical practice a significant minority remain undiagnosed but these illnesses generally have a benign course.

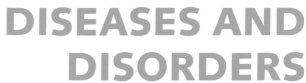

DISEASES AND DISORDERS

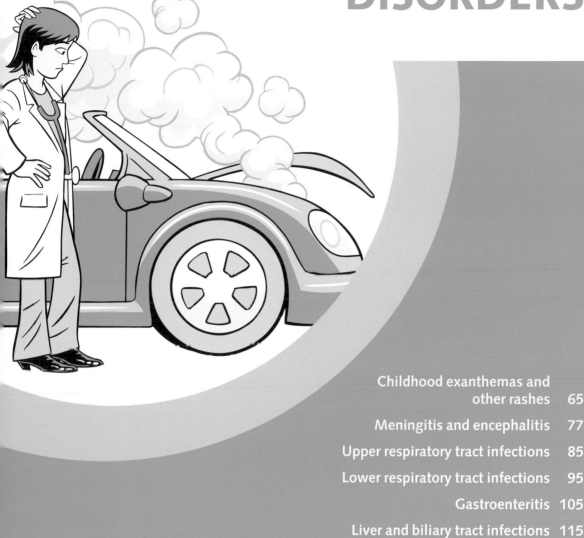

Childhood exanthemas and other rashes

Objectives

In this chapter you will learn:

- Who should receive antiviral treatment for chickenpox
- How shingles arises
- Why a child may not have received MMR immunization
- For whom rubella is a threatening infection and what the result can be
- For whom erythema infectiosum is a threatening infection and why
- Whether rheumatic fever is an infection.

An exanthema is a rash, i.e. a temporary skin eruption. The childhood exanthemas (Fig. 14.1) are very contagious and hence usually contracted in early childhood, although adults who have not been exposed when younger are susceptible. Immunity, either derived from infection or immunization, is usually lifelong.

CHICKENPOX (VARICELLA ZOSTER VIRUS)

Chickenpox is a highly contagious illness with up to 90% of children contracting the disease after coming into contact with an infected individual. It is spread via direct person-to-person contact or from infected objects such as bedding and toys or via inhaled airborne droplets. It is most common in children less than 10 years old.

Clinical features

Chickenpox presents with a prodromal illness of ~ 48 hours, comprising fever and malaise that precedes the rash. The rash starts on the face and trunk before extending to the limbs. It consists of pruritic lesions that arrive in crops. The lesions progress from papules through vesicles and pustules to then become crusted over. At any one stage in the illness there is a variety of lesions depending on the maturity of each crop. Cropping and the distribution of the rash are important features that help to differentiate chickenpox from smallpox.

Diagnosis

The diagnosis is made clinically since the rash is very distinctive. Vesicular fluid can be taken for culture or electron microscopy (EM) identification of the virus but this is not done routinely. PCR (polymerase chain reaction) is becoming the most common mode of diagnosis confirmation, if required.

Treatment

Most patients just require supportive treatment. Calamine lotion topically on the lesions is used for symptomatic relief of pruritus without much evidence of efficacy. Immunocompromised patients, however, receive aciclovir, and if the patient is aged over 16 years, this should be considered because the infection tends to be more severe and there is a greater risk of complications. Secondary bacterial infection of the skin lesions may require antibiotic therapy.

Complications

In children, secondary bacterial infection of the skin lesions with staphylococcus and streptococcus is the most likely complication to occur, often as a result of itching. Varicella pneumonia, whilst being very uncommon in children, does occur more frequently in adults and pregnant women. Thrombocytopenia, meningitis and encephalitis are rare. There is a significant mortality in immunocompromised patients. Reactivation of the dormant virus in sensory ganglia results in shingles in the affected dermatomes.

Fig. 14.1 Infectious childhood exanthemas

Disease	Incubation	Duration of rash	Recommended isolation
Chickenpox	14–17 days	6–10 days	Until all lesions are crusted (usually 5–6 days)
Measles	10–14 days	5 days	From onset of coryza to day 5 of rash
Rubella	14–21 days	2–3 days	None, except non-immune pregnant women in first trimester
Scarlet fever	2–4 days	5 days	1 day after start of treatment
Erythema infectiosum	4–14 days	Weeks	None
Mumps*	16–21 days	None	Until swelling subsides (usually 5–10 days)

* Mumps is included for completeness but does not feature a rash
Source: Rudolf M, Levene M. Paediatrics and Child Health. Oxford: Blackwell Science; 1999: Table 5.31, p. 193.

Immunization

There is a vaccine which has been in use in Japan and the USA for some time. It has recently been licensed in the UK but its place in routine immunization is not yet clear. Immunocompromised patients and pregnant women, in the peripartum period, with no previous history of chickenpox are sometimes given varicella zoster immunoglobulin (VZIG) post-exposure.

SHINGLES OR HERPES ZOSTER (VARICELLA ZOSTER VIRUS)

Shingles can occur at any age but is mainly an adult disease, only rarely seen in children. The probability of developing shingles increases with age.

Pathophysiology

Following chickenpox, the varicella zoster virus lies dormant in the sensory nerve ganglia. Many years later the virus can be reactivated in a sensory ganglion, producing shingles vesicles in the dermatome of that particular ganglion. It is unusual for more than one dermatome to be involved unless the patient is immunocompromised.

Clinical features

Painful vesicles appear in a dermatomal distribution, i.e. stop in the midline, which is very distinctive, as shown in Figure 14.2. The pain in the dermatomal area precedes the appearance of the vesicles. Children tend to suffer less pain than adults.

Diagnosis

Recognition of the rash and its distribution is the mainstay of diagnosis. As with chickenpox, vesicular fluid can be examined to identify the virus although this is not routine practice.

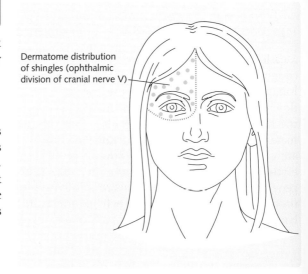

Dermatome distribution of shingles (ophthalmic division of cranial nerve V)

Fig. 14.2 Shingles affecting the ophthalmic division of the right fifth cranial nerve.

Treatment

Aciclovir, or drugs like valaciclovir or famciclovir, can be used to shorten the course of the rash if the patient presents promptly and aciclovir is given intravenously in immunocompromised patients. Good analgesia is required for pain control. Sometimes, antibiotics are necessary for secondary bacterial infection of the vesicles.

Complications

The most important complication is post-herpetic neuralgia, which can last for a prolonged period and can be severe. Antiviral treatment may limit acute pain but has little impact on the development of post-herpetic neuralgia. Ophthalmic sequelae result from involvement of the first branch of the trigeminal nerve. As with chickenpox, secondary infection of the vesicles can occur, usually with staphylococcus and streptococcus.

MEASLES (MORBILLIVIRUS)

Like chickenpox, measles is highly contagious with up to 90% of contacts becoming infected. It is spread by droplet transmission. Prior to the introduction of the MMR vaccine there were 2-yearly measles epidemics, which ceased following the introduction of the immunization programme. Measles is a notifiable disease, i.e. all cases need to be reported to the Consultant of Communicable Disease Control (CCDC).

Clinical features

Measles presents with the three Cs: coryzal symptoms, cough and conjunctivitis, followed by a maculopapular rash which starts on the face and spreads downwards. The lesions become more confluent as the illness progresses and may ultimately desquamate. The pathognomonic sign of Koplik spots, which are classically described as 'grains of salt' on the erythematous background of the buccal mucosa, generally heralds the rash. The child usually feels unwell, cries inconsolably and is irritable. Cervical lymphadenopathy is palpable.

Diagnosis

Usually the diagnosis is made from the clinical picture. This can be confirmed by viral isolation from nasopharyngeal secretions or serology but these are not performed routinely.

Treatment

The treatment is supportive only. Paracetamol can be helpful in reducing the fever. Antibiotics are required if pneumonia or otitis media develop. Vitamin A is given in developing countries to malnourished children, as vitamin A deficiency confers an increased mortality risk.

Complications

Although measles can be a relatively benign disease in healthy children there is a risk of mortality, which is highest in those less than 1 year of age, with immunocompromise, and in vitamin A deficiency. Most of the complications result from secondary bacterial infections, namely pneumonia, otitis media and gastroenteritis. Less common are myocarditis and hepatitis. Less than 1 in 1000 patients with measles will develop encephalitis but 25% of those suffer brain damage. Very rarely, subacute sclerosing panencephalitis (SSPE) can result from measles infection early in life. Typically this presents in puberty with a progressive decline in mental function and seizures until death.

Immunization

Immunization is available as either a combined preparation with mumps and rubella (MMR) or as a single immunization. All children receive routine immunization in their pre-school years unless there is a specific contraindication. MMR is given at 12–15 months and the second dose pre-school at 3–5 years.

There has been marked controversy over the MMR vaccine and a potential link to autism. The current evidence does not support a link but immunization uptake has fallen markedly (up to 10% decline), with some parents opting to give the three components separately. This has led to an increase in cases of mumps and measles.

RUBELLA (RUBELLA VIRUS)

Rubella occurred in epidemics every 6–9 years before the introduction of the MMR immunization programme in 1988. Previously only teenage girls were immunized with the single rubella vaccine to prevent transmission of infection to the fetus during pregnancy but young males who were not immunized were a source of infection for pregnant women and it was therefore felt that the immunization programme should include males as well as females. Rubella is spread by droplets or direct contact. There tends to be a seasonal variation in infection rates, highest in winter and spring. It is a notifiable disease, i.e. all cases need to be reported to the Consultant of Communicable Disease Control (CCDC). Rubella is also known as German measles.

Clinical features

Rubella is a mild illness with low-grade fever, generalized lymphadenopathy and a macular rash. The macular rash appears on the face and trunk initially and spreads peripherally to the limbs. It is not itchy. Rubella in adults commonly presents with arthralgia and arthritis.

Diagnosis

Rubella can be confirmed with serology or rarely viral culture of throat swabs. The diagnosis is made on clinical grounds.

Treatment

There is no specific therapy required for rubella.

Complications

The most important complication is transplacental infection resulting in fetal death or abnormalities, such as congenital heart disease, mental retardation, cataracts and sensorineural deafness. The risk of transmission is greatest in the first 11 weeks of pregnancy. Rubella can also cause thrombocytopenia, encephalitis, myocarditis and arthritis.

Immunization

Rubella can either be given as part of the MMR immunization or given individually.

SCARLET FEVER (*STREPTOCOCCUS PYOGENES*, I.E. GROUP A BETA-HAEMOLYTIC STREPTOCOCCUS)

Group A streptococcus can cause a wide range of infections from the more benign such as pharyngitis to severe infections like necrotizing fasciitis and septicaemia. The rash of scarlet fever results from the ability of the streptococcus to produce an erythrogenic toxin. Scarlet fever is transmitted by aerosol. It is a notifiable disease, i.e. all cases need to be reported to the Consultant of Communicable Disease Control (CCDC).

Clinical features

The precipitant for scarlet fever is a sore throat due to *Streptococcus pyogenes*. Fever, headache, vomiting and lymphadenopathy precede the rash by about a day. The rash is initially over the neck area and rapidly spreads down over the body, although it spares the palms of the hands and the soles of the feet. It is a fine punctate rash which blanches and has a predilection for skin fold areas, i.e. neck, axillae and groins. After 5 days the rash desquamates. The tongue also goes through a transformation: initially it has a white coating through which the papillae are seen ('red strawberry' appearance) then the coating is lost to leave a bright red tongue ('raspberry' appearance).

Diagnosis

A streptococcal infection can be confirmed by bacterial isolation from throat swab and blood cultures. Antistreptolysin O titre (ASOT) is a quantifiable antibody detection test that remains positive for a more prolonged period than cultures, which can be useful to confirm the streptococcal precipitant for the complications of rheumatic fever and acute glomerulonephritis.

Treatment

Antibiotics are the treatment of choice for scarlet fever. Streptococcal infections respond to penicillin, or if the patient is allergic to penicillin then erythromycin is used.

Complications

The local effects of a streptococcal pharyngitis are peritonsillar or retropharyngeal abscesses and otitis media. Streptococcal antigen–antibody immune complexes can be deposited in the glomeruli and this results in acute glomerulonephritis. This is not commonly seen, nor is rheumatic fever (see below).

Immunization

There is no vaccine available currently.

ERYTHEMA INFECTIOSUM (PARVOVIRUS B19)

Parvovirus B19 infections tend to have a seasonal peak in the first half of the year. Epidemics occur on a 3- to 4-yearly basis. Erythema infectiosum is commonest in children aged 6–10 years. The virus can be transmitted via respiratory secretions, contaminated blood products and transplacentally. Thirty to forty percent of infections are asymptomatic.

Clinical features

Erythema infectiosum initially presents with just an erythematous rash across the face, described as 'slapped cheek' (see Fig. 14.3). There is sometimes a low-grade fever associated with this, but in general the child feels very well. Subsequently a lacy-patterned maculopapular rash develops on the trunk, buttocks and limbs with a symmetrical distribution. The rash can wax and wane over several weeks and may be itchy.

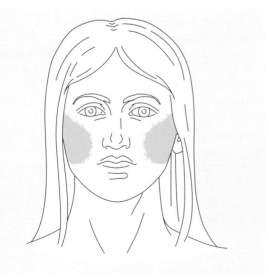

Fig. 14.3 'Slapped cheek' appearance of acute parvovirus infection.

Diagnosis

Parvovirus B19 can be detected by serology. Given that erythema infectiosum is a benign infection and can be diagnosed clinically, there is not usually a need to check the serology.

Treatment

There is no specific therapy required for an erythema infectiosum infection.

Complications

Patients can develop arthritis following parvovirus B19 infection. The complications which create much concern are those following infection in pregnant women when the virus can be transmitted transplacentally. The risk of complications in the fetus is greatest in the first 9 weeks of pregnancy. If the virus replicates in the bone marrow of the fetus then the resultant anaemia leads to hydrops fetalis (anaemia, oedema, hepatosplenomegaly) which is not compatible with life. It can also cause spontaneous abortions. Parvovirus infection can also cause aplastic anaemia in those with sickle cell anaemia.

Parvovirus B19 replicates in rapidly dividing erythroid progenitor cells. Aplastic anaemia can occur in patients who already suffer with a haemoglobinopathy, e.g. sickle cell anaemia, thalassaemia trait or hereditary spherocytosis, as they are unable to tolerate a brief termination of red cell production given that they normally have a compensatory increased red cell turnover.

Immunization

There is no immunization available.

MUMPS (PARAMYXOVIRUS)

Mumps is included in this section on childhood infections for completeness but it is important to remember that there is in fact no rash involved. Mumps is less contagious than chickenpox and measles, and is spread by direct contact with saliva. There is a seasonal variation in infection rate with the peaks occurring in winter and spring. Prior to the introduction of the MMR immunization programme, epidemics of mumps occurred in 3-yearly cycles. Recently, an increase in cases of mumps in susceptible young adults has been noted because this age group only received one dose of vaccine in childhood. Mumps is a notifiable disease, i.e. all cases need to be reported to the Consultant of Communicable Disease Control (CCDC).

Clinical features

Mumps presents with fever, headache and malaise initially, followed 1–2 days later by facial swelling. The latter results from either unilateral or bilateral parotid swellings that are extremely painful (Fig. 14.4). Some patients can have no salivary gland involvement and present with one of the complications such as orchitis, and 30% of infections are asymptomatic altogether.

Diagnosis

The parotid swellings are generally very characteristic for mumps and the diagnosis is therefore made clinically. If there is particular doubt, then serology or tissue cell culture for viral isolation can be performed to identify the mumps virus.

Treatment

There is no specific treatment for mumps; however, good mouth care and adequate analgesia are necessary for symptomatic relief.

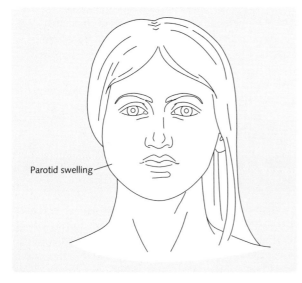

Parotid swelling

Fig. 14.4 Mumps parotitis.

Complications

Mumps was the most common cause of viral meningitis before the introduction of the MMR immunization. Patients can also have a combined meningoencephalitis. The other important concern in post-pubertal males is that 20% develop orchitis and there is a small risk of sterility. Less well known is that post-pubertal females can develop oophoritis, from which there is the same small possibility of sterility. The other potential complications include sensorineural deafness, pancreatitis, myocarditis and thyroiditis.

Immunization

Mumps immunization can either be given as part of the MMR triple vaccine or given individually.

OTHER RASHES

Neisseria meningitidis (Gram-negative diplococci) (see Ch. 15)

Neisseria meningitidis is carried by 10% of the population in their nasopharynx. The highest rates of carriage are in teenagers: 25% of 15- to 19-year-olds are carriers. Transmission is achieved by inhaling respiratory secretions and from direct contact such as kissing, although there needs to be prolonged contact usually. Infections with *N. meningitidis* show two peaks: one in those < 1 year old and the second in the group aged 15–19 years. Infection rates also tend to be higher in the winter months. There are several serotypes of *N. meningitidis*, with the UK having mostly serotypes B and C (85% of cases). Since the introduction of routine childhood immunization with serotype C in November 1999, the proportion of cases of meningitis or meningococcal septicaemia due to serotype C has fallen markedly. Both meningitis, from any cause, and meningococcal septicaemia are notifiable diseases, i.e. all cases need to be reported to the Consultant of Communicable Disease Control (CCDC).

Clinical features

Infection with *N. meningitidis* can present as either meningitis or the purpuric rash of meningococcal septicaemia or the two combined. Meningococcal meningitis is discussed in Chapter 15. The important characteristic of a purpuric rash is that it does not blanch since it results from bleeding into the skin. The purpuric rash is usually predominantly on the limbs but as the number of lesions increases it extends to cover the trunk. The more extensively the rash appears on the body the worse is the prognosis in general. The rash indicates that the patient has meningococcal septicaemia and hence the signs of shock will be present, i.e. tachycardia, hypotension or postural hypotension and reduced urine output.

It is critical not to miss the deadly combination of a purpuric rash and shock, as meningococcal septicaemia can be rapidly fatal in a matter of hours. Patients need immediate treatment with antibiotics and close monitoring in an intensive care setting, as they can deteriorate extremely rapidly.

Diagnosis

Suspicion of the diagnosis of meningococcal septicaemia should prompt treatment with no delay. The diagnosis can be confirmed by blood culture or by PCR performed on blood.

Treatment

Any patient suspected of having meningococcal septicaemia, even in the absence of any signs of meningitis, must be given an immediate dose of penicillin and urgently transferred to hospital. Once in hospital, if the suspicion continues, nothing must delay the rapid administration of a third-generation cephalosporin, e.g. cefotaxime. Patients who are treated for a full course of antibiotics with just penicillin will require rifampicin to eradicate *N. meningitidis* carriage, but this is not necessary if a third-generation cephalosporin is used for treatment.

Complications

The complications of meningococcal septicaemia are severe. They include renal failure, disseminated intravascular coagulation (DIC), adrenal haemorrhage leading to necrosis and failure, which is known as Waterhouse–Friderichsen syndrome, petechial haemorrhage and necrotic purpura of digits requiring amputation. The mortality is 10% from meningococcal septicaemia, which is more frequently fatal than meningococcal meningitis alone.

Immunization

Meningococcal immunization with serotype C is given to all children as part of their 2, 3 and 4 months of age immunization schedule. Students about to attend college are offered immunization if under 24 years of age, since they are a high-risk group.

An important differential diagnosis of a purpuric rash and fever is neutropenic sepsis resulting from chemotherapy given for a haematological malignancy. The malignancy itself or the chemotherapy may cause thrombocytopenia and hence a purpuric rash. Chemotherapy can produce neutropenia and thereby a vulnerability to infection that would give rise to the fever.

RHEUMATIC FEVER

Rheumatic fever is an immune-mediated inflammatory disease that results from the cross-reaction of a group A beta-haemolytic streptococcal cell wall antigen and an antigen of cardiac muscle. The patient initially suffers with a streptococcal infection, most commonly streptococcal pharyngitis, and develops rheumatic fever up to 3 weeks later. It is important to appreciate that this condition is not a direct streptococcal infection of the heart. It typically affects children and teenagers, aged 5–15 years. The incidence of rheumatic fever has dramatically declined in the UK since the introduction of antibiotics to treat streptococcal infections, although it remains a common complication in developing countries.

Pathophysiology

All three layers of the heart are involved in rheumatic fever, i.e. pancarditis. The cardiac lesion which typifies rheumatic fever is called an 'Aschoff nodule': this is a granulomatous lesion with central necrosis that arises in the myocardium with a predilection for the left ventricle. Non-infective vegetations can develop on the endocardium and may result in valvular incompetence. Inflammation of the pericardium usually induces a serous pericardial effusion in addition.

The inflammatory process also affects the synovial membranes of joints which become inflamed giving rise to the polyarthritis seen. If the skin is affected, there can be granulomatous nodules subcutaneously that are similar to the Aschoff nodules of the myocardium.

Clinical features

The patient typically presents with a sudden onset of fever, malaise, anorexia and arthritis. The symptoms suffered by each patient depend on what has been affected by the inflammation, which may include the heart, skin, joints and central nervous system. Cardiac involvement can manifest as chest pain, arrhythmias or cardiac failure and clinically a new or changed heart murmur may be detected. The skin signs are painless subcutaneous nodules, occurring particularly over joints and tendons, and the rash erythema marginatum. This is characteristic for rheumatic fever. It appears as pink coalescent rings on the trunk and may come and go. The arthritis is described as 'flitting' because one joint becomes hot, red and inflamed and just as that is resolving after a few days another joint is affected. Usually the arthritis targets larger joints such as knees, elbows, ankles and wrists. The last component of rheumatic fever to occur is the neurological symptom of Sydenham's chorea, also known as St Vitus' dance. This is a jerky, fidgeting movement that the patient cannot control and is usually unilateral. Occasionally, a patient's speech may be affected, or the patient can be confused.

Diagnosis

The first component of making the diagnosis for rheumatic fever involves proving the preceding streptococcal infection. This could be in one of several ways: either by the clinical diagnosis of a streptococcal infection, e.g. recent scarlet fever or a positive throat culture or an ASOT > 200 U/ml. In addition the patient needs to demonstrate two major, or one major and more than one minor criteria from the Duckett Jones criteria detailed in Figure 14.5.

Treatment

If there could still be an active streptococcal infection then penicillin antibiotics are given to treat it. Carditis and arthritis require bed rest until the temperature, symptoms and inflammatory markers have settled back to normal. Both of these are treated with NSAIDs (non-steroidal anti-inflammatory drugs), preferably aspirin, at high dose. Carditis may be treated with steroids. Haloperidol is used for relief of chorea.

Fig. 14.5 The revised major and minor Duckett Jones criteria for diagnosing rheumatic fever

Major criteria	Minor criteria
Pancarditis (pericarditis, myocarditis with Aschoff nodules, endocarditis)	Raised CRP, ESR
Flitting polyarthritis	Arthralgia
Sydenham's chorea (St Vitus' dance)	Fever
Subcutaneous nodules	Previous rheumatic fever or rheumatic heart disease
Erythema marginatum	Prolonged PR interval on ECG

Complications

Up to 60% of patients who had carditis as part of their rheumatic fever illness will subsequently (10–20 years later) suffer with chronic rheumatic valvular disease. The risk is obviously higher if there are repeated episodes of rheumatic fever, hence the importance of prophylactic antibiotics. If the heart valves are permanently damaged then there is a predisposition to both recurrent rheumatic fever and bacterial endocarditis, which can further damage the valves. Valvular stenosis can be a late complication of rheumatic valve disease. The majority of cases of mitral stenosis are due to rheumatic valve disease.

The mitral valve is most commonly affected by rheumatic fever, followed in frequency by combined mitral and aortic valve involvement and then to a lesser extent the aortic valve alone.

Prophylaxis

Oral penicillin antibiotics are essential until the age of 20, or for 5 years after the illness if this occurred as an adult, to prevent recurrent episodes. If the patient is penicillin allergic then erythromycin is used. All invasive procedures which could result in bacterial release into the bloodstream, e.g. dental work leading to gingival bleeding, upper respiratory tract surgery, instrumentation or surgery of the gastrointestinal (GI) or genitourinary (GU) tracts, obstetric or gynaecological procedures, must be covered by prophylactic antibiotics. Usually, diagnostic upper GI endoscopy, flexible bronchoscopy, transoesophageal echocardiography, cardiac catheterization and caesarean sections do not require antibiotic cover prophylactically.

LYME DISEASE *(BORRELIA BURGDORFERI)*

Lyme disease is a tick-borne infection, with the ticks living on deer and sheep. It was named Lyme disease due to the description of a cluster of cases occurring in Old Lyme in Connecticut, USA. It would be a mistake, however, to presume that this infection is only acquired in the USA, as it is found in many of the forested areas across the UK, e.g. New Forest, South Downs, Thetford forest and Exmoor. There are 1000–2000 cases reported annually in the UK.

Clinical features

Lyme disease presents 7–10 days after the tick bite with erythema chronicum migrans. This is a papule at the site of the tick bite that enlarges to a ring and develops central pallor. There is local lymphadenopathy related to the lesion. The rash is accompanied by fever, malaise, myalgia and arthralgia forming the first stage of the illness. Many patients are unable to remember the tick bite, so even if there is no history of a tick bite this does not exclude the possibility of Lyme disease. Weeks to months after the initial symptoms the second stage of Lyme disease occurs, comprising neurological and cardiac complications, and finally the third stage develops years later, which involves the joints.

Diagnosis

The combination of the symptoms described by the patient, the signs on examination and a history of travel to a forested area is used to make the diagnosis of Lyme disease. The causative organism is only rarely isolated from blood or CSF cultures or the skin lesions. Serology may be helpful.

Treatment

Doxycycline or amoxicillin is given for the first stage of Lyme disease and may shorten the course of the illness. Complications are treated with penicillin or a third-generation cephalosporin such as cefotaxime or ceftriaxone.

Complications

The second stage of Lyme disease includes the neurological and cardiac features. Neurologically, a patient can suffer with meningitis, cranial nerve palsies, neuropathy and amnesia. The cardiac features comprise myocarditis and conduction abnormalities such as complete heart block. The third stage of Lyme disease consists of arthritis and ataxia.

Prevention

The best way of avoiding acquiring Lyme disease is to prevent bites by ticks. In tick-infested areas, especially forests, it is recommended to use insect repellent and wear garments that cover ones limbs.

ERYTHEMA MULTIFORME

The hallmark of erythema multiforme is the target lesion. It consists of a ring of erythema with a central erythema spot and normal skin between the two, so that it appears like an archery target, hence the name. These lesions can occur anywhere on the body including the palms of the hands and the soles of the feet. Sometimes the lesions develop blisters and not all of the lesions have the central target. There are multiple causes of erythema multiforme but only the infective ones are included in the list below:

- Herpes simplex virus (most common cause)
- *Mycoplasma pneumoniae*
- Orf (maculopapular lesion occurring on hands after contact with sheep)
- Epstein–Barr virus
- HIV.

The clinical picture and symptoms occurring in addition to the erythema multiforme are used to guide the investigations to identify the cause.

Stevens–Johnson syndrome describes the more serious version of erythema multiforme when vesicles and ulcers develop on the oral mucosa and conjunctivae. There is systemic involvement with fever, arthralgia, and myalgia as well.

ERYTHEMA NODOSUM

Erythema nodosum consists of raised erythematous lesions, typically on the shins. The lesions can occur on the thighs and forearms but this is not seen commonly. The erythematous nodules are painful. Again, there are multiple causes but only the infective ones are included in Figure 14.6.

Figure 14.7 provides a summary of childhood exanthemas and other rashes.

Further reading

Smeeth L, Cook C, Fanbonne E, Heavey L, Rodrigues LC, Smith PG, Hall AJ. MMR vaccination and pervasive development disorders: a case-control study. Lancet 2004; 364:963–969.

Steere AC. Medical progress: Lyme disease. NEJM 2001; 345:115–125.

van der Poll T. Immunotherapy of sepsis. Lancet Infect Dis 2001; 1:165–174.

Fig. 14.6 The infective causes of erythema nodosum

Common causes	Less frequent causes
Streptococcus	Leptospirosis
Mycobacterial, e.g. tuberculosis, leprosy	Yersinia
	Viral infections
	Fungal infections

Fig. 14.7 Summary of childhood exanthemas and other rashes

Disease	Rash type	Other clinical features	Diagnosis	Treatment	Complications	Immunization
Chickenpox (varicella zoster virus)	Crops of papules, vesicles and pustules; pruritic	Prodromal illness	Clinical	Supportive; aciclovir in some cases	Secondary bacterial infection of skin lesions; varicella pneumonia; shingles	Yes, not routine
Shingles/herpes zoster (varicella zoster virus)	Dermatomal vesicles; painful		Clinical	Aciclovir, valaciclovir or famciclovir	Post-herpetic neuralgia	N/a
Measles (morbilliform)	Maculopapular	Koplik spots. Coryzal symptoms, cough, conjunctivitis. Cervical lymphadenopathy	Clinical	Supportive; vitamin A in developing countries	Secondary bacterial infection, e.g. pneumonia; encephalitis	Yes, routine
Rubella (rubella virus)	Macular	Low-grade fever, lymphadenopathy. Arthralgia, arthritis	Clinical	None	Transplacental infection resulting in fetal abnormalities	Yes, routine
Scarlet fever (Streptococcus pyogenes)	Macular	Fever, headache, vomiting, lymphadenopathy. Tongue involvement	Throat swab, blood cultures, ASOT	Penicillin (erythromycin if penicillin allergic)	Pharyngitis, peritonsillar or retropharyngeal abscesses. Rheumatic fever, glomerulonephritis	No
Erythema infectiosum (parvovirus B19)	'Slapped cheeks'. Maculopapular; pruritic		Clinical	None	Transplacental infection resulting in fetal death; arthritis, anaemia	No
Mumps (paramyxovirus)	None	Parotid swellings, prodromal illness	Clinical	Supportive	Meningitis; orchitis or oophoritis; sensorineural deafness, pancreatitis	Yes, routine
Neisseria meningitidis	Purpuric	Meningitis, septicaemia	Blood microscopy and culture, blood PCR	Immediate penicillin; third-generation cephalosporin, e.g. cefotaxime	Death, renal failure, DIC, adrenal haemorrhage, Waterhouse-Friderichsen syndrome, necrotic purpura of digits	Yes, routine
Rheumatic fever (immune-mediated)	Erythema marginatum; subcutaneous nodules	Pancarditis, polyarthritis, Sydenham's chorea, fever, malaise, anorexia	Throat swab/ASOT and Duckett Jones criteria	NSAIDs, steroids, haloperidol. Bed rest	Rheumatic heart disease, bacterial endocarditis	N/a
Lyme disease (Borrelia burgdorferi)	Erythema chronicum migrans	Fever, malaise, arthralgia, myalgia	Clinical; serology	Doxycycline or amoxicillin. Penicillin or cefotaxime/ceftriaxone for later stages	Second stage – neurological and cardiac features. Third stage – arthritis and ataxia	No

Meningitis and encephalitis

Objectives

In this chapter you will learn:

- How to distinguish between meningitis and encephalitis at the bedside
- What to do if you suspect meningococcal infection
- The empiric treatment for meningitis
- Who should be immunized to protect them against meningitis
- How to manage encephalitis.

MENINGITIS

Meningitis is an inflammation of the meninges. These are the three layers of membranes overlying the brain that continue down over the spinal cord. Symptoms arise from any irritation of the meninges, which can be infective such as bacterial or viral infections, or blood, e.g. from a subarachnoid haemorrhage, or infiltrative, e.g. from a CNS lymphoma. In this chapter only the infective causes of meningitis will be covered.

In the infective causes of meningitis, there is a range of severity of the illness: bacterial meningitis tends to be a more serious, potentially life-threatening infection, whereas viral meningitis tends to be a more benign illness that is often self-limiting. The likely organisms causing meningitis vary, depending on the age and immune status of the patient. Neonates and children under the age of 1 year are particularly vulnerable to meningitis because their blood–brain barrier is not as robust as in older individuals; for this reason a 'septic screen' looking for the cause of a fever in neonates should routinely include a lumbar puncture to obtain CSF (cerebrospinal fluid) for microscopy and culture.

Meningitis is a notifiable disease in the UK. Close contacts of a case of meningitis need to be traced by the public health team and given prophylactic antibiotics. In cases of meningococcal and *Haemophilus influenzae* meningitis, rifampicin or ciprofloxacin are the antibiotics given.

Common bacterial causes in adults and children:
- *Neisseria meningitidis*
- *Streptococcus pneumoniae*
- *Haemophilus influenzae* type b (now rare).

Common bacterial causes in neonates:
- Group B beta-haemolytic streptococcus
- *Escherichia coli*
- *Listeria monocytogenes*.

Viral causes:
- Enteroviruses
- Paramyxovirus (mumps)
- Herpes simplex viruses
- Varicella zoster virus
- HIV
- Epstein–Barr virus.

Causes in immunocompromised patients:
- *Mycobacterium tuberculosis*
- Fungal e.g. *Cryptococcus neoformans*
- *Listeria monocytogenes*.

For further details of tuberculous meningitis see Chapter 26, and for information on the infections suffered by those with HIV and immunocompromise see Chapter 25.

Clinical features

Meningitis presents with the triad of symptoms: headache, neck stiffness and photophobia. These features are a consequence of inflammation or irritation of the meninges. The clinical sign for meningeal inflammation is neck stiffness. Sometimes Kernig's sign is used, which involves stretching the meninges (see Ch. 2 for how to perform this) thereby producing pain if there is meningitis. Vomiting can be a feature, and may reflect raised intracranial pressure. There is not usually any reduction in the level of consciousness or any focal neurological deficits, in contrast to encephalitis, or unless there is a meningo-encephalitis. The onset of symptoms is more rapid with bacterial meningitis and the patient appears more unwell. In cases of meningitis due to a viral aetiology there is often a flu-like illness that precedes the meningitis symptoms.

Meningococcal septicaemia gives rise to a purpuric rash in about 50% of cases, which can be with or without meningitis. In both cases immediate treatment with intravenous penicillin is imperative. In a septicaemic patient there might be signs of shock; namely tachycardia, hypotension or postural hypotension in the early stages, and reduced urine output.

Diagnosis

The essential investigation to make a diagnosis of meningitis and elucidate the causative organism is a lumbar puncture to obtain CSF. The differential biochemistry and microscopy results from the CSF are given in Chapter 2. Gram staining of any bacteria seen in the CSF can identify the organism, which should be confirmed by culture. PCR on both CSF and blood can help discover the cause in culture negative cases. PCR is used to detect *Neisseria meningitidis*, *Streptococcus pneumoniae* and viral causes. Blood cultures can isolate the bacterial causes of meningitis if there is concomitant bacteraemia.

Treatment

If the lumbar puncture reveals cloudy CSF then empirical antibiotic therapy should be started immediately. Initial blind therapy in adults and children is an intravenous third-generation cephalosporin such as cefotaxime or ceftriaxone. Once the organism has been identified, therapy can be tailored, e.g. penicillin used in sensitive pneumococcal meningitis. In immunocompromised patients, pregnant women or in those who appear encephalitic, ampicillin to cover *Listeria monocytogenes* should be added to the empirical therapy. Neonatal therapy consists of intravenous penicillin combined with an aminoglycoside (gentamicin) or a third-generation cephalosporin.

Meningococcal infection can present with either meningitis or septic shock; therefore, if a petechial rash is seen, even in the absence of any neck stiffness, the patient should be given intramuscular benzylpenicillin immediately by the GP prior to urgent transfer to hospital.

The use of steroids has recently been shown to improve mortality and morbidity, in particular with respect to sensorineural deafness in children. The steroids need to be given empirically with the first dose of antibiotics and continued for 4 days. If the patient has been given benzylpenicillin prior to admission, then the steroids should start with the first in-hospital dose of antibiotics. If the diagnosis is subsequently found not to be bacterial meningitis, then the steroids can be stopped.

Penicillin therapy does not eradicate nasopharyngeal carriage of the meningococcus, so treated cases should be given rifampicin or ciprofloxacin to eradicate carriage at the end of treatment. However, treatment with third-generation cephalosporins, e.g. ceftriaxone, does eliminate carriage, in which case rifampicin and ciprofloxacin are not required.

Complications

Meningitis can result in sensorineural deafness, venous sinus thrombosis, severe cerebral oedema and hydrocephalus.

Bacterial causes

Neisseria meningitidis (Gram-negative diplococci)

Neisseria meningitidis is found in the nasopharynx of 10% of the population, although in the high-risk group of 15- to 19-year-olds the carriage rate can reach 25%. Transmission is via respiratory secretions either from inhalation or by direct contact, e.g. kissing (more than fleeting contact needed). Meningococcus can give rise to meningitis as well as septicaemia. Meningococcal meningitis occurs in children and young adults more commonly, which is why these groups are now immunized. Infants in the UK receive three doses of the meningococcus serotype C vaccine at monthly intervals from 2 months of age. Students about to attend college can elect to receive a dose of the vaccine if aged under 24 years (no benefit has been shown for those aged > 24 years). Travellers to high-risk areas, e.g. Hajj pilgrimage to Saudi Arabia, are advised to receive immunization covering the four most common serotypes to cause infection, i.e. A, C, W135 and Y. Until recently, travellers to the tropics were advised to have the meningococcal vaccine against serotypes A and C but current recommendations are that they should receive the quadrivalent vaccine as well. It is important to remember that this immunization requires a booster after 3–5 years for continued protection. In patients who have had their spleen removed or in cases of hyposplenism, e.g. in sickle cell anaemia, there may be an increased risk of meningococcal infections.

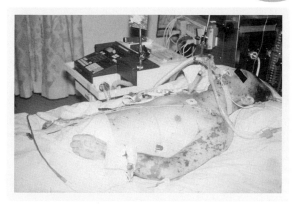

Fig. 15.1 This patient developed shock with meningococcal meningitis, requiring intensive care support.
Source: Conlon CP, Snydman DR. Mosby's Colour Atlas and Text of Infectious Diseases. Edinburgh: Mosby; 2000: Fig. 1.3.

> When patients recover from meningococcal meningitis, especially if they have more than one episode, they should be checked for complement (C5–9) deficiency as this predisposes to infection with *Neisseria meningitidis*.

Additional clinical details

The critical aspect to remember is to check for a purpuric rash when the meningitic symptoms are present because meningococcal septicaemia confers a higher mortality rate than meningitis without septicaemia (Fig. 15.1). Further details of the purpuric rash are found in Chapter 14. Ten to fifteen percent of cases of meningococcal meningitis will result in permanent hearing loss, mental retardation, limb loss or other serious sequelae.

> Meningococcal septicaemia can result in infarction of the distal extremities, which may require digit or limb amputation depending on the severity, and haemorrhagic necrosis of the adrenal glands, which is known as Waterhouse–Friderichsen syndrome. Recent trials involving activated protein C have shown improved outcomes.

Diagnosis

Microscopy and culture of the CSF are the mainstay of isolating the meningococcus. Blood cultures will be positive if there is septicaemia or bacteraemia. PCR of both the blood and CSF can identify *Neisseria meningitidis*.

Streptococcus pneumoniae (Gram-positive cocci, seen as diplococci or short chains)

Streptococcus pneumoniae is a commensal of the upper respiratory tract. If someone sustains a skull fracture then the pneumococcus has direct access to the meninges and infection can arise. The second route for acquiring pneumococcal meningitis is from pneumococcal septicaemia, which could have originated from a respiratory tract infection. The group of people at highest risk for contracting pneumococcal meningitis include patients without a spleen, the elderly and children usually less than 2 years of age. As a result, asplenic patients, the elderly and those who have sustained a skull fracture are offered pneumococcal immunization to protect against pneumococcal infections including meningitis. Children older than 2 months of age can be successfully immunized with the pneumococcal vaccine but this is not routinely performed.

> Asplenic patients are at an increased risk of infection from encapsulated bacteria, i.e. pneumococcus, meningococcus and *Haemophilus influenzae*, because the organisms cannot be opsonized and phagocytosed in the spleen. Asplenic patients should all be immunized with pneumococcal, Hib and meningococcal vaccines and take daily prophylactic penicillin antibiotics (erythromycin if penicillin allergic) at least until aged 16.

Additional clinical details

Sensorineural deafness is a more common complication than with other causes of meningitis. No prophylaxis is required for contacts of the index meningitis case.

Diagnosis

Microscopy and culture of the CSF is the best way to identify *Streptococcus pneumoniae* as the cause of a meningitis. If there is a bacteraemia then the blood cultures will be positive in addition. PCR on blood can be used to identify the pneumococcus as the cause.

Haemophilus influenzae **type b (Hib) (Gram-negative bacilli)**

It is widely accepted that since the introduction in 1992 of Hib immunization, Hib had largely been eliminated as a cause of either upper respiratory tract infections, where it is a commensal, and meningitis. Unfortunately there seems to be a small resurgence in the number of cases since 2000: pre-Hib immunization there were > 850 cases/year, which dropped to 37 cases in 1998, but since 2000 there have been > 100 cases/year. The reason for this is not clear. Hib typically infects children less than 5 years old and asplenic patients.

Additional clinical details

Hib meningitis can result in serious complications: 20% of cases suffer with permanent hearing loss or other long-term neurological sequelae. Rifampicin prophylaxis is required for contacts of the index meningitis case.

Diagnosis

Microscopy and culture of CSF is the usual method to identify the Hib bacteria. Blood cultures may also be positive.

Listeria monocytogenes **(Gram-positive bacilli)**

Listeria monocytogenes exists ubiquitously in the environment and can be found as a commensal of the gastrointestinal tract in some healthy people. It tends to only cause severe disease in pregnant women, neonates, the elderly and immunocompromised patients. Infection can be acquired from foodstuffs: pregnant women are advised to avoid soft, unpasteurized cheeses and pâtés in particular.

Additional clinical details

Listeria infection is more likely to present as a meningo-encephalitis, than solely meningitis. There is often a flu-like illness in the days preceding the onset of meningitic symptoms. Importantly the maternal infection may be asymptomatic but the neonate can become infected either across the placenta or during birth or from direct person-to-person contact immediately after delivery.

Diagnosis

Listeria monocytogenes can be isolated from both CSF and blood cultures.

Escherichia coli **(Gram-negative bacilli)**

E. coli is a very common gastrointestinal commensal and usually causes infections related to the gastrointestinal or urinary tracts. Meningitis due to *E. coli* is only really seen in neonates. It is particularly the K1 serotype that causes neonatal meningitis. The gentamicin or cephalosporin part of the antibiotic treatment is the element that treats *E. coli* meningitis.

Additional clinical details

In most cases, whilst the neonate becomes infected with *E. coli* the mother would be asymptomatic. The transmission is usually from commensal carriage rather than a maternal infection.

Diagnosis

E. coli can be identified from CSF and blood cultures.

Group B beta-haemolytic streptococcus (Gram-positive cocci)

Group B beta-haemolytic streptococcus is the most common cause of meningitis in neonates, affecting 0.8 per 1000 live births. 70% of cases occurring within the first 6 days of life are due to group B streptococcus. The source of infection is thought to vary depending on when the infection is acquired during the first few weeks of the neonate's life. Meningitis presenting in the first week occurs as a result of passage down the birth canal: 30% of mothers will have group B streptococcus as part of their genital flora. Cases of meningitis developing more than 1 week after birth are more likely to be due to cross-infection, for instance in a neonatal intensive care unit. The Royal College of Obstetrics and Gynaecology produced a set of guidelines in November 2003 to target the prevention of early-onset group B streptococcal infection in neonates.

Additional clinical details

In most cases the mother is an asymptomatic carrier of group B streptococcus rather than being infected when the neonate develops meningitis.

Diagnosis

Group B streptococcus can be cultured from CSF and blood specimens.

Viral causes

The viruses that cause meningitis can also lead to encephalitis; usually there is a combined infection, i.e. meningo-encephalitis. The viruses involved will be discussed further below.

ENCEPHALITIS

Encephalitis describes infection of the brain parenchyma itself and is often in conjunction with meningitis. The aetiology is viral in the majority of cases (Fig. 15.2); it can, however, be a complication of bacterial or fungal meningitis. In many instances the exact viral cause is not clarified by serology, culture or PCR but the causative organism is still assumed to be a virus. The incidence of encephalitis is 1.5 cases per 100 000 population in the UK. It can be a serious infection with a mortality rate of 20% despite treatment; most of these more severe cases are due to HSV. Like meningitis, encephalitis is a notifiable disease and therefore all cases must be reported to the CCDC.

Clinical features

The triad of meningitis symptoms, i.e. headache, neck stiffness and photophobia, are present with encephalitis also. This reflects the joint involvement of meninges and brain parenchyma. The differentiating factor is that patients with encephalitis usually have a reduced level of consciousness and focal neurological deficits, e.g. ophthalmoplegia, dysphasia, hemiparesis. Fever, vomiting and seizures are common in the presentation of encephalitis. Initially the patient may be non-specifically unwell and confused, before the more localizing symptoms are apparent.

Diagnosis

Given the presence of focal neurology, reduced consciousness or seizures, a scan, either CT or MRI, is indicated to exclude a space-occupying lesion and ensure it is safe to proceed with a lumbar puncture. A CT or MRI scan of the brain showing diffuse oedema, particularly in the temporal lobes, would be suggestive for encephalitis (Fig. 15.3).

A lumbar puncture to obtain CSF for microscopy and culture is the definitive investigation to make the diagnosis. The CSF results seen in encephalitis are detailed in Chapter 2. An EEG can demonstrate the

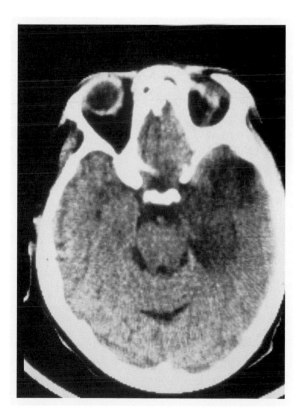

Fig. 15.3 CT scan of the brain showing herpes simplex virus involvement of the temporal lobe.
Source: Conlon CP, Snydman DR, 2000: Fig. 7.17.

Fig. 15.2 Viral causes of encephalitis

Most common causes	Less common causes	Rare causes
Herpes simplex 1 and 2	Echoviruses Coxsackie A and B Mumps and measles viruses Epstein–Barr virus	Varicella zoster virus Adenovirus Enteroviruses Influenza viruses

slow wave changes typical of encephalitis. Serology and PCR are used to attempt to identify the exact viral cause, although this is not always found. PCR has replaced viral isolation by culture because it is more rapid and sensitive as a test. Positive serology results would be indicated by a fourfold rise in antibodies between acute and convalescent samples.

Treatment

In suspected cases of HSV encephalitis prompt treatment with intravenous aciclovir can improve the prognosis. There is no specific antiviral therapy for the other types of viral encephalitis. Otherwise, treatment is supportive and in severe cases transfer to the intensive care unit is appropriate. Anticonvulsants should be considered not just for treating seizures but also as prophylaxis to prevent them. Cerebral oedema may require dexamethasone and mannitol therapy to reduce intracranial pressure increases.

Complications

The prognosis is poor with 20% mortality even with treatment and there is a significant risk of severe long-lasting brain injury.

Viral causes

Clinically it is not possible to distinguish one virus from another as the cause of a case of encephalitis. All the viruses mentioned are capable of causing meningitis and encephalitis, usually seen as a combined meningo-encephalitis.

Herpes simplex viruses 1 and 2

HSV-1 and -2 are the most common causes of encephalitis and also tend to cause the most severe infections. The most crucial aspect of management is to suspect that there may be encephalitis as part of the infection picture and give aciclovir promptly.

Mumps and Measles viruses

Before the introduction of MMR, mumps was the commonest viral cause of meningitis. It causes mild meningitis in 5% of cases and less frequently encephalitis. Measles only leads to encephalitis in less than 1 in 1000 cases but children less than 1 year of age, immunocompromised patients or those with vitamin A deficiency are at an increased risk. Very rarely, measles occurring in children less than 18 months old can develop into subacute sclerosing panencephalitis (SSPE), which presents in the teenage years with a progressive decline in mental functioning and seizures, to coma and eventually death.

Enteroviruses genus

The enteroviruses genus includes polioviruses, Coxsackie A and B viruses, echoviruses and enteroviruses types. All of these can cause both meningitis and encephalitis. The infections tend to be fairly mild and self-limiting.

Epstein–Barr virus

Glandular fever caused by EBV can become a more disseminated infection leading to meningo-encephalitis as well as hepatitis and myocarditis.

Varicella zoster virus

Chickenpox only rarely causes meningitis and encephalitis in healthy children. Immunocompromised patients and adults who acquire chickenpox are at a greater risk of suffering a more severe illness and developing the complications.

Figure 15.4 summarizes information on meningitis and encephalitis.

Further reading

Chaudhuri A. Adjunctive dexamethasone treatment in acute bacterial meningitis. Lancet Neurol 2004; 3:54–62.

Quagliarello VJ, Scheld WM. Drug therapy: treatment of bacterial meningitis. N Engl J Med 1997; 336:708–716.

Royal College of Obstetricians and Gynaecologists. Guidelines for group B streptococcus. Website: www.rcog.org.uk/guidelines.asp?PageID=106&GuidelineID=56.

Solomon T. Current concepts: flavivirus encephalitis. N Engl J Med 2004; 351:370–378.

Fig. 15.4 Summary of meningitis and encephalitis

	Meningitis	Encephalitis
Clinical features	Triad: headache, neck stiffness and photophobia. Vomiting. Purpuric rash and shock with meningococcal meningitis. Preceding flu-like illness with viral meningitis	Meningitis triad: headache, neck stiffness and photophobia. Reduced level of consciousness and focal neurological deficits. Fever, vomiting and seizures
Diagnosis	CSF for microscopy, culture and biochemistry. PCR on blood and CSF. Blood cultures	Diffuse oedema, especially in the temporal lobes, on CT or MRI scan. CSF for microscopy, culture and biochemistry. PCR; acute and convalescent serology. Slow wave changes on EEG
Treatment	Adults and children: intravenous third-generation cephalosporin, e.g. cefotaxime, ceftriaxone. Additionally ampicillin in some cases. Concomitant steroid therapy in children. Neonates: intravenous penicillin and gentamicin, or third-generation cephalosporin. Intensive care unit support may be necessary	Intravenous aciclovir for HSV encephalitis. Anticonvulsant therapy for treatment and prophylaxis of seizures. Dexamethasone and mannitol therapy for cerebral oedema. Intensive care unit support
Complications	Sensorineural deafness, venous sinus thrombosis, severe cerebral oedema and hydrocephalus. Death	Mortality 20%. Severe prolonged brain injury

Upper respiratory tract infections

16

Objectives

In this chapter you will learn:

- The differential diagnoses for glandular fever
- Which infections give rise to stridor
- Which upper respiratory tract infections can be immunized against
- The infections that need to be notified to the CCDC and Public Health Department
- Why influenza epidemics arise.

The upper respiratory tract extends from the point of entry at either the nostrils or the oral cavity down to the trachea. Each of us is normally colonized by bacteria throughout the respiratory tract, but these bacteria do not cause an infection unless they manage to penetrate the mucosal barrier. A variety of viral and bacterial infections can affect the upper respiratory tract as detailed below.

VIRAL INFECTIONS

The severity of the viral infections is highly variable: from the benign common cold to more serious infections such as influenza and glandular fever.

Common cold

Viruses

The majority of infections resulting in a common cold are caused by rhinoviruses but many others can be implicated, such as coronaviruses, influenza viruses, coxsackie viruses, para-influenza viruses, adenoviruses and echoviruses.

Transmission

Sneezing results in an aerosol of droplets containing the causative viruses, which is a highly effective method of transmission, especially in crowded environments. Spread by direct contact with virus-containing droplets can also occur. The incubation period is usually 1–4 days.

Clinical features

The illness involves rhinorrhoea (runny nose), headache and malaise. Collectively these are known as 'coryza'. The person affected is not usually unwell enough to feel the need to retire to bed.

Investigations

In the majority of cases the cost of identifying the exact virus responsible for the infection is not justified, particularly since treatment is not influenced by the virus involved.

Treatment

No antiviral therapy is given for the common cold. Treatment is purely supportive, with paracetamol or aspirin usually used for the headache. Over-the-counter preparations for symptomatic relief of rhinorrhoea are used by many sufferers.

Complications

In a child a common cold can be the initial precipitant for otitis media (see below).

Glandular fever

Virus

Glandular fever is caused by Epstein–Barr virus (EBV).

Transmission

EBV is transmitted by direct saliva contact such as via kissing. This is the most common route amongst

85

teenagers, who are the most frequently affected age group, although any age can be infected. The incubation period is not clearly known but can be up to 1 month.

Clinical features

Glandular fever presents with tonsillar enlargement which is associated with an exudate over the tonsils, a sore throat and cervical lymphadenopathy in combination with a fever and malaise. The latter two symptoms may remain for a prolonged period of months. Some patients become jaundiced, and splenomegaly can occur. If the patient is given ampicillin for the sore throat, on the assumption that it is due to a streptococcal pharyngitis, a maculopapular rash develops.

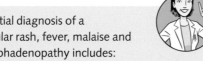

The differential diagnosis of a maculopapular rash, fever, malaise and cervical lymphadenopathy includes:

- HIV seroconversion
- Cytomegalovirus (CMV) infection
- Toxoplasmosis infection
- EBV treated with ampicillin.

If there is also jaundice and splenomegaly present then the differential diagnosis includes the viral hepatitis infections, A to E.

Investigations

The blood film of a patient suffering with glandular fever shows an increased lymphocyte count with atypical lymphocytes and signs of a haemolytic anaemia, i.e. reduced numbers of mature red blood cells and increased numbers of reticulocytes (immature red blood cells). A monospot test (or Paul–Bunnell test), which detects the heterophile antibodies that are common in glandular fever, is positive. The liver function tests may show a hepatitic derangement, i.e. high aspartate transaminase (AST) and alanine transaminase (ALT), and raised bilirubin if there is an associated hepatitis.

Treatment

There is no specific treatment for glandular fever. The management is just supportive: paracetamol can be used as an antipyretic; throat gargles can be useful for symptomatic relief of the sore throat. Many patients feel sufficiently unwell in the initial stages to require bed rest.

Complications

An EBV infection can result in thrombocytopenia, haemolytic anaemia and hepatitis, and if the spleen is enlarged, there is an increased risk of traumatic rupture. The other complications of glandular fever are rare but include aseptic meningitis, encephalitis, pericarditis, pneumonitis, Guillain–Barré syndrome and lymphoma.

There are a number of tumours associated with an EBV infection, namely: Burkitt's lymphoma, Hodgkin's lymphoma, large B cell lymphoma and nasopharyngeal carcinoma.

Croup (viral laryngotracheobronchiolitis)

Virus

Croup can be caused by parainfluenza viruses, respiratory syncytial virus and measles.

Transmission

Croup is spread by aerosolization of droplets containing the virus, e.g. sneezing. There is a seasonal variation in infection rates with higher numbers of cases occurring in the autumn and spring months.

Clinical features

Croup presents with a cough that is classically described as 'bovine' or 'barking', with the additional features of a sore throat and fever. The symptoms develop over several days. The child, typically less than 3 years old, can also suffer with inspiratory stridor and dyspnoea due to oedema of the vocal cords and epiglottis causing airway narrowing. In severe cases the child may become cyanosed.

Investigations

The diagnosis is made clinically and it is unusual for investigations to be performed. Virus identification is not routinely carried out as it has no bearing on management.

Treatment

Traditionally, children are given mist inhalations to improve their symptoms. In severe cases of inspiratory stridor, especially when the child is becoming cyanosed, ventilatory support in hospital may be required but in the majority of cases admission to hospital is not necessary.

Influenza

Virus

Influenza (colloquially known as flu) is caused by influenza A viruses, responsible for epidemics and pandemics, and influenza B viruses, causing smaller outbreaks. More recently, there has been concern about avian influenza that has affected humans; the viruses affecting humans and birds are very similar.

Transmission

Influenza viruses are transmitted by aerosol spread of droplets and via direct contact with virus-containing fluid from droplets. The incubation period is 2–3 days. Seasonal epidemics and pandemics typically occur in the winter months. On average there are about 60 consultations with the GP per 100 000 population at the peak of the winter period outbreaks in the UK. Any age group can be affected but typically the elderly and those suffering from systemic illnesses are the most vulnerable.

Clinical features

Influenza presents with rhinorrhoea, a dry cough and sore throat combined with fever, headache, myalgia and malaise. The myalgia and malaise can be quite marked. The severity tends to be greatest in those at the extremes of age.

Investigations

The diagnosis is made clinically. The expense of identifying the exact virus involved is not usually justified, except for surveillance and during outbreaks, as it does not influence treatment.

Treatment

In the majority of cases treatment is supportive and usually involves drinking plenty of fluids, bed rest and paracetamol. Paracetamol is good as it combines antipyretic effects for the fever with analgesia for the headache and myalgia. There are numerous over-the-counter preparations for symptomatic relief of flu which can be beneficial. Oseltamivir and zanamivir (viral neuraminidase inhibitors) are licensed for use within 48 hours of the onset of symptoms of influenza in high-risk patients and act to shorten the course of the illness. The NICE guidelines on influenza treatment specifically state that these drugs should not be used as a substitute for vaccination nor should they be prescribed to otherwise healthy individuals. Oseltamivir can be used as treatment in children if indicated. Amantadine is licensed for the treatment of influenza A infections but is no longer recommended by the NICE guidelines.

Complications

Secondary bacterial pneumonia is the most common complication of influenza infections, especially in those who have a pre-existing lung disease, e.g. COPD. *Staphylococcus aureus* is often the causative organism. Otitis media and sinusitis can be sequelae of influenza as detailed below. More rarely, influenza infection can lead to the development of encephalitis, pericarditis and Guillain–Barré syndrome.

Prophylaxis

Influenza immunization is given to high-risk groups. Those deemed at high risk are the elderly (> 65 years old), health workers and anyone over the age of 6 months with chronic diseases such as renal failure, heart disease, diabetes mellitus and lung disease, including asthma. In addition, patients with immuno-suppression resulting from disease or treatment, including those without a spleen or with splenic dysfunction, should receive immunization. Vacci-nation is the most effective method of prevention and is offered to high-risk patients via their GPs or via Occupational Health for health workers in the autumn months in preparation for the seasonal outbreaks over winter.

Oseltamivir is licensed for prophylactic use in high-risk individuals over the age of 13 years. It can be given if started within 48 hours of exposure to influenza and when there is an influenza outbreak in the local community. It is also licensed for exceptional circumstances, e.g. when the influenza circulating is not covered by the current vaccination, for those who are unable to be immunized or who only received the vaccine within the preceding 2 weeks, and therefore may not have yet developed immunity. Amantadine is licensed for prophylactic use during an influenza outbreak but is no longer recommended by the NICE guidelines.

Influenza viruses are capable of antigenic shift (major change) and drift (minor change), so vaccines need to be constantly updated. These alterations are to the viral antigenic structures of haemagglutinins and neuraminidases. Epidemics and pandemics occur when there has been a significant antigenic shift so that the virus is able to evade the host immune system.

BACTERIAL INFECTIONS

Bacterial infections can affect the tonsils, throat, middle ear and sinuses as detailed below:

Streptococcal pharyngitis

Bacteria

Streptococcus pyogenes, also known as a group A beta-haemolytic Streptococcus, is responsible for throat infections. Streptococcus is a Gram-positive coccus that tends to occur in chains when viewed on microscopy. This can be remembered by thinking that 'strep occurs in a strip', whereas staphylococci appear in clumps.

Transmission

Strep. pyogenes is a commensal of the upper respiratory tract in up to 10% of the population, with higher rates in children. It is transmitted by aerosol droplets and via direct contact. There is seasonal variation in infection rates, with increased cases in winter months.

Clinical features

Streptococcal pharyngitis consists of tonsillar enlargement with an associated purulent exudate giving rise to a sore throat and reactive cervical lymphadenopathy. The patient also complains of fever and general malaise.

Investigations

Streptococcus can be confirmed as the cause of the pharyngitis with throat swabs taken for microscopy and culture. Antistreptolysin O titre (ASOT) is not routinely checked in the acute phase but may be useful later to confirm that a resultant complication, e.g. glomerulonephritis, did originate from a streptococcal infection.

Treatment

Streptococcal infections are treated with an oral course of penicillin, or erythromycin if the patient is allergic to penicillin.

Complications

The local complications arising from a streptococcal pharyngitis include a peritonsillar abscess (known as quinsy), otitis media (due to blocking of the Eustachian tube – see below) and sinusitis (see below). There are also a number of complications from a streptococcal infection that are independent of the location of the original infection, e.g. scarlet fever (see Ch. 14), rheumatic fever, acute glomerulonephritis and septicaemia. Rheumatic fever is not an infective complication but results from a cross-reaction between a streptococcal bacterial antigen and a heart muscle antigen (see Ch. 14). Acute glomerulonephritis occurs due to immune complex deposition in the glomeruli and subsequent complement activation. Septicaemia is the consequence of any local infection entering the bloodstream so that it is distributed throughout the circulation, and hence the bacteria are then detectable on blood culture.

Diphtheria

Bacteria

Diphtheria, which is a rare disease nowadays, is caused by *Corynebacterium diphtheriae*. This is a spore-forming Gram-positive bacillus that has the ability to produce an exotoxin.

Transmission

Diphtheria is transmitted by aerosol spread of droplets from the nose and throat. It has largely been eradicated in countries that have managed to implement a successful immunization programme. There is still a significant prevalence in Russia, Southeast Asia, India and Brazil. The incubation period is 2–5 days but can be longer, and typically adolescents and adults are affected.

Clinical features

Diphtheria presents with a sore throat from pharyngitis and tonsillar enlargement. Classically the tonsils are covered with a firmly adherent 'false membrane', which is the profuse exudate resulting from necrosis of mucosal cells due to the effects of the toxin. There is pronounced tender cervical lymphadenopathy and oedema, which is described as giving the patient a 'bull neck'. Occasional cases present with wounds or skin ulcers that have become infected with *Corynebacterium diphtheriae* and these patients suffer with the toxin-mediated complications listed below.

Investigations

Throat swabs are taken for microscopy and culture to identify *Corynebacterium diphtheriae*. Most important though is to ascertain if the strain causing infection is toxin-producing, as the complications of diphtheria arise from the effects of the toxin. The toxin used to be detected by the Elek test but now PCR (polymerase chain reaction) is used to detect the gene encoding the toxin.

Diphtheria is a notifiable disease. All case contacts should have throat swabs taken and if these are found to be positive the individuals should receive antibiotics (penicillin or erythromycin) and immunization.

Treatment

Antitoxin must be given rapidly if diphtheria infection is suspected, i.e. before bacteriological confirmation, in order to minimize the toxin-mediated effects. Clinicians administering the antitoxin must be alert to the hypersensitivity reactions which can occur because the antitoxin is derived from horse serum. In addition penicillin or erythromycin (if the patient is penicillin allergic) is given intravenously. The antibiotic therapy eradicates carriage of *C. diphtheriae* from the upper respiratory tract but is not a substitute for antitoxin. The immunization status of the patient should be ascertained and vaccination given if required. Bed rest and isolation are advised.

Complications

The complications of diphtheria are due to toxin production, and include myocarditis, palatal or pharyngeal paralysis, polyneuropathy, cranial nerve palsies and rarely encephalitis.

Immunization

In countries which operate an effective immunization programme, all children should receive their immunizations at 2, 3 and 4 months followed by several boosters throughout their schooling (see Ch. 1 for schedule).

Epiglottitis

Bacteria

Epiglottitis is caused by *Haemophilus influenzae* type b (Hib) infection. This is a Gram-negative bacillus.

Transmission

Hib is spread by aerosolized droplets. It is a commensal of the upper respiratory tract but only causes infections when it breaches the respiratory tract mucosa. Infection rates had dramatically declined since the introduction of Hib immunization in 1992 but there has been a small resurgence in the number of cases since 2000, the reasons for which are not totally clear.

Clinical features

Epiglottitis presents with fever and an acute onset of respiratory distress and stridor. The child looks ill and is often irritable. Generally, epiglottitis only occurs in children less than 5 years old. The epiglottis, when seen, is swollen and erythematous.

Only someone able to intubate should examine a child with suspected epiglottitis as airway obstruction can occur rapidly. *Any* distress can trigger airway obstruction in epiglottitis, so the child needs to be kept as calm as possible.

Investigations

Hib can be isolated from throat swabs and blood cultures for microscopy and culture. It is important that these samples should only be obtained by a person able to intubate as the procedure or upset to the child could precipitate airway obstruction.

Treatment

Epiglottitis is best treated with a second- or third-generation cephalosporin, e.g. cefuroxime or cefotaxime, since 15% of strains of Hib are resistance to ampicillin. The deterioration of the child to the point of requiring intubation and ventilation can be very rapid and therefore these patients are best looked after in a high-dependency area or the intensive care unit. Rifampicin is used to eradicate nasopharyngeal carriage and may be given as prophylaxis to vulnerable household contacts of an index case.

Immunization

Hib immunization is given routinely in childhood (see Ch. 1 for schedule) and to all asplenic patients since they are at increased risk of infection (see Ch. 15).

Whooping cough

Bacteria

Whooping cough results from infection with *Bordetella pertussis*. This is a Gram-negative coccobacillus.

Transmission

Bordetella pertussis is acquired from aerosol spread of droplets containing the organism. The incubation period is 7–10 days. Whooping cough is a notifiable disease in the UK, so all cases must be reported to the Consultant of Communicable Disease Control and the Public Health Department. In 1975 there was a health scare over the safety of the pertussis vaccine and immunization uptake plummeted to 30%; as a result there were two epidemics following this. Immunization uptake steadily rose from then to the current level of 94% and notifications of whooping cough are at a nadir.

Clinical features

Whooping cough starts initially with coryzal symptoms and malaise. After a week there is the development of the distinctive paroxysms of coughing followed by a 'whoop' which is a sudden huge inspiratory effort against a narrowed glottis. These paroxysms of coughing often induce vomiting and conjunctival suffusion. There may be associated dyspnoea and stridor. It is principally an illness of childhood and may last for 2–3 months; hence its name as the '100-day cough'.

Investigations

The diagnosis is largely made clinically but is confirmed by culturing *Bordetella pertussis* from nasopharyngeal swabs or a nasopharyngeal aspirate.

Treatment

Erythromycin is the antibiotic of choice for treating whooping cough. It shortens the course and lessens the severity of the illness if given early.

Complications

Whooping cough can precipitate the development of inguinal hernias from the force of such repeated coughing. Damage to the respiratory airways can result in secondary infections including bronchopneumonia and bronchiectasis. The 'whoop' phenomenon can lead to apnoea, convulsions and ultimately death. The severe complications, including death, are more common in those aged < 6 months, while the infection tends to be less serious in older children and adults. Preventing infection in older children and adults is important though, because otherwise they form a potential source of infection for young children.

Immunization

Bordetella pertussis is one of the infections covered by the recommended childhood immunization programme in the UK (see Ch. 1 for schedule).

Otitis media

Bacteria

Otitis media is most commonly caused by:

- *Streptococcus pneumoniae* (Gram-positive diplococci)
- *Streptococcus pyogenes* (Gram-positive cocci, seen in chains)
- *Staphylococcus aureus* (Gram-positive cocci, seen in clumps)
- *Haemophilus influenzae* type b (Gram-negative bacilli).

Aetiology

Otitis media is an infection of the middle ear. It generally follows from an upper respiratory tract infection when the Eustachian tube becomes blocked, thereby inhibiting drainage of fluid from the middle ear (Fig. 16.1), which is then liable to infection.

Clinical features

Otitis media manifests with fever, earache and impaired hearing. Some patients report that they feel unable to clear their ears, i.e. equalize the pressure either side of their eardrum. Since otitis media follows from an upper respiratory tract infection, the patient will initially have suffered the symptoms of the prodromal illness. On examination, the eardrum is

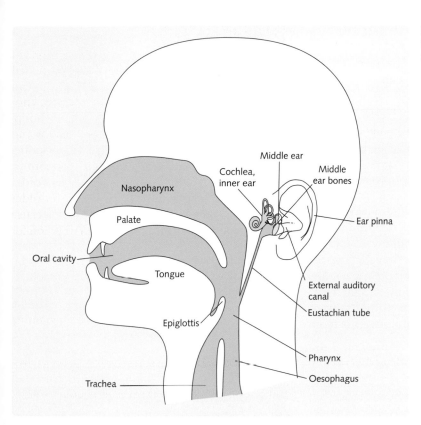

Fig. 16.1 The relationship between the middle ear, Eustachian tube and upper respiratory tract.

reddened and bulging and a fluid level may be visible behind it. The eardrum is liable to rupture; hence a perforation and purulent discharge along the ear canal may also be seen.

Investigations

The diagnosis is formed from the otoscopy appearances of the eardrum but the causative organism will only be established from culture of any discharging or aspirated fluid from the ear.

Treatment

The organisms causing otitis media will in the majority of cases be covered by co-amoxiclav, or erythromycin if the patient is allergic to penicillins. If the infection does not resolve, then the sensitivities of the organisms cultured need to be checked or empirical therapy with a second- or third-generation cephalosporins initiated. Chronic or repeated episodes of otitis media may require the placement of grommets to allow drainage of fluid from the middle ear (Fig. 16.2).

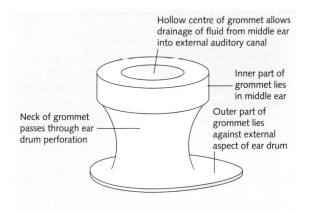

Fig. 16.2 A grommet.

Complications

Otitis media can give rise to a perforated eardrum and impaired hearing. The latter will be a conductive hearing loss. Mastoiditis was a significant consequence of otitis media before the ready availability of antibiotics but it is now rare.

Sinusitis

Bacteria

Sinusitis can result from infection with:

- *Streptococcus pneumoniae* ⎫
- *Haemophilus influenzae* type b ⎬ most commonly
- *Streptococcus pyogenes* ⎭
- *Staphylococcus aureus*.

Aetiology

Sinusitis follows from an upper respiratory tract infection when a sinus cavity or cavities become blocked and therefore unable to drain any fluid, which subsequently becomes infected. The frontal sinuses are most likely to be affected since their drainage occurs from the superior aspect of the sinus and therefore gravity does not naturally help with drainage. Maxillary sinusitis can follow dental abscesses or tooth root infections.

Clinical features

Sinusitis presents with fever, headache and facial pain over the relevant sinuses. These areas are also tender to palpation. Symptoms of the preceding infection will have occurred prior to the development of facial pain.

Investigations

The involvement of the sinuses can be confirmed using plain radiographs of the skull or an MRI scan, each of which will show a fluid level within the affected sinuses (see Fig. 16.3). Any infected fluid obtained should be cultured to identify the causative organism and check antibiotic sensitivities.

Treatment

Sinusitis is treated with co-amoxiclav or erythromycin (for patients with a penicillin allergy) since there is significant resistance to amoxicillin in strains of Hib. Those cases which do not resolve with appropriate antibiotic therapy require surgical sinus drainage and washout.

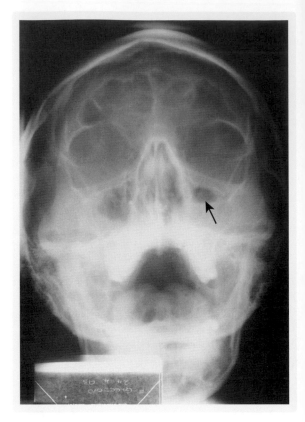

Fig. 16.3 Plain X-ray of fluid level in maxillary sinus in acute sinusitis.
Source: Conlon CP, Snydman DR. Mosby's Colour Atlas and Text of Infectious Diseases. Edinburgh: Mosby; 2000: Fig. 6.26.

Upper respiratory tract infections are summarized in Figure 16.4.

Further reading

Bisno AL. Primary care: acute pharyngitis. N Engl J Med 2001; 344:205–211.

Bonnet JM, Begg NT. Control of diphtheria: guidance for consultants in communicable disease control. Commun Dis Pub Health 1999; 2:242–249.

ENT UK. Further information on grommets. Website: www.entuk.org/patient_info/ear/surgery_glue_html.

NICE. Guidelines on influenza prophylaxis and treatment. Website: www.nice.org.uk.

Fig. 16.4 Summary of upper respiratory tract infections

Infection	Clinical features	Investigations	Treatment	Complications	Immunization
Common cold (mainly rhinoviruses)	Rhinorrhoea, headache, malaise	Clinical diagnosis	Supportive	Otitis media in children	No
Glandular fever (Epstein–Barr virus)	Tonsillar enlargement, sore throat, cervical lymphadenopathy, fever and malaise. Jaundice, splenomegaly	Blood film, monospot test for diagnosis. Liver function tests	Supportive	Thrombocytopenia, haemolytic anaemia, hepatitis and splenic rupture if enlarged. Tumours	No
Croup (viral laryngo-tracheobronchiolitis)	'Bovine' cough, sore throat and fever. Inspiratory stridor, dyspnoea	Clinical diagnosis	Supportive. Severe inspiratory stridor may require ventilatory support	Respiratory failure	No
Influenza (influenza A and B viruses)	Rhinorrhoea, dry cough, sore throat, fever, headache, myalgia and malaise	Clinical diagnosis	Supportive. Oseltamivir and zanamivir in high-risk patients	Secondary bacterial pneumonia, otitis media and sinusitis	Yes, in high-risk groups
Streptococcal pharyngitis (Streptococcus pyogenes)	Tonsillar enlargement, sore throat, cervical lymphadenopathy, fever and malaise	Throat swabs for microscopy and culture	Oral penicillin (or erythromycin if allergic to penicillin)	Peritonsillar abscess, otitis media, sinusitis. Scarlet fever, rheumatic fever, acute glomerulonephritis and septicaemia	No
Diphtheria (Corynebacterium diphtheriae)	Tonsillar enlargement with 'false membrane', sore throat, tender cervical lymphadenopathy – 'bull neck'	Throat swabs for microscopy and culture. PCR for toxin detection	Antitoxin, also penicillin (or erythromycin) intravenously	Myocarditis, palatal or pharyngeal paralysis, polyneuropathy, cranial nerve palsies and encephalitis	Yes, routine in children
Epiglottitis (Haemophilus influenzae type b)	Fever, respiratory distress and inspiratory stridor. Irritable, ill-looking child	Throat swabs and blood cultures for microscopy and culture	Second- or third-generation cephalosporin, e.g. cefuroxime or cefotaxime. ITU support	Airway obstruction	Yes, routine in children
Whooping cough (Bordetella pertussis)	Coryza, malaise, then paroxysms of coughing ending with a 'whoop'. Dyspnoea, stridor	Clinical diagnosis. Nasopharyngeal swabs or aspirate for culture	Erythromycin	'Whoop' can lead to apnoea, convulsions, death. Coughing can lead to inguinal hernias. Secondary broncho-pneumonia and bronchiectasis	Yes, routine in children
Otitis media	Fever, earache and impaired hearing. Purulent discharge from ear canal if eardrum perforates	Clinical diagnosis from otoscopy. Culture of discharge for causative organism	Co-amoxiclav or erythromycin. Grommets for chronic or repeated cases	Perforated eardrum and conductive hearing loss. Mastoiditis	No
Sinusitis	Fever, headache and pain over the relevant sinuses	Plain radiograph or MRI of sinuses. Infected fluid for culture	Co-amoxiclav or erythromycin. Sinus drainage and washout	Local or cerebral abscesses	No

Lower respiratory tract infections

17

Objectives

In this chapter you will learn:

- The signs associated with consolidation
- The features that would make you suspicious of an atypical pneumonia
- What types of jobs or hobbies have exposure risk for atypical pneumonias
- Who is at risk of aspiration pneumonia.

Infections of the lung parenchyma result in pneumonia, which can be typical or atypical and community- or hospital-acquired. The importance of these distinctions is that they alter the likelihood of different organisms causing the infection and therefore the antibiotic cover required. Atypical pneumonia refers to infection caused by the so-called 'atypical organisms'. These intracellular bacteria have cell walls that are not susceptible to penicillin and other beta-lactam antibiotics, so antibiotics that work on protein synthesis, e.g. tetracyclines or macrolides, are the drugs of choice. It is usually impossible to differentiate typical and atypical pneumonia at the bedside. Tuberculosis is also an infection of the lung tissue but is considered separately as its presentation and treatment are different from those of other bacterial infections (see Ch. 26).

COMMUNITY-ACQUIRED TYPICAL PNEUMONIA

Every medical take, especially over the winter months, will include several cases of community-acquired pneumonia, most of which will be caused by the 'typical' bacteria. These include:

- *Streptococcus pneumoniae*
- *Haemophilus influenzae* type b
- *Klebsiella pneumoniae*
- *Staphylococcus aureus*.

But by far the most common cause is *Streptococcus pneumoniae*, accounting for up to 80% of all cases of pneumonia.

Clinical features

Pneumonia commonly presents with a high fever and a cough productive of purulent (yellow or green) sputum. There may also be some haemoptysis, although this is more common in tuberculosis. Pleuritic chest pain, caused by inflammation of the pleura from the infected lung, can accompany the cough. Rigors may occur with the fevers. In elderly patients, confusion with an increased respiratory rate may be the predominant symptoms and often precede the productive cough. On examination there may be signs of consolidation: reduced expansion on the affected side; a dull percussion note, crepitations on auscultation with or without a pleural rub; and increased vocal resonance with bronchial breathing heard over the affected area.

Investigations

The presentation of community-acquired pneumonia does not generally give an indication of the bacterial organism responsible. This requires isolation of the bacteria itself, which is achieved in less than 30% of cases. Sputum microscopy and culture are often not particularly helpful due to the high rate of contamination from commensal bacteria of the oral cavity. Blood cultures are more reliable at identifying the causative organism, but few patients are bacteraemic. A chest radiograph is important for confirming the diagnosis and assessing the extent and distribution of a pneumonia (Fig. 17.1). It can also illustrate potential complications such as lung abscesses and an empyema.

The full blood count demonstrates a leucocytosis or leucopenia, and with a bacterial infection the

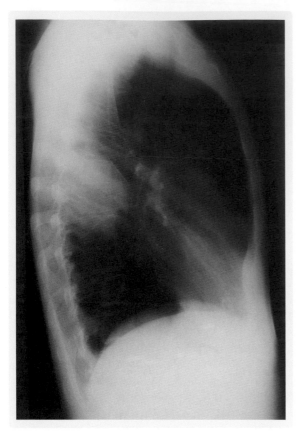

Fig. 17.1 Lobar consolidation in pneumococcal pneumonia. *Source:* Conlon CP, Snydman DR. Mosby's Colour Atlas and Text of Infectious Diseases. Edinburgh: Mosby; 2000: Fig. 6.37.

raised white cell count is a neutrophilia. The biochemistry shows a raised CRP (C-reactive protein) and with a severe infection the urea is elevated and the albumin reduced.

The investigation of a case of pneumonia should include an assessment of the severity. As described in Chapter 4, the British Thoracic Society have devised the CURB-65 score for severity which requires an Abbreviated Mental Test Score to gauge confusion, checking the urea and blood pressure, counting the respiratory rate and the age of the patient.

Chest radiograph changes can lag by several days behind the clinical picture so may not be very impressive at presentation.

Complications

Pneumonia can result in lung abscesses (see Fig. 17.2), especially in cases due to *Staphylococcus aureus* or *Klebsiella pneumoniae* as they have a tendency to cause cavitation. If the pneumonia is slow to resolve on the appropriate antibiotic therapy, an empyema should be suspected. On a chest radiograph the pleura appears thickened due to the pus in the pleural space, (see Fig. 17.3). An empyema requires drainage in addition to antibiotic therapy.

Causative organisms

Streptococcus pneumoniae (Gram-positive diplococci, also known as pneumococcus)

Incidence

Pneumococcus is by far the most common cause of community-acquired pneumonia in the UK. In 2000 there were just over 4700 cases of *Streptococcus pneumoniae* identified. It can also be responsible for hospital-acquired infections but accounts for a smaller proportion of cases. Pneumococcus is a commensal of the respiratory tract but only causes infections when it breaches the respiratory mucosa.

Risk groups

Pneumococcal infections occur more readily in patients who have previously damaged lung parenchyma, e.g. those with chronic lung disease such as chronic obstructive pulmonary disease (COPD) or prior infection with either of the influenza viruses. People with HIV and those without spleens are more susceptible to the pneumococcus and to other encapsulated bacteria.

Specific clinical features

Pneumococcal pneumonia is often accompanied by high fevers, >39°C, which then return quickly to normal after the administration of appropriate antibiotics.

Specific investigations

Streptococcus pneumoniae is the most likely bacteria causing pneumonia to appear in the blood; about 30% of cases will have positive blood cultures. Sputum samples are rarely helpful but antigen detection using blood or urine samples is increasingly used.

Treatment

Pneumococcus is treated with penicillin, or erythromycin if the patient is penicillin allergic, in cases of non-severe pneumonia. It should be noted,

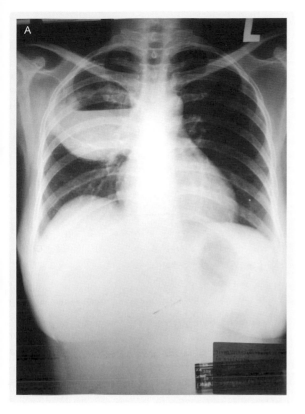

Fig. 17.2 Lung abscess: (A) PA view; (B) lateral view.

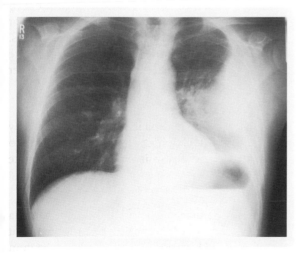

Fig. 17.3 Pleural empyema with pneumococcal pneumonia. Source: Conlon CP, Snydman DR, 2000: Fig. 6.41.

however, that in some parts of the world antibiotic resistance is increasing, so intravenous second-generation cephalosporins, e.g. cefuroxime, are used for severe cases (see Ch. 4 for severity scoring).

Prophylaxis

Pneumococcal immunization is advised for high-risk groups. These are patients with chronic diseases, e.g. lung disease, renal disease, heart disease, liver disease; those who are immunodeficient and patients with impaired or absent splenic function. Asplenic patients under the age of 16 years or within 3 years of being rendered asplenic are given prophylactic penicillin to take daily. There is not a consensus over antibiotic prophylaxis for adults but those who are happy to take antibiotics daily should be advised to do so. The new conjugate pneumococcal vaccines look very promising.

Haemophilus influenzae **type b (Hib) (Gram-negative bacilli)**

Incidence

Hib infection rates have dramatically declined since the introduction of routine immunization to children in 1992, although since 2000 there has been a small resurgence, the reasons for which are not clear. Hib is a commensal of the respiratory tract but only causes infection when it breaches the mucosal barrier.

Risk groups

Children less than 5 years old are particularly susceptible to Hib infections. Since *Haemophilus influenzae* is an encapsulated bacterium, asplenic patients are at an increased risk of infection because they have a reduced capacity to deal with encapsulated bacteria.

Treatment

Many strains, up to 19% (highest rates in children), of Hib in the UK are now resistant to ampicillin, hence the initial treatment recommended is a second- or third-generation cephalosporin, e.g. cefuroxime or cefotaxime respectively, until ampicillin sensitivities are known.

Prophylaxis

Hib immunization is given to all children routinely in their pre-school years (see Ch. 1 for schedule). Immunization is also recommended for asplenic patients or those with splenic dysfunction from whatever cause.

Klebsiella pneumoniae (Gram-negative bacilli)

Incidence

Klebsiella is widespread in the environment as well as being a commensal of the gastrointestinal tract. It is usually more opportunistic in causing infections than pneumococcus or Hib and hence more commonly causes nosocomial infections than community-acquired ones.

Risk groups

Elderly patients with heart or lung disease, malignancy or diabetes mellitus are at an increased risk of *Klebsiella pneumoniae* infections due to their general poor state of health.

Specific clinical features

Klebsiella pneumoniae infections typically tend to affect the upper lobes.

Treatment

Klebsiella bacteria often produce beta-lactamases, thereby rendering penicillin therapy ineffective. Good Gram-negative cover for klebsiella is achieved using second-generation cephalosporins, e.g. cefuroxime, or aminoglycosides, e.g. gentamicin. In hospital-acquired infections there can be problems with

multidrug resistant strains of klebsiella and this can make the choice of antibiotic therapy difficult. There is in fact a large regional variation in the resistance patterns for klebsiella, with London having the highest rates of resistance to gentamicin in the UK.

> Abscesses and cavitation on the chest radiograph are complications particularly associated with *Staphylococcus aureus* and *Klebsiella pneumoniae* infections. With *Staph. aureus* there tend to be multiple lesions in the lung resulting from septic emboli arising from the original site of infection (see Fig. 17.4). An important differential diagnosis to remember for lung cavitation is tuberculosis.

Staphylococcus aureus (Gram-positive cocci)

Incidence

Staph. aureus is a rarer cause of pneumonia, accounting for 2% of all cases. It usually arises following a previous influenza infection or as septic emboli spread haematogenously from the site of original

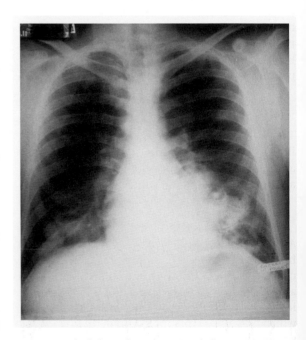

Fig. 17.4 Multiple lung abscesses in *Staphylococcus aureus* pneumonia.
Source: Conlon CP, Snydman DR, 2000: Fig. 6.38.

infection, e.g. osteomyelitis or tricuspid valve endocarditis.

Risk groups

Classically, *Staph. aureus* pneumonia occurs following influenza or in intravenous drug users (IVDUs) when it is secondary to tricuspid valve endocarditis or embolization from abscesses at the sites of injection. Those individuals with chronically damaged lungs are also susceptible to *Staph. aureus* infection.

Treatment

Staph. aureus is treated with flucloxacillin, or erythromycin if the patient is allergic to penicillin. It is obviously important to check for methicillin-resistant *Staphylococcus aureus* (MRSA), especially in emboli resulting from haematogenous spread since 40% of all *Staph. aureus* bacteraemias in 2000 in the UK were due to MRSA.

COMMUNITY-ACQUIRED ATYPICAL PNEUMONIAS

Community-acquired atypical pneumonias are generally only diagnosed if the attending physician actively considers the possibility. The suspicion of an atypical pneumonia should be raised if the respiratory symptoms are slow to resolve on conventional antibiotic therapy or there is a recent travel history or an outbreak of community-acquired pneumonia.

Clinical features

The patient is more likely to present with a flu-like illness and then develop a dry cough. Myalgia, arthralgia and diarrhoea as associated symptoms are also more common than with a typical pneumonia.

Investigations

Acute and convalescent serology are often used to help in identifying the causative organism in atypical cases, but the tests are not very reliable and the results are often only available after the acute event. An important exception is with legionella urinary antigen which gives a rapid result, although this only detects serotype 1 (responsible for 80% of cases). Newer molecular methods to detect atypical organisms are leading to more rapid identification.

Causative organisms

Mycoplasma pneumoniae (cell wall deficient bacteria)

Incidence

Mycoplasma pneumoniae infections tend to occur in 4-yearly epidemics. The incubation period is 12–14 days.

Risk group

Young adults are the group particularly affected by *Mycoplasma pneumoniae*, especially if they are living in institutions, e.g. college campus, army barracks.

Clinical features

Mycoplasma pneumoniae infection presents with a dry, persistent cough following a flu-like prodrome. Diarrhoea and vomiting are seen in association with the cough. Patients also complain of arthralgia and myalgia.

Investigations

Acute and convalescent serology can be used to identify the *Mycoplasma pneumoniae* organism but these complement fixation tests are not reliable and are now being replaced by molecular methods. On biochemistry there is classically low sodium and abnormal liver function tests (LFTs) with a hepatitic picture, i.e. raised aspartate transaminase (AST) and alanine transaminase (ALT). On a blood film in addition to the leucocytosis, there may be evidence of haemolysis (e.g. fragmented red blood cells) and thrombocytopenia. Cold agglutinins are associated with mycoplasma infections. The chest radiograph shows bilateral patchy consolidation, usually affecting the lower lobes (see Fig. 17.5).

Treatment

Mycoplasma pneumoniae is treated with a macrolide, e.g. erythromycin or clarithromycin. A tetracycline, such as doxycycline, can be used as an alternative.

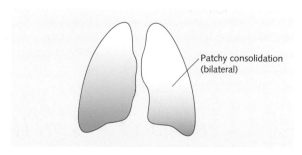

Fig. 17.5 Diagram of mycoplasma on chest radiograph.

Complications

Mycoplasma infections are one of the commoner causes of erythema multiforme (see Chs 1 and 14) and the closely linked Stevens–Johnson syndrome. The other complications associated with *Mycoplasma pneumoniae* are meningoencephalitis, haemolytic anaemia, myocarditis, pericarditis and Guillain–Barré syndrome.

Atypical pneumonias are often classically described as having more multilobar involvement on the chest radiograph than typical pneumonias. This probably has more to do with the delayed diagnosis and hence later commencement of appropriate antibiotic therapy than with an inherent difference between the two groups.

Legionella pneumophila (Gram-negative bacilli)

Incidence

Legionella pneumophila usually causes sporadic cases of pneumonia but does occur in outbreaks, classically when an air-conditioning system's water supply becomes contaminated, particularly if this occurs in a public or highly populated building. In England there are about 200 cases per year of pneumonia due to *Legionella pneumophila*, i.e. Legionnaire's disease. The incubation period is 2–10 days.

Risk group

Legionella pneumophila tends to affect males twice as often as females and has a preponderance for smokers. Point source outbreaks occur when a group of people is exposed to the organism in aerosols from contaminated cooling systems or air-conditioning. Immunocompromised patients are particularly vulnerable to developing legionella pneumonia.

Clinical features

With legionella infections there is a prodromal flu-like illness with high fevers, e.g. up to 40°C before the dry cough develops. Subsequently confusion, diarrhoea and vomiting are the prominent symptoms. In elderly patients particularly the mortality can be 10–15%.

Investigations

Like with mycoplasma infections, the biochemistry may show a low sodium and deranged LFTs with a raised AST and ALT. Classically the blood film shows a lymphopenia. The identification of *Legionella pneumophila* can be achieved by several methods, the most rapid being the urinary legionella antigen or direct immunofluorescence on sputum, pleural fluid or bronchoalveolar lavage (BAL) specimens; other options include acute and convalescent serology and sputum cultures, although these require special media to grow. The chest radiograph typically shows a lobar pattern of consolidation, which may become multilobar.

Treatment

Legionella pneumophila is treated with macrolide antibiotics: erythromycin or clarithromycin. Ciprofloxacin can be used as an alternative and in severe cases rifampicin may be added to the initial therapy.

Chlamydia pneumoniae (chlamydia family)

Incidence

Chlamydia pneumoniae causes 5–10% of community-acquired pneumonias. It tends to occur in outbreaks within families or institutions.

Risk group

Young adults are the most likely to acquire *Chlamydia pneumoniae* infections, but elderly patients are susceptible to particularly severe infections.

Clinical features

Chlamydia pneumoniae can present with either upper respiratory tract symptoms such as a sore throat or a flu-like illness or lower respiratory tract symptoms like a dry cough.

Investigations

The causative organism is identified from acute and convalescent serology.

Treatment

Chlamydia pneumoniae is treated with erythromycin or a tetracycline such as doxycycline.

Chlamydia psittaci (chlamydia family)

Incidence

Chlamydia psittaci causes about 3% of all pneumonias. The incubation period is 7–14 days.

Risk group

Classically *Chlamydia psittaci* results from contact with birds, especially parrots and pigeons, although not all cases can remember the bird contact.

Clinical features

Chlamydia psittaci presents with fever, malaise, myalgia and cough. Occasionally there is hepatosplenomegaly.

Investigations

Chlamydia psittaci is clarified as the causative organism from acute and convalescent serology. The chest radiograph typically shows diffuse or segmental shadowing.

Treatment

As with *Chlamydia pneumoniae, Chlamydia psittaci* is treated with erythromycin or doxycycline.

Coxiella burnetii (rickettsia family, Gram-negative bacilli)

Transmission

Coxiella burnetii is transmitted via inhaled faecal matter from domesticated animals or less commonly via tick bites, or from unpasteurized milk from infected cows. There are about 100 cases of *Coxiella burnetii* infection (Q fever) per year in the UK. The incubation period is 2–3 weeks.

Risk group

Those who have an occupation involving close work with farm animals are most at risk, for example vets, and farm and abattoir workers.

Clinical features

Coxiella burnetii presents with a high fever and a flu-like illness involving headaches, myalgia and sweats. These symptoms are followed by cough and nausea, vomiting and diarrhoea. Many of the infections also result in hepatitis.

Investigations

Acute and convalescent serology are performed to ascertain the causative organism. The chest radiograph may show multifocal consolidation. The LFTs may be deranged as a consequence of an associated hepatitis.

Treatment

As with the other atypical pneumonias, macrolide, e.g. erythromycin, or tetracycline, e.g. doxycycline, antibiotics are recommended. Rifampicin can be used in severe cases.

Complications

The most important complication of Q fever is 'culture-negative' endocarditis, i.e. the organism is not grown from blood cultures. Less commonly epididymo-orchitis, myocarditis and osteomyelitis can result from *Coxiella burnetii* infection.

VIRAL INFECTIONS

Influenza viruses A and B do not solely cause upper respiratory tract infections but can extend to involve the lung parenchyma as well, thereby causing pneumonia (see Ch. 16). An influenza infection is often the preceding event to a bacterial community-acquired pneumonia, with the organisms mentioned above.

HOSPITAL-ACQUIRED INFECTIONS

A hospital-acquired infection is defined as any infection developing in a patient after 2 or more days in hospital. Pneumonia is the third most common hospital-acquired infection, after infections from intravenous cannulas and urinary tract infections. Pneumonia accounts for 15% of nosocomial infections, which is highly significant given the mortality of 20–33%. Many of the nosocomial causes of pneumonia are the same as for community-acquired infections. The typical bacteria *Strep. pneumoniae* and *H. influenzae* type b detailed above are frequent causes of hospital-acquired infections although their proportion of the infections is less than with community-acquired infections. *Klebsiella pneumoniae* and *Staph. aureus* can also cause a nosocomial pneumonia. The main difference is the prevalence of Gram-negative bacteria usually found in the gastrointestinal tract as the organisms causing the pneumonia.

> An aspiration pneumonia is more commonly acquired in hospital. Patients with a reduced level of consciousness are particularly at risk as are stroke patients due to loss of their gag reflex. Epileptics might aspirate if unconscious following a seizure and alcoholic patients might aspirate while intoxicated.

Causative organisms

Escherichia coli **and other coliforms (Gram-negative bacilli)**

Risk groups

Patients who are liable to aspirate their gastric contents and those with septicaemia from a gastrointestinal tract source are prone to pneumonia from Gram-negative bacilli since these bacteria are gastrointestinal commensals.

Clinical features

In addition to the infective pneumonia, there can be marked corrosive damage to the lung parenchyma from any gastric acid aspirated. This results in an acute lung injury which prolongs the recovery period and may heal with scarring.

Investigations

Blood cultures can identify the causative organism. With an aspiration pneumonia the chest radiograph typically shows consolidation in the right lower zone since aspirated material is more likely to descend the right main bronchus, as it branches first and is a straighter route.

Treatment

Good Gram-negative cover is achieved with a second- or third-generation cephalosporin, e.g. cefuroxime or ceftriaxone. Most oral anaerobes are penicillin susceptible, so there is no need to add metronidazole if the aspiration has occurred in the community. In hospitals, prior exposure to antibiotics (and hence a risk of penicillin resistance) may warrant the addition of metronidazole or clindamycin.

Pseudomonas aeruginosa **(Gram-negative bacilli)**

Risk groups

Pseudomonas aeruginosa is a particular problem for immunocompromised patients, those with cystic fibrosis and bronchiectasis, and ventilated patients. In all these patients it can colonize the respiratory tract and be very difficult if not impossible to eradicate. It is a commensal of the gastrointestinal tract.

Investigations

Pseudomonas aeruginosa can be isolated from cultures of sputum, BAL washings and blood.

Treatment

Only a limited range of antibiotics are effective against *Pseudomonas aeruginosa*. Examples include the anti-pseudomonal penicillins, ticarcillin and piperacillin; the third-generation cephalosporin, ceftazidime; the beta-lactams, imipenem, meropenem and aztreonam; and the aminoglycosides, amikacin, gentamicin and tobramycin. A popular regimen is an antipseudomonal penicillin given in combination with an aminoglycoside such as gentamicin because they have a synergistic effect.

INFECTIONS IN IMMUNOCOMPROMISED PATIENTS

Patients who are immunocompromised are vulnerable to a much wider range of organisms resulting in pneumonia (see Chs 12 and 25).

Lower respiratory tract infections are summarized in Figure 17.6.

Further reading

British Thoracic Society. BTS Guidelines for the Management of Community Acquired Pneumonia in Adults. Thorax 2001; 56(suppl IV):iv1–iv64. Note: 2004 update. Online. Available: www.brit_thoracic.org.uk.

Fig. 17.6 Summary of lower respiratory tract infections

Community-acquired typical pneumonia

Organism	Risk groups	Distinguishing clinical features	Diagnosis	Treatment	Other
Streptococcus pneumoniae	Patients with chronic lung disease, e.g. COPD; prior infection with influenza viruses; HIV and asplenic patients	High fevers (> 39°C)	Blood cultures. Antigen detection from blood or urine samples. Sputum cultures less useful	Penicillin or erythromycin (if patient allergic to penicillin) if non-severe. Second-generation cephalosporin, e.g. cefuroxime if severe	Pneumococcal immunization is available for high-risk groups
Haemophilus influenzae type b	Children less than 5 years of age and asplenic patients		Blood and sputum cultures	Second- or third-generation cephalosporin, e.g. cefuroxime or cefotaxime	Routine immunization for children
Klebsiella pneumoniae	Elderly patients with heart and lung disease, malignancy and diabetes mellitus	Typically upper lobes affected	Blood and sputum cultures	Second-generation cephalosporin, e.g. cefuroxime or an aminoglycoside, e.g. gentamicin	Abscesses and cavitation on chest radiograph are complications
Staphylococcus aureus	Following influenza infection; in IVDUs (from septic emboli) and those with chronically damaged lungs	Source of septic emboli may be clinically apparent	Blood and sputum cultures	Flucloxacillin or erythromycin (if patient allergic to penicillin). Vancomycin for MRSA	Abscesses and cavitation on chest radiograph are complications

Community-acquired atypical pneumonia

Organism	Risk groups	Distinguishing clinical features	Investigations	Treatment	Complications
Mycoplasma pneumoniae	Young adults, especially in institutions	Prodromal flu-like illness then a dry cough. Diarrhoea, vomiting, myalgia and arthralgia	Molecular methods replacing acute and convalescent serology. Bilateral patchy consolidation in lower lobes on CXR. Leucocytosis, haemolysis and thrombocytopenia on blood film. Cold agglutinins. Low sodium and hepatitic LFTs	Macrolide, e.g. erythromycin, clarithromycin or tetracycline, e.g. doxycycline	Erythema multiforme, Stevens–Johnson syndrome, meningo-encephalitis, myocarditis, pericarditis and Guillain–Barré syndrome
Legionella pneumophila	Males, smokers; exposure to contaminated air conditioning system	Prodromal flu-like illness with high fevers then a dry cough. Confusion, diarrhoea and vomiting	Urinary legionella antigen, direct immunofluorescence on sputum; acute and convalescent serology; sputum culture. Lobar consolidation on CXR. Leucopenia on blood film. Low sodium and hepatitic LFTs	Macrolide, e.g. erythromycin, clarithromycin or the quinolone ciprofloxacin. In severe cases rifampicin used as an adjunct	Mortality up to 10–15%

(Continued)

Fig. 17.6 Summary of lower respiratory tract infections—continued

Community-acquired atypical pneumonia

Organism	Risk groups	Distinguishing clinical features	Investigations	Treatment	Complications
Chlamydia pneumoniae	Young adults	Sore throat, flu-like illness or dry cough	Acute and convalescent serology	Erythromycin or doxycycline	
Chlamydia psittaci	Bird contact	Fever, cough, myalgia and malaise. Hepatosplenomegaly	Acute and convalescent serology. Diffuse or segmental shadowing on CXR	Erythromycin or doxycycline	
Coxiella burnetii	Close contact with farm animals	High fever, flu-like illness with headaches, myalgia and sweats. Cough, diarrhoea and vomiting	Acute and convalescent serology. Multifocal consolidation on CXR. Hepatitic LFTs	Macrolide, e.g. erythromycin, clarithromycin or tetracycline, e.g. doxycycline. Rifampicin used in severe cases	'Culture-negative' endocarditis. Epididymo-orchitis, myocarditis and osteomyelitis

Hospital-acquired pneumonia

Organism	Risk groups	Distinguishing clinical features	Investigations	Treatment
Streptococcus pneumoniae	As with community-acquired typical pneumonia but lesser proportion of cases			
Haemophilus influenzae type b	As with community-acquired typical pneumonia but lesser proportion of cases			
Klebsiella pneumoniae	As with community-acquired typical pneumonia			
Staphylococcus aureus	As with community-acquired typical pneumonia			
E. coli and other coliforms	Patients liable to aspirate gastric contents or those with Gram-negative septicaemia	Acute lung injury from corrosive damage to lungs in addition to infective process	Blood cultures. Right lower zone consolidation on CXR	Second- or third-generation cephalosporin, e.g. cefuroxime or ceftriaxone. Metronidazole or clindamycin for additional anaerobic cover
Pseudomonas aeruginosa	Immunocompromised patients, those with cystic fibrosis or bronchiectasis. Ventilated patients		Blood, sputum and BAL washings cultures	Antipseudomonal penicillins, e.g. ticarcillin, piperacillin; third-generation cephalosporin ceftazidime; beta-lactams, e.g. imipenem, meropenem, aztreonam; aminoglycosides, e.g. amikacin, gentamicin, tobramycin

Objectives

In this chapter you will learn:

- The differential diagnosis for bloody diarrhoea
- The ways in which toxins can give rise to diarrhoea
- Which infections may be complicated by toxic dilatation of the colon
- The mainstay of treatment for gastroenteritis.

Gastroenteritis is an infection of the gastrointestinal tract, which usually causes diarrhoea and/or vomiting. As described in Chapter 5, diarrhoea is defined as > 300 g of loose stool passed in a 24-hour period. It is an extremely common infection which most people will experience during their lifetime. The origin of the infection along the gastrointestinal tract is reflected in the nature of the diarrhoea: watery diarrhoea results from an infection of the small intestine, whereas bloody diarrhoea indicates colonic mucosal damage.

Food poisoning relates to diarrhoea and/or vomiting resulting from the ingestion of infected foodstuffs. It is a notifiable disease and all cases should be reported to the Consultant of Communicable Disease Control (CCDC). There are > 70 000 cases per year of food poisoning in the UK, and only half of these are formally notified currently.

Many organisms can cause gastroenteritis and they are detailed below:

BACTERIAL CAUSES

The bacteria causing gastroenteritis affect different regions of the bowel and their modes of action vary as detailed in Figure 18.1. The diarrhoea from small bowel infections is generally due to toxin production, which can occur in food prior to consumption or in vivo, and is watery in nature. The cholera toxin is the paradigm for all infectious small bowel diarrhoea. The diarrhoea from large bowel infections results from colonic mucosal damage and is usually bloody in nature, hence presenting as dysentery.

Vibrio cholerae (Gram-negative comma-shaped rods)

Transmission

Vibrio cholerae is transmitted via the faecal–oral route, particularly picked up from contaminated water although infected foodstuffs and direct person-to-person contact can be responsible for infection. Cholera is especially prevalent after natural disasters where drinking water supplies become polluted with sewage. Currently the seventh cholera pandemic is affecting India, South-east Asia, Africa and South America. Cholera is a notifiable disease; therefore all cases must be reported to the CCDC. It is rarely isolated in travellers returning to the UK: there have been < 21 reports per year in the UK since 1990.

Pathogenesis

The diarrhoea from cholera is due to the action of an exotoxin. The exotoxin has two subunits, A and B: the B subunit is responsible for *b*inding to specific cell membrane receptors; and the A subunit then *a*ctivates the intracellular enzyme adenylate cyclase (Fig. 18.2). The effect is increased production of cAMP (cyclic adenosine monophosphate), which results in the marked loss of water and electrolytes (sodium and chloride) into the lumen of the small intestine.

Clinical features

Patients with cholera present with profuse, can be up to 20 litres per day, watery diarrhoea, which is known as 'rice water stools'. Given the totally liquid nature of the stools, the patient is usually incontinent. The main risk is that the patient can very quickly become

Fig. 18.1 The aetiology of the bacterial causes of gastroenteritis

Small bowel Preformed toxin i.e. ingested	Small bowel In-vivo-formed toxins	Large bowel Colonic mucosal damage
Vibrio cholerae	Clostridium perfringens	Salmonella enteritidis
Staphylococcus aureus	Clostridium difficile	Campylobacter jejuni
Bacillus cereus		Shigella species
E. coli (ETEC and VTEC)		E. coli (EIEC)
Campylobacter jejuni		Yersinia enterocolitica
Shigella species		

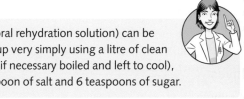

dehydrated from the profound fluid loss. The incubation period is a few hours to 5 days.

In countries where cholera is endemic some hospitals have what is called a 'Cholera bed'. This is a bed with a hole in the centre under which a bucket is kept in order to collect and measure the volume of the diarrhoea. This emphasizes how profuse the diarrhoea is.

Investigations

V. cholerae can be detected from microscopy and culture of stool.

Treatment

Intensive rehydration therapy with ORS (oral rehydration solution) and/or intravenous fluid replacement is essential given the large volumes of fluid lost as diarrhoea. In severe cases of cholera antibiotic therapy is used to decrease the stool frequency, shorten the course of the illness and help eradicate the infection. The drugs of choice are oral tetracycline, doxycycline and ciprofloxacin. The latter is being used more commonly as resistance to tetracycline increases.

ORS (oral rehydration solution) can be made up very simply using a litre of clean water (if necessary boiled and left to cool), 1 teaspoon of salt and 6 teaspoons of sugar.

Complications

The fluid loss is so profound in cholera that the major risk is death from dehydration.

Prevention

Clean supplies of drinking water, good sanitation and meticulous hand-washing are essential to prevent outbreaks of cholera. There is currently no effective immunization available.

Staphylococcus aureus (Gram-positive cocci)

Transmission

Gastroenteritis due to *Staphylococcus aureus* occurs as a consequence of eating contaminated food, in which there are enterotoxins produced by *Staph. aureus* that endure heating. The bacteria gain access to the food usually from an open skin wound infected with *Staph*.

Fig. 18.2 Diagram showing the action of cholera exotoxin.

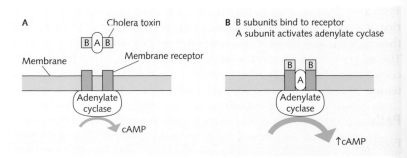

aureus of someone preparing the food. The types of food often involved include meat and dairy products.

Pathogenesis

Staphylococcus aureus produces enterotoxins that induce severe vomiting, and diarrhoea to a lesser extent.

Clinical features

There is a rapid onset of symptoms, only 2–6 hours after eating, because these are toxin-induced symptoms. Vomiting combined with severe abdominal pain are the predominant features and diarrhoea is commonly not present. Some patients can also suffer with a fever. The symptoms tend to be short-lived, usually resolving within 12–24 hours.

Investigations

A sample of the suspected food is required both to look for the organism and for detection of the enterotoxin.

Treatment

There is no specific treatment for *Staph. aureus* food poisoning just supportive care, as the illness tends to be self-limiting.

Prevention

Strict hygiene practices within the kitchen can reduce the risk of *Staph. aureus* food poisoning. It is vital that all skin lesions are covered whilst preparing food.

Food poisoning resulting from toxin production has a rapid onset and vomiting is a more prominent feature.

Bacillus cereus (Gram-positive bacilli)

Transmission

Typically *Bacillus cereus* is acquired from eating rice, although cases have been reported following the consumption of pasta, meat and dairy products. The spores produced by the bacteria can survive cooking and once the food, e.g. rice, is left at room temperature the spores can germinate.

Pathogenesis

Food poisoning from *Bacillus cereus* results from the production of enterotoxins.

Clinical features

Since the symptoms are due to toxin production they occur with a rapid onset: just 1–6 hours for the commencement of vomiting and 8–12 hours for the diarrhoea to appear. *Bacillus cereus* food poisoning can either present as watery diarrhoea or severe vomiting. Abdominal pain and fever do not occur.

Investigations

Both faecal and food cultures can be used to identify *Bacillus cereus* as the causative organism.

Treatment

There is no specific therapy for *Bacillus cereus*. Supportive care including ORS to prevent dehydration is recommended.

Prevention

Careful preparation and storage of rice is important in preventing infection.

Escherichia coli (EPEC, ETEC, VTEC, EIEC) (Gram-negative bacilli)

Transmission

E. coli is spread via the faecal–oral route from contaminated food. The *E. coli* 0157:H7 strain is specifically acquired from undercooked beef or unpasteurized cow's milk. *E. coli* is a commensal of the gastrointestinal tract.

Pathogenesis

There are four types of *E. coli*, each with their own mode of action as detailed:

- Enteropathic *E. coli* (EPEC): attaches to and damages the intestinal villi directly, e.g. O111 and O127 strains. EPEC is particularly seen in children less than 2 years old; outbreaks in nurseries are seen.
- Enterotoxigenic *E. coli* (ETEC): has an enterotoxin which acts on cAMP in a similar manner to the cholera toxin produced by *Vibrio cholerae* (see above) and causes traveller's diarrhoea.
- Verotoxigenic *E. coli* (VTEC): possesses a toxin, like the shigella toxin, that acts locally on the mucosa to cause a haemorrhagic colitis or systemically resulting in renal failure from haemolytic-uraemic syndrome (HUS), e.g. O157 strain.

- Enteroinvasive *E. coli* (EIEC): invades the mucosa in a manner similar to shigella (see below).

Clinical features

A presentation with watery diarrhoea occurs if the cause is an ETEC infection, whereas all the other types of *E. coli*, i.e. EPEC, EIEC and VTEC, cause bloody diarrhoea. Pain can be associated with bloody diarrhoea. Fever may occur with VTEC and EIEC infections.

Investigations

Stool microscopy and cultures are essential to isolate the *E. coli* bacteria. Serotyping can be performed to identify EPEC and VTEC strains. It is possible to demonstrate toxin production in order to distinguish ETEC.

Treatment

Supportive therapy with ORS is useful to prevent dehydration. Antibiotics are usually reserved for severe systemic infections, when ciprofloxacin is the drug of choice. There are some data to suggest that antibiotics may worsen outcomes in disease due to *E. coli* 0157.

Complications

VTEC infection is associated with HUS, especially in children. It occurs in 5% of VTEC infections, but is significant because there is a 10% mortality rate.

Prevention

Transmission of *E. coli* is eliminated with good personal hygiene, in particular the washing of hands, and the correct preparation of food.

Clostridium perfringens (Gram-positive bacilli)

Transmission

Clostridium perfringens is a commensal of the colon in many animals as well as humans. Meat can become contaminated with spores and these are able to withstand boiling. If the meat is then left at room temperature the spores germinate and replication occurs.

Pathogenesis

Once the infected meat or poultry is consumed, *Clostridium perfringens* produces an enterotoxin (an alpha toxin). This toxin is able to induce diarrhoea. The enterotoxin is not able to reproduce in food itself, only after ingestion.

Clinical features

Clostridium perfringens presents 8–24 hours after ingestion, usually 12–18 hours, with explosive watery diarrhoea in association with cramping abdominal pain. The symptoms are very short-lived, usually resolving within 6 hours. Fever is typically not present.

Investigations

Microscopy and culture of both the suspected food and faeces can demonstrate *Clostridium perfringens* as the causative organism.

Treatment

Supportive therapy with ORS to prevent dehydration is recommended. There is no specific antibiotic treatment.

Prevention

Maintaining high standards of hygiene within the kitchen and appropriate preparation and storage of meats can help reduce cases of food poisoning from *Clostridium perfringens*.

Clostridium difficile (Gram-positive bacilli)

Transmission

C. difficile is a commensal of the colon, particularly in neonates and the elderly. Eighty percent of cases of *C. difficile* diarrhoea occur in the over-65-year-old age group. Person-to-person contact is responsible for outbreaks in hospitals. It is a significant problem: there are > 28 800 diagnosed cases of *C. difficile* reported each year in the UK.

Pathogenesis

Broad-spectrum antibiotic therapy, e.g. the cephalosporin, cefuroxime, alters the natural flora of the gut and allows overgrowth of *C. difficile*. Some strains of *C. difficile* have the ability for toxin production. The colitis seen is a result of toxin activity.

Clinical features

C. difficile can produce a spectrum of disease ranging from mild diarrhoea through to the more severe bloody diarrhoea and systemic upset of pseudomembranous colitis.

Investigations

Microscopy and culture of the faeces tends not to be informative as healthy individuals can be carriers of *C. difficile*. Detection of the toxin in stool is the preferred method for diagnosis.

Treatment

Antibiotic therapy is required for diarrhoea due to *C. difficile*. The first-line therapy is oral metronidazole, and if the diarrhoea fails to resolve after a 10- to 14-day course then oral vancomycin is used. Equally important is stopping the causative broad-spectrum antibiotics. An alternative approach is to give probiotic agents, e.g. yeasts and lactobacilli; this is more commonly adopted in less unwell patients.

Complications

Pseudomembranous colitis can result in toxic megacolon and colonic perforation.

Prevention

Selective antibiotic therapy is desirable whenever possible to prevent *C. difficile* infections and of course to impede the development of antibiotic resistance. Once an organism has been isolated and the antibiotic resistance pattern ascertained, then the initial broad-spectrum antibiotic therapy should be rationalized to the simplest appropriate antibiotic. Thorough hand-washing, barrier nursing and patient isolation in hospitals help to control outbreaks of *C. difficile*.

Clostridium botulinum is a rare cause of food poisoning but it does not result in gastroenteritis. The bacteria are able to produce spores that can survive heating and then generate a neurotoxin whilst in the anaerobic conditions generated after canning the food. Within 12–36 hours of ingesting the toxin, the patient develops a flaccid paralysis due to the toxin blocking the neuromuscular junctions globally throughout the body and consequently a respiratory arrest. Patients require antitoxin and respiratory support in an intensive care unit in order to survive. There is a 5–10% mortality rate.

Salmonella enteritidis (Gram-negative bacilli)

Transmission

Salmonella enteritidis is transmitted via the faecal–oral route, frequently involving contaminated chicken, although any undercooked meat or foodstuff may be a source of disease. A high infecting dose is required to cause infection, i.e. there need to be many bacteria in the food for the person consuming it to actually become infected. It is also possible to spread salmonella directly from person to person.

Pathogenesis

Salmonella enteritidis damages the mucosal wall of the gastrointestinal tract resulting in increased fluid in the bowel lumen. The extra fluid increases the volume of the stool to the extent that the liquid content overwhelms the absorptive capacity of the colon, resulting in diarrhoea. The damage to the mucosal wall also means that the diarrhoea can contain blood.

Clinical features

In cases of salmonella food poisoning, 12–24 hours after eating the contaminated food, patients present with an abrupt onset of diarrhoea and abdominal pain, and they may vomit. Fever is a commonly associated feature. The symptoms usually resolve within 2–3 days.

Investigations

Salmonella enteritidis can be isolated from stool cultures, and if the patient is systemically unwell the bacteria will also be found in blood cultures. Positive blood cultures are more common in the elderly and the immunocompromised.

Treatment

In the majority of cases of salmonella food poisoning the diarrhoea is self-limiting and so no antibiotic therapy is required. However, if the patient is septicaemic or at high risk of disseminated disease, e.g. infection in the elderly, neonates or immunocompromised patients, then ciprofloxacin or co-trimoxazole is given. Most important is supportive treatment in the form of ORS or intravenous fluids, which can prevent dehydration and speed recovery.

Complications

If the *Salmonella enteritidis* successfully manages to invade through the mucosal wall and enter the bloodstream then it can result in septicaemia, meningitis, osteomyelitis and septic arthritis. Toxic megacolon is a rare but extremely serious local complication of a salmonella infection. Suspicion should be raised if pain is a prominent feature, the abdomen is distended, the patient is systemically unwell and the symptoms do not seem to settle over a couple of days. A plain abdominal radiograph is the investigation of choice which will demonstrate a grossly dilated colon (see Fig. 18.3). The upper limit of normal for the diameter of the large bowel in an adult is taken as 5 cm.

Patients with sickle cell anaemia are at an increased risk of developing salmonella osteomyelitis. It tends to occur in bone that is necrotic from previous sickling crises.

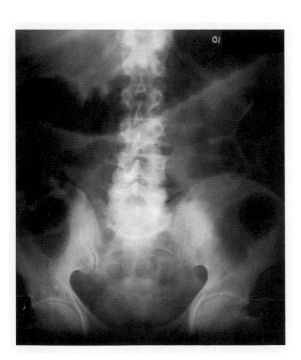

Fig. 18.3 Plain abdominal X-ray showing toxic dilatation in salmonella infection.
Source: Conlon CP, Snydman DR. Mosby's Colour Atlas and Text of Infectious Diseases. Edinburgh: Mosby; 2000: Fig. 9.14.

Prevention

Salmonella food poisoning can be prevented with good hand and kitchen hygiene. This is even more crucial in commercial kitchens. Hand-washing before preparing any food, not using the same utensils for uncooked and cooked meat, thorough cooking and proper storage of meat are essential elements of eliminating food poisoning.

Campylobacter jejuni (Gram-negative bacilli)

Transmission

Campylobacter jejuni is contracted via the faecal–oral route. It is typically acquired from undercooked meat, especially chicken, unpasteurized milk and contaminated water supplies. Large outbreaks are usually associated with the latter two, i.e. inadequately pasteurized milk or contaminated water supplies rather than from chicken. A relatively low infecting dose is needed to cause infection and it can also be spread directly from person to person. *Campylobacter jejuni* is the most common bacterial cause of sporadic gastroenteritis in the UK, whereas *Salmonella enteritidis* is more associated with outbreaks.

Pathogenesis

The cell wall of *Campylobacter jejuni* contains an endotoxin. Enterotoxins have also been identified but as yet their mechanism of action is unclear. The bacteria are able to invade the mucosa of both the small and large bowel, producing bloody diarrhoea.

Clinical features

Campylobacter jejuni presents 48–96 hours (but can be up to 11 days) after eating the contaminated food and results in diarrhoea that has associated blood, mucus and pus. The abdominal pain, malaise and fever are more marked than with other causes of gastroenteritis. Vomiting is uncommon.

Investigations

Stool sent for microscopy and culture can isolate *Campylobacter jejuni* as the cause of the gastroenteritis. Bacteraemia is uncommon.

Treatment

The diarrhoea from *Campylobacter jejuni* is usually self-limiting, resolving within 3–5 days, so no antibiotic therapy is required. If the symptoms are prolonged or the patient immunocompromised then erythromycin is used. Supportive therapy with ORS is helpful to prevent dehydration.

Complications

By invading through the mucosal wall the bacteria can access the bloodstream, which may result in septi-caemia, especially in immunocompromised patients. Like *Salmonella enteritidis* infections, *Campylobacter jejuni* can rarely lead to toxic megacolon. Guillain–Barré syndrome occurring secondary to a *Campylobacter jejuni* infection tends to be at the more severe end of the spectrum with an increased risk of requiring ventilatory support for respiratory muscle involvement.

Prevention

The risk of acquiring food poisoning from *Cam-pylobacter jejuni* is reduced by special attention paid to hand-washing and good kitchen hygiene practices.

Severe cases of salmonella and campylobacter gastroenteritis can closely mimic inflammatory bowel disease (Crohn's disease and ulcerative colitis) with their bloody diarrhoea, abdominal pain and risk of toxic dilatation of the colon. It is critical to differentiate the infective causes from the inflammatory causes, as the management and long-term prognosis are quite different.

Shigella (Gram-negative bacilli)

Transmission

Shigella is transmitted via the faecal–oral route from contaminated food but only a small infective dose is required.

Pathogenesis

There are four *Shigella* species that cause gas-troenteritis: *Shigella dysenteriae*, *Sh. flexneri*, *Sh. boydii* or *Sh. sonneri*. All the *Shigella* species are capable of invading the colonic mucosa and hence giving rise to bloody diarrhoea. A toxin is produced by some strains of *Sh. dysenteriae*, *Sh. flexneri* and *Sh. sonneri* which results in a more watery diarrhoea. In general *Sh. sonneri*, which is endemic in the UK, gives rise to a

milder form of diarrhoea, whereas the other three species are more likely to cause a severe colitis and lead to complications. These three species tend to be acquired whilst outside the UK and brought in.

Clinical features

Shigella presents about 28 hours after the con-sumption of contaminated food, although it can take up to 7 days, with watery and then bloody diarrhoea that has mucus associated with it. There is associated cramping abdominal pain, malaise and fever. Patients also describe tenesmus (the sensation of stool in the rectum, even after defecation).

Investigations

Stool microscopy and cultures are required in order to identify shigella and the species.

Treatment

ORS as supportive therapy to prevent dehydration is the mainstay of treatment. If the infection is severe then ciprofloxacin is given.

Complications

Since the *Shigella* species are all able to invade the mucosal wall, an infection can be complicated by colonic perforation and septicaemia. This infection can result in Reiter's syndrome with gastroenteritis as the precipitant infection rather than a non-specific urethritis, combined with a reactive arthritis and conjunctivitis to complete the triad. Like VTEC infection, shigella can be associated with haemolytic-uraemic syndrome.

Prevention

Since only a small infecting dose is required for infection meticulous care needs to be taken over personal hygiene and the preparation of food to prevent transmission and avert an outbreak.

Yersinia enterocolitica (Gram-negative bacilli)

Transmission

Yersinia enterocolitica can be contracted from con-taminated food, especially undercooked pork and pork products. It can also be transmitted from person to person directly.

Pathogenesis

The Gram-negative bacilli invade the terminal ileum and can give rise to a terminal ileitis resulting in watery diarrhoea or mesenteric adenitis.

Clinical features

Yersinia enterocolitica presents 3–7 days after consumption, with fever, watery diarrhoea and severe abdominal pain in adults, reflecting the terminal ileitis. Children tend to suffer with abdominal pain due to a mesenteric adenitis. In both cases the abdominal pain can be mistaken for an appendicitis.

Investigations

Yersinia enterocolitica can be isolated from both stool and blood cultures. Serology can be a more reliable method for making the diagnosis.

Treatment

Most cases of *Yersinia enterocolitica* only require supportive management with ORS. In very severe infections tetracycline or ciprofloxacin can be used.

Complications

Local complications due to the invasive nature of the bacteria include colonic dilatation and perforation. Septicaemia can also be a consequence. A reactive polyarthritis can result from *Yersinia enterocolitica* infection, which may be part of Reiter's syndrome if it occurs in combination with conjunctivitis as well. Erythema nodosum can be triggered by *Yersinia enterocolitica* infection.

Prevention

The careful preparation of food and hand-washing can reduce *Yersinia enterocolitica* infections. Proper storage of pork and pork products is essential, since *Yersinia enterocolitica* is able to multiply at just 4 °C.

VIRAL CAUSES

Rotavirus (double-stranded RNA virus, reovirus family)

Transmission

Rotavirus is passed from person to person, and only a small infecting dose is needed for successful transmission. Epidemics tend to occur in the winter months, particularly affecting child nurseries and geriatric wards in hospitals. Worldwide, rotavirus infections are a significant cause of diarrhoea in children less than 5 years old, with many in the developing world dying as a result. Children who are bottle-fed are at an increased risk compared to those who receive breast milk.

Pathogenesis

Rotavirus impairs water and electrolyte transport across the gastrointestinal mucosa resulting in significant losses and hence watery diarrhoea.

Clinical features

Rotavirus infections present after about 48 hours with watery diarrhoea, vomiting and fever. The diarrhoeal illness may be preceded by upper respiratory tract symptoms.

Investigations

The diagnosis is usually not confirmed but the virus can be identified by electron microscopy (EM) or enzyme-linked immunosorbent assay (ELISA) of the faeces.

Treatment

There is no specific antiviral therapy and management should be supportive. ORS can be helpful to prevent dehydration.

Prevention

Hand-washing is the mainstay of limiting infections, especially as only a small infecting dose is required. Cases identified in hospital should be strictly barrier-nursed to prevent further spread on the ward. Recent trials of a vaccine resulted in an excess of cases of intussusception and were abandoned.

Other viruses

The calcivirus family which includes novovirus, Norwalk-like virus and small round structured viruses can cause outbreaks of gastroenteritis, particularly in hospitals, nursing homes, schools and other confined communities such as on a cruise ship. The immunity to these viruses tends not to be very long-lasting and therefore any age group can be affected. Sapoviruses are also in the calcivirus family and typically cause diarrhoea in children less than 5 years of age. Astroviruses and adenoviruses can also cause diarrhoea.

As with rotavirus infections, there are no specific antiviral treatments and patients should just be kept well hydrated. Identification of the specific virus responsible is possible using EM of a faecal sample.

'Winter vomiting disease' is associated with the caliciviruses, e.g. Norwalk and small round viruses.

PROTOZOAL CAUSES

Entamoeba histolytica **(amoeba)**

Transmission

Entamoeba histolytica is transmitted via the faecal–oral route when food and water supplies become contaminated with cysts. It can also be contracted through direct person-to-person contact and oral–anal sexual practices. Although *Entamoeba histolytica* is found worldwide there are higher incidence rates of infection in the tropics. In the UK there have been < 200 cases detected per year since 2002.

Pathogenesis

Entamoeba histolytica has two forms: motile trophozoites and sessile cysts. People can harbour cysts asymptomatically and these are released in faeces. After cysts containing trophozoites are ingested, the cysts are digested in the small intestine and release the trophozoites. These multiply in the colon and in some cases invade the colonic mucosa resulting in ulceration and necrosis. The trophozoites may penetrate through the colon wall into the bloodstream from where they travel to the liver via the portal vein and can result in hepatic abscesses (Fig. 18.4).

Clinical features

Amoebiasis presents with bloody diarrhoea, abdominal pain, nausea and loss of appetite. The diarrhoea varies in severity between cases. A low-grade fever is associated with more severe cases.

Investigations

Stool microscopy for cysts and trophozoites can identify *Entamoeba histolytica*. Serology can be helpful in imported disease but is less useful in endemic areas; the detection rate is higher in those with liver involvement than in those with purely gastroenteritis.

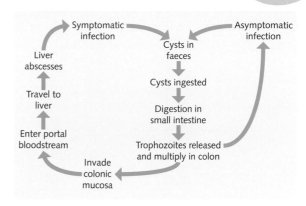

Fig. 18.4 *Entamoeba histolytica* life cycle.

If there is a hepatic abscess, then microscopy can be performed on the aspirated abscess contents (classically described as looking like 'anchovy sauce') to confirm the diagnosis.

Treatment

Metronidazole is the most commonly used antibiotic treatment for *Entamoeba histolytica*; an alternative is tinidazole. Adjunct therapy for the eradication of cysts and hence also asymptomatic carriage is achieved with diloxanide furoate. The management of liver abscesses is covered in Chapter 19.

Complications

Erosion through the colonic wall by the amoebae so that they gain access to the bloodstream can result in liver abscesses and less commonly lung and brain abscesses. Chronic infection with *Entamoeba histolytica* can result in colonic strictures due to the damage to the mucosa. Rarely, toxic dilatation of the colon, perforation and haemorrhage can occur.

Giardia lamblia **(see Ch. 24)**

Cryptosporidium parvum **(see Ch. 25)**

Isospora belli **(see Ch. 25)**

Gastroenteritis is summarized in Figure 18.5.

Further reading

Thielman NM. Acute infectious diarrhea. N Engl J Med 2004; 350:38–47.

Fig. 18.5 Summary of gastroenteritis

Organism	Type of diarrhoea	Associated symptoms	Investigations for diagnosis	Antibiotics (if required)	Complications
Vibrio cholerae	Watery	Severe dehydration	Stool for microscopy and culture	Tetracycline, doxycycline, ciprofloxacin	Severe dehydration and death
Staphylococcus aureus	Watery, not always present	Severe vomiting, fever and abdominal pain	Food sample for microscopy and toxin detection	N/a	Self-limiting
Bacillus cereus	Watery	Severe vomiting	Food and stool for microscopy and culture	N/a	Self-limiting
Escherichia coli	Watery (ETEC); bloody (EIEC, VTEC, EPEC)	Fever (VTEC, EIEC); abdominal pain (EIEC, VTEC, EPEC)	Stool for microscopy and culture; serotyping	Ciprofloxacin	Haemolytic-uraemic syndrome (VTEC)
Clostridium perfringens	Watery	Abdominal pain	Food and stool for microscopy and culture	N/a	Self-limiting
Clostridium difficile	Watery/bloody	Systemic illness	Stool for toxin isolation	Oral metronidazole, oral vancomycin	Toxic megacolon and colonic perforation
Salmonella enteritidis	Bloody	Abdominal pain, fever and vomiting	Stool and blood for microscopy and culture	Ciprofloxacin, co-trimoxazole	Septicaemia, meningitis, osteomyelitis, septic arthritis. Toxic megacolon
Campylobacter jejuni	Bloody (and mucus, pus)	Abdominal pain, fever and malaise	Stool for microscopy and culture	Erythromycin	Septicaemia, Guillain–Barré syndrome. Toxic megacolon
Shigella species	Watery then bloody (and mucus)	Abdominal pain, fever, malaise and tenesmus	Stool for microscopy and culture	Ciprofloxacin	Septicaemia, Reiter's syndrome, haemolytic-uraemic syndrome. Colonic perforation
Yersinia enterocolitica	Watery	Fever and severe abdominal pain	Stool and blood for microscopy and culture; serology	Tetracycline, ciprofloxacin	Septicaemia, Reiter's syndrome, erythema nodosum. Colonic dilatation and perforation
Rotavirus	Watery	Preceding upper respiratory tract symptoms. Fever and vomiting	Stool for ELISA or EM	N/a	Self-limiting
Entamoeba histolytica	Bloody	Abdominal pain, nausea, fever and anorexia	Stool for microscopy; serology	Metronidazole, tinidazole. (Cyst eradication with diloxanide furoate)	Liver, lung and brain abscesses. Colonic strictures. Toxic megacolon and perforation

Objectives

In this chapter you will learn:

- Which infections can result in fulminant liver failure
- The investigations that can be used to assess liver damage
- The risk factors for hepatitis C
- The organisms that may be responsible for an abscess in the liver
- Which zoonoses affect the liver
- The symptoms that suggest a biliary tract infection.

Broadly speaking, infections of the liver cause either a generalized inflammation resulting in jaundice or space-occupying lesions due to an abscess or cysts that present as right upper quadrant pain with or without jaundice. Infections affecting the biliary tree are a differential diagnosis of right upper quadrant pain.

HEPATITIS

Inflammation of the liver, known as hepatitis, can arise from a number of viruses: the hepatitis viruses A to E as well as Epstein–Barr virus (EBV) and cytomegalovirus (CMV) (Fig. 19.1). The inflammation can also be non-infectious, caused by alcohol, drugs and autoimmune disorders. Viral hepatitis is a notifiable disease in the UK therefore all cases should be reported to the CCDC (Consultant of Communicable Disease Control).

Hepatitis A virus (HAV)

Hepatitis A gives rise to an acute hepatitis but can rarely cause fulminant liver failure.

Epidemiology

Hepatitis A is the most common type of viral hepatitis. It is present throughout the world but there is a higher incidence of cases in the developing world. This reflects the poorer quality of sanitation in those areas. Children are at a greater risk of infection.

Transmission

Hepatitis A is transmitted via the faecal–oral route. Shellfish are a particular risk because if they live in estuaries where there is sewage effluent they can become contaminated. Since hepatitis A is excreted in the faeces of an infected person before the symptoms appear, they can unwittingly spread the infection if they are not meticulous about hand-washing before preparing food. Outbreaks tend to occur when an infected person is preparing food commercially or from contaminated batches of shellfish.

Clinical features

After an incubation period of 2–6 weeks the patient presents with nausea, anorexia and malaise. There is tender hepatomegaly and some patients have splenomegaly in addition. The jaundice appears about 1 week after the onset of symptoms and lasts for several weeks or occasionally longer. Not all patients, however, are jaundiced.

Investigations

The hepatitis A aetiology is confirmed with serology, detecting the IgM anti-HAV. The presence of IgG anti-HAV indicates immunity due to previous infection or immunization. HAV can also be detected in faeces using electron microscopy (EM), although this is not done in routine practice. The liver function tests (LFTs) show a hepatitic picture, i.e. the aspartate transaminase (AST) and alanine transaminase (ALT) are much more markedly elevated than the alkaline phosphatase (ALP) and gamma glutamyl transpeptidase (GGT). The bilirubin will be raised if there is jaundice. The synthetic function of the liver is determined by the serum albumin and prothrombin time (PT), which give a more accurate reflection than the LFTs of the insult to

Fig. 19.1 The different viruses causing hepatitis

Virus	RNA/DNA virus	Transmission	Incubation	Serology	Chronicity
Hepatitis A	RNA	Faecal-oral	2–6 weeks	IgM anti-HAV	No
Hepatitis B	DNA	Sexual, vertical, blood-borne	6 weeks to 6 months	HBsAg, anti-HBs, IgM and IgG anti-HBc, HBeAg, anti-HBe, HBV DNA	In < 10% of adults but 90% of neonates
Hepatitis C	RNA	Blood-borne, IVDUs, sexual	2–6 months	Anti-HCV, viral RNA PCR	Up to 50% cases
Hepatitis D	RNA	Blood-borne, sexual		Anti-HDV, HDV Ag, HDV RNA	Yes, with HBV
Hepatitis E	RNA	Faecal-oral	6–8 weeks	Anti-HEV, HEV RNA	No
EBV	DNA	Saliva contact	Uncertain, up to 1 month	IgM anti-EBV, EBV DNA, monospot test	No
CMV	DNA	Blood transfusion, transplantation, droplet spread	Uncertain as most asymptomatic	IgM anti-CMV, CMV DNA	Remains latent

the liver by any cause. The synthetic function is usually only deranged in cases that are severe enough to cause fulminant liver failure. Haematological blood tests demonstrate a lymphocytosis and a raised erythrocyte sedimentation rate (ESR).

> The inflammatory process of hepatitis affects the hepatocyte cells of the liver. When damaged, these release the transaminase enzymes AST and ALT. Hence a 'hepatitic picture' of LFT impairment describes the transaminase levels being more elevated comparatively to the ALP and GGT.

Treatment

There is no specific antiviral therapy for hepatitis A. Except in cases of liver failure, patients usually do not require admission to hospital.

Complications

The majority of cases of hepatitis A resolve completely. Rarely, in less than 1 in 1000 patients, the infection can result in fulminant liver failure and patients die from liver necrosis. Hepatitis A does not lead to chronic liver disease, however. Extrahepatic complications of HAV are rare but include vasculitis, myocarditis and renal failure.

Prevention

There is a vaccination for those travelling to high-risk areas in the developing world. Hepatitis A immunization is recommended for those travelling outside of Northern and Western Europe, North America, Japan, Australia and New Zealand. In addition, care needs to be taken over food hygiene and sanitation. Other groups who are advised to be immunized are haemophiliacs, those already suffering with chronic liver disease, people who work with untreated sewage, and staff and residents of institutions caring for people with learning difficulties. Studies show that vaccination can prevent infection in recent contacts of people with hepatitis A. The HAV immunoglobulin is no longer routinely used but may be indicated for some immunocompromised patients post-exposure.

Hepatitis B virus (HBV)

Hepatitis B infection can cause acute hepatitis but asymptomatic infection also occurs. Infection can progress to a chronic infection that does not resolve.

Epidemiology

Worldwide the prevalence of HBV is variable with developed countries having rates less than 1% whereas countries in sub-Saharan Africa and Asia can have chronic infection rates of HBV up to 20%. In the UK the prevalence is 0.3%, as estimated by the WHO (World Health Organization).

Transmission

The predominant route of transmission is dependent on the local population prevalence of HBV. In developing countries with a high prevalence of HBV the most important route of transmission is vertically from mother to baby. In contrast in developed countries where lower chronic infection rates exist, sexual and blood-borne modes of spread account for the majority of cases. Blood-borne routes cover intravenous transmission, such as intravenous drug abuse, tattoo needles or accidentally as needle-stick injuries to health professionals, or via blood products, although the latter is extremely rare in countries that operate a screening programme for infections in all blood products.

Clinical features

Following the incubation period of 6 weeks to 6 months patients present with malaise, anorexia and jaundice. In fact many of the infections are asymptomatic.

Investigations

The serology results for hepatitis B and the differing states of infection or immunity are described in Chapter 6 (see Fig. 6.3). There are three HBV antigens that can be detected: hepatitis B surface antigen, HBsAg; hepatitis B e antigen, HBeAg; and hepatitis B core antigen, HBcAg. The order of their rise and fall is shown in Figure 19.2. The e antigen reflects higher infectivity when present. An inability to clear the HBsAg denotes chronic hepatitis B.

The LFTs have a hepatitic pattern of derangement. The bilirubin will be raised in those with jaundice. Like with hepatitis A, there may be a lymphocytosis and raised ESR in acute infections.

Treatment

There is no antiviral therapy available for acute hepatitis B infections. Interferon alpha is used in chronic hepatitis B infection but the response rate is only 50% and relapses occur frequently. As a result, if there is no improvement seen after 3–4 months of therapy it should be discontinued. Lamivudine and adefovir are alternative treatment options for chronic hepatitis B infections but the development of resistance is a problem.

Patients with chronic hepatitis should also be advised to minimize their alcohol consumption, as that predisposes to liver cirrhosis in addition.

Patients who are co-infected with HIV should only receive lamivudine if it is part of a combination of antiretroviral drugs, otherwise the HIV will quickly become lamivudine-resistant.

Complications

Immune complexes can result in arthralgia, vasculitis, skin rashes and glomerulonephritis (usually membranous GN). Chronic hepatitis is the consequence of about 10% of hepatitis B infections. It is defined as persistently detectable HBsAg for more than 6 months. Patients with chronic hepatitis are at risk of developing cirrhosis and subsequently hepatocellular carcinoma many years later. Some patients fail to clear the HBV and permanently have HBsAg detectable but do not have any ongoing liver disease and are considered carriers. There is a spontaneous clearance rate of HBsAg of 1–2% per year in carriers. Acute

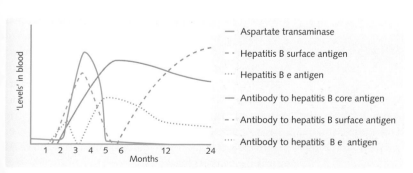

— Aspartate transaminase

-- Hepatitis B surface antigen

···· Hepatitis B e antigen

— Antibody to hepatitis B core antigen

-- Antibody to hepatitis B surface antigen

···· Antibody to hepatitis B e antigen

'Levels' in blood

1 2 3 4 5 6 12 24

Months

Fig. 19.2 Graph of markers of hepatitis B.
Source: Conlon CP, Snydman DR. Mosby's Colour Atlas and Text of Infectious Diseases. Edinburgh: Mosby; 2000: Fig. 9.35.

hepatitis B is much more likely to result in fulminant liver failure than is hepatitis A.

Prevention

Screening all blood products for HBV helps to eliminate these as a potential source of infection. Thorough sterilization of medical equipment and the use of disposable needles by healthcare professionals, tattoo artists and acupuncturists, and needle exchange programmes for (and vaccination of) intravenous drug users (IVDUs) are measures aimed at reducing other blood-borne routes of transmission.

Vertical transmission is controlled by checking the hepatitis B status of all mothers antenatally. Babies born to HBeAg-positive mothers should receive passive immunity with HBV immunoglobulin at birth. All babies deemed to be at high risk of hepatitis B should be vaccinated at birth. The vaccine against hepatitis B is also recommended for healthcare professionals, IVDUs, sex workers, close contacts of an index case, haemophiliacs, patients with chronic renal failure and travellers to endemic areas who intend to stay for a prolonged period. A course of three injections is given followed by boosters every 3–5 years, depending on the individual's response to the vaccine, to maintain immunity. It is a requirement that all healthcare professionals have their hepatitis B status checked before starting work and are able to provide documentation of their antibody titre.

Healthcare professionals who are chronically infected with hepatitis B are not permitted to perform any invasive procedures (exposure-prone procedures) where there is a potential risk they could infect the patient.

Hepatitis C virus (HCV)

Like hepatitis B, hepatitis C can lead to both acute and chronic liver infections.

Epidemiology

Hepatitis C was only identified as an entity in 1990. HCV accounts for most of the cases of what had previously been known as 'non-A, non-B hepatitis'. In the UK more than 40% of the IVDU population are infected with HCV so even very limited needle sharing is a high-risk option.

Transmission

Hepatitis C is transmitted via similar routes to hepatitis B but the relative proportions in the various modes differ. The majority of cases of HCV in the UK have been acquired from blood, either blood products pre-1990 or from sharing needles as an IVDU. Hepatitis C is only rarely transmitted vertically from mother to child or sexually.

Patients who received blood products before 1990, which is when screening for hepatitis C was introduced, are at risk from having contracted hepatitis C. The patients at greatest risk were those who required multiple transfusions of blood products, such as haemophiliacs, patients with haematological disorders and those undergoing major surgery.

Clinical features

The incubation period for hepatitis C is 2–6 months. Acute hepatitis is rare and is usually mild but there is a much greater risk of chronic infection than with hepatitis B.

Investigations

The diagnosis is confirmed by detecting anti-HCV antibodies and the presence of HCV RNA detected by PCR (polymerase chain reaction). The presence of antibody with negative HCV PCR implies the virus has been cleared. The genotype of hepatitis C and the viral load should be ascertained, as this has treatment implications. The LFTs show a hepatitic picture in acute infection but may be normal in chronic infection.

Treatment

Interferon alpha has been used as an early treatment in acute hepatitis C in an attempt to prevent chronic infection but at present this is an unlicensed indication. The NICE guidelines for the treatment of chronic hepatitis C in adults recommend the use of pegylated interferon alpha in combination with ribavirin for moderate to severe infections. The length of treatment is determined by the genotype and response to therapy. As with chronic hepatitis B, the consumption of alcohol can hasten the progression to cirrhosis and therefore patients should be advised to minimize their intake.

Genotype 1 is the most common in western Europe. Genotypes 1 and 4 are the least amenable to treatment, whereas genotypes 2 and 3 show good responses to therapy.

Transmission

HDV is transmitted via contaminated blood and sexual intercourse.

Clinical features

Coinfection with HDV worsens the clinical picture of hepatitis B.

Complications

Hepatitis C persists as a chronic infection in 70% of cases. It is also more likely than hepatitis B to result in cirrhosis and hepatocellular carcinoma. However, HCV does not cause fulminant liver failure as an acute infection. Coinfection with HIV and HCV is an important problem. Trials suggest that those with HIV can clear the HCV with pegylated interferon and ribavirin but the response rates are significantly lower than in HIV-negative individuals.

Investigations

Hepatitis D is diagnosed by detecting the anti-HDV antibody or more rarely the HDV antigen. HDV RNA can be measured using PCR. There is a hepatitic picture of LFTs.

Complications

The combined infection of HBV and HDV is also more likely to result in fulminant liver failure than HBV alone.

Prevention

There is currently no vaccine against hepatitis C. Healthcare workers need to be vigilant against needle-stick injuries to prevent infection. Needle exchange programmes to discourage IVDUs from sharing needles are essential in the battle against that route of transmission. In a survey of IVDUs, 90% of those who had been in contact with any healthcare or rehabilitation services reported that they had used needle exchange facilities. All blood products in the UK are screened for HCV.

Treatment

There is no specific antiviral therapy for hepatitis D.

Prevention

There is no vaccination available against HDV currently. Blood products in the UK are screened for hepatitis, and barrier contraception can help prevent sexual transmission.

Hepatitis E (HEV)

Hepatitis E generally causes a mild acute hepatitis, although the infection can progress to fulminant liver failure. Chronic hepatitis E infection has not been described.

Aetiology

Hepatitis E is more prevalent in the developing world. There have been large outbreaks in India.

The relative risks of contracting hepatitis B, C and HIV from a needle-stick injury involving a patient with the infection are significantly different. Roughly, the risks are HBV 30%, HCV 3% and HIV 0.3%. This should be of concern to healthcare workers because they are immunized against HBV, and post-exposure prophylaxis is available for HIV, but currently there is no proven prevention for HCV infection.

Transmission

Hepatitis E is transmitted via the faecal–oral route, like hepatitis A. The usual source is contaminated water supplies, although seafood can be implicated. The incubation period is 6–8 weeks.

Hepatitis D (HDV)

Hepatitis D cannot occur as an independent infection. It coexists with hepatitis B, since HDV can only replicate in hepatitis B infected cells.

Clinical features

Hepatitis E presents in a very similar manner to hepatitis A. The patient suffers with nausea and vomiting in addition to being jaundiced.

Investigations

Hepatitis E is diagnosed from the detection of anti-HEV antibodies. HEV RNA can also be found in stool and serum samples by PCR.

Treatment

Hepatitis E infections require supportive therapy but there is no specific antiviral treatment.

Complications

Fulminant liver failure from HEV infection has a mortality of 1–2% but this can increase to as high as 20% in pregnant women.

Prevention

There is no immunization available against HEV. Hand-washing, good sanitation and the provision of clean drinking water are the mainstays of limiting hepatitis E infections.

Epstein–Barr virus (EBV)

This virus is classically known for causing glandular fever (see Ch. 16). One of the complications of EBV infection is hepatitis.

Cytomegalovirus (CMV)

CMV can cause a disseminated infection, including hepatitis, in immunocompromised individuals (see Ch. 25).

Yellow fever

Yellow fever is caused by a flavivirus that can result in jaundice (see Ch. 24).

OTHER LIVER INFECTIONS

Leptospirosis (Weil's disease)

Leptospirosis comprises a group of infections caused by the Gram-negative coiled bacterium *Leptospira interrogans*, of which there are over 200 serotypes. Weil's disease is caused by *Leptospira interrogans icterohaemorrhagiae*. It is a zoonosis because the infection is transmitted from animals to humans.

Aetiology

Leptospira interrogans icterohaemorrhagiae is found in freshwater contaminated with rat urine or urine from other wild animals. Hence, those people at risk of contracting Weil's disease are sewage workers, farmers and anyone in contact with water from their occupation or hobbies. An open skin wound or abrasion and intact mucosal surfaces including the conjunctivae are the potential ports of entry for the bacteria, from the water.

Clinical features

The incubation period for Weil's disease is 10 days on average. The classical triad of Weil's disease is jaundice, haemorrhage and renal impairment. In fact, this classical picture is only seen in severe infections, accounting for 10–15% of cases. The majority of cases merely result in a non-specific febrile illness that is self-limiting. The severe infection has two distinct phases:

- Leptospiraemic stage which occurs initially and lasts for a week. The patient suffers with a severe headache, malaise, fever, myalgia and anorexia. The more specific symptoms are suffusion of the conjunctivae, hepatosplenomegaly and generalized lymphadenopathy. Patients may also develop arthralgia and skin rashes.
- Immune stage which occurs with a delay of 1–3 days after the leptospiraemic phase. The patients suffer with meningitis, i.e. the triad of headache, neck stiffness and photophobia. In a small number the hepatomegaly becomes tender and the patient appears jaundiced. The patient may develop renal complications with microscopic haematuria and oliguric renal failure or cardiac sequelae with dysrhythmias and cardiac failure.

Investigations

Leptospira interrogans icterohaemorrhagiae can be isolated from blood, urine and CSF (cerebrospinal fluid) cultures; PCR or identified from serology. On routine blood testing the full blood count may show a haemolytic anaemia in addition to the neutrophilia indicating a bacterial infection. The inflammatory markers ESR and CRP (C-reactive protein) will be raised. The renal function and liver function may be deranged depending on the severity of the illness.

Treatment

Penicillin and tetracycline are effective against *Leptospira interrogans icterohaemorrhagiae*. The other management involves supportive care for the complications that arise, e.g. anti-arrhythmic drugs for dysrhythmias and renal replacement therapy if the impairment is severe.

Complications

Only a minority of the severe infections will be affected by complications such as renal impairment, arrhythmias and congestive cardiac failure. The mortality is variable but can be up to 20% in the elderly.

Prevention

The mainstay of preventing Weil's disease is to avoid high-risk water contact but if this is not possible then shower thoroughly in clean water post-exposure and ensure any skin abrasions are covered. Doxycycline can be used as prophylaxis on a short-term basis.

Liver abscesses – pyogenic

Liver abscesses caused by bacteria are known as pyogenic. There are more likely to be multiple pyogenic abscesses in a liver than there are with amoebic abscesses.

Aetiology

Liver abscesses can arise from direct local spread from the biliary tract, e.g. in cholangitis (see below), or via the portal vein from the gastrointestinal (GI) tract. Therefore abscesses can occur secondary to GI tract infections, e.g. dysentery or diverticulitis. Spread of infection to the liver from the systemic circulation may also occur.

Organisms

The predominant bacteria to cause pyogenic liver abscesses are commensals from the GI tract:

- *E. coli* (commonest cause)
- *Enterococcus faecalis*
- *Streptococcus milleri*
- Proteus vulgaris
- Anaerobes, such as *Bacteroides fragilis*.

It is not uncommon to find a mixed growth of bacteria in the abscess, including anaerobes.

Clinical features

Liver abscesses can present either acutely with an unwell patient or chronically as a non-specific febrile illness, which may be investigated as a PUO (pyrexia of unknown origin). Classically the fever of an abscess is swinging in nature. Acutely, patients tend to be generally unwell with fever, rigors, sweating, vomiting and anorexia. They may also complain of right upper quadrant pain and be jaundiced. On examination of these patients the liver is tender. Since many of the GI tract commensals are Gram-negative bacteria, e.g. *E. coli* and *Proteus vulgaris*, the patient may develop Gram-negative septicaemia and shock. The chronic presentation of a pyogenic abscess includes malaise and fevers over a prolonged period. With some cases of pyogenic liver abscesses a reactive right-sided pleural effusion develops.

Investigations

The safest method used to detect abscesses in the liver is an ultrasound scan (see Fig. 19.3). If an abscess is detected, then an aspiration procedure under ultrasound guidance can be done at the same time. If the underlying source of infection is from the biliary tract, it can be assessed simultaneously. Particularly in patients with a high body mass index (BMI), a CT (computerized tomography) scan of the abdomen may be a more sensitive test with the additional benefit of also imaging the whole of the abdomen, which may elucidate the origin of the infection.

Microscopy and culture of the aspirated abscess contents is ideal for identifying the causative organism or organisms. Abscesses that have resulted from haematogenous spread are more likely to give positive blood cultures but the yield is still low.

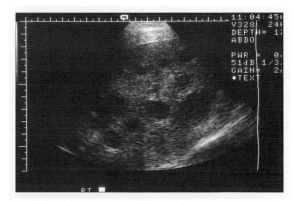

Fig. 19.3 Ultrasound scan of pyogenic liver abscess. *Source:* Conlon CP, Snydman DR, 2000: Fig. 9.40.

The liver function tests may not be abnormal, especially in mild chronic cases. Most commonly there will be a raised alkaline phosphatase level, which suggests an obstructive aetiology that could be an abscess. A leucocytosis and raised inflammatory markers, CRP and ESR, are usually seen. A right pleural effusion would be seen on a plain chest radiograph as the loss of definition of the right costophrenic angle and a fluid level. The hemidiaphragm may also be raised due to the abscess.

> An abscess is a space-occupying lesion which can occlude the biliary canaliculi causing an increase in the levels of alkaline phosphatase and GGT released into the bloodstream. The hepatocyte damage is minimal in comparison, so lower levels of AST and ALT are seen. This gives rise to the 'obstructive picture'.

Treatment

The initial antibiotic cover should be broad-spectrum, e.g. the second-generation cephalosporin cefuroxime with metronidazole for anaerobic cover, until the organisms responsible are identified. Most abscesses require drainage in addition to antibiotics for resolution and this can be performed under ultrasound guidance.

Liver abscesses – amoebic

Amoebic liver abscesses are usually single.

Organism

Amoebic liver abscesses are caused by *Entamoeba histolytica*. This protozoon occurs worldwide with a higher prevalence in the tropics. In the UK there have been less than 200 cases per year since 2002.

Pathophysiology

Entamoeba histolytica is able to invade through the mucosal wall to enter the portal bloodstream and hence reach the liver (see Ch. 18 for life cycle).

Clinical features

The patients are often remarkably asymptomatic. The presentation can be more acute though, with patients experiencing right upper quadrant pain and tender hepatomegaly on examination. This can be accompanied with fevers, malaise, anorexia and weight loss. There may be oedema and redness of the skin overlying superficial abscesses. There may not be a history of preceding bloody diarrhoea.

Investigations

The abscess is usually discovered by performing an ultrasound scan of the liver. The right lobe of the liver is most commonly involved. This finding should be followed up by an aspiration of the abscess contents under ultrasound guidance, both for diagnostic and therapeutic reasons. Microscopy and culture of the aspirated abscess contents, classically described as looking like 'anchovy sauce', is an excellent way of elucidating the organism responsible. *Entamoeba histolytica* can also be confirmed as the cause by examining stool specimens for cysts or using serology. An abdominal CT scan can also detect abscesses (see Fig. 19.4). The liver function tests may be mildly deranged with an obstructive picture.

Treatment

Metronidazole antibiotics combined with aspiration of the abscess contents is the optimal treatment for amoebic abscesses.

Hydatid disease

Hydatid disease is a zoonosis acquired from ingesting the eggs of the dog tapeworm, *Echinococcus granulosus*. It is particularly a problem in sheep farming areas such as Wales, the Middle East, Australasia, South and North America.

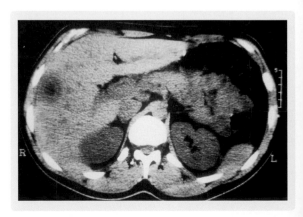

Fig. 19.4 CT scan of amoebic liver abscess.
Source: Conlon CP, Snydman DR, 2000: Fig. 9.44.

Pathophysiology

Humans are an inadvertent host of *Echinococcus granulosus*, acquired by ingestion of the eggs from contaminated food or direct contact with infected dog faeces (Fig. 19.5). Once ingested, the eggs hatch into larvae that are able to penetrate the gut wall and enter the portal bloodstream. Therefore hydatid cysts most commonly develop in the liver, in about two-thirds of cases, but dissemination to other sites also occurs, such as to the lungs, bone and the brain. The second most frequent site for cysts to occur is in the lungs.

Clinical features

Hydatid disease tends to have an insidious presentation or be entirely asymptomatic. The patient can become jaundiced, and may develop a slowly progressive right upper quadrant swelling and pain due to the hepatomegaly resulting from cysts within the liver. Hydatid disease may be discovered as part of the investigations for a PUO. Symptoms can also arise from cysts found elsewhere, such as in the lungs, bone and the brain. Dyspnoea, chest pain and haemoptysis can result from cysts in the lung, which is the most common site for symptomatic disease. Seizures may be the consequence of cysts in the brain.

Investigations

The cysts are usually diagnosed from imaging of the affected area: abdominal ultrasound or CT scans for liver cysts; plain chest radiographs or chest CT for pulmonary cysts; CT or MRI scans of the head for brain cysts; and plain radiographs of the limbs for bone cysts. The cysts may be found entirely incidentally. The characteristic appearance of hydatid cysts is to have many daughter cysts within the parent one. Serological tests can also be used for diagnosis. Microscopy of the daughter cysts can identify the immature tapeworm heads which are produced on the inner surface of the cyst. There may be an eosinophilia seen on the full blood count.

> An anaphylactic reaction can occur from contamination with released cyst contents. Cysts should not, therefore, be aspirated unless scolicidal agents are used first (see Treatment).

Treatment

Asymptomatic cysts usually do not require any treatment, especially once the outer layer has calcified. A combination therapy using albendazole and praziquantel gives good penetration into the cysts and may obviate the need for surgery. A technique known as 'PAIR' (Puncture, Aspiration, Injection, Re-aspiration) is commonly used to treat cysts that are not easily resectable. This involves injecting a scolicidal agent, such as alcohol or hypertonic saline, into the cyst under imaging guidance. This is best done after a cycle or two of albendazole and praziquantel therapy. Surgical resection of the cysts may be required for symptomatic relief.

Schistosomiasis

The blood flukes, *Schistosoma mansoni* and *Schistosoma japonicum*, cause granuloma in the liver and subsequent obstructive complications (see Ch. 24).

Liver flukes

Organisms

Clonorchis sinensis (also known as *Opisthorchis sinensis*), found in the Far East, and *Fasciola hepatica*, occurring worldwide, are liver flukes.

Aetiology

Clonorchis sinensis is transmitted to humans via raw fish, whereas *Fasciola hepatica* is acquired

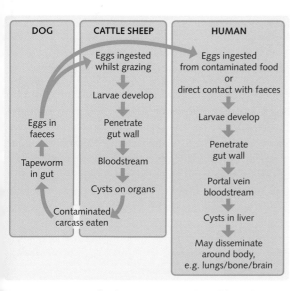

Fig. 19.5 Diagram of *Echinococcus granulosus* life cycle.

Fig. 19.6 Life cycle of *Fasciola hepatica* and *Clonorchis sinensis*.

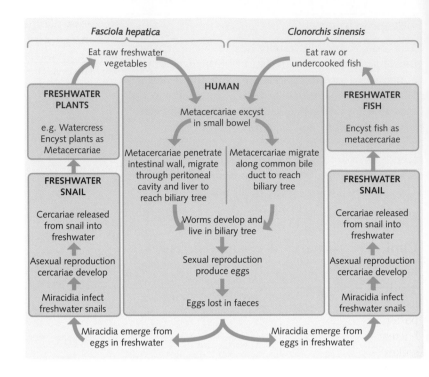

from eating watercress. The life cycles are shown in Figure 19.6.

Clinical features

As the immature flukes migrate through the liver, the patient can experience fevers, malaise, right upper quadrant pain and urticaria, although this stage may be asymptomatic. Symptoms generally arise from obstruction of the biliary tract. This can result in jaundice and cholangitis.

Investigations

During the migration stage there is usually an eosinophilia. The flukes can be visualized in the liver or biliary tract on ultrasound, CT and MRI scans. Detection of the ova in faeces or duodenal aspirates confirms the diagnosis. Serology can also be used to make the diagnosis.

Treatment

Clonorchiasis is treated with a 2-day course of praziquantel. Fascioliasis is treated with triclabendazole as a single dose, although some patients may require a repeated dose.

Complications

Clonorchiasis can give rise to secondary liver abscesses and is a risk factor for cholangiocarcinoma. Fascioliasis can be complicated by flukes settling in ectopic sites, such as the brain or lungs.

BILIARY TRACT INFECTIONS

Cholecystitis is an infection of the gallbladder, resulting from inflammation due to the presence of gallstones.

Cholangitis is an infection of the hepatic and common bile ducts. A mild cholangitis generally accompanies cholecystitis, whereas a severe infection tends to occur secondary to bile duct obstruction which may be due to gallstones, strictures (e.g. in sclerosing cholangitis) or tumours. In both cases there is a stagnation of bile, which is then vulnerable to becoming infected with gastrointestinal tract commensals. Ascending cholangitis (i.e. tracking up towards the gall bladder) can complicate pancreatitis and manipulation of the bile duct as occurs with an ERCP (endoscopic retrograde cholangiopancreatography).

Organisms

The organisms that typically cause infections of the biliary tract are the Gram-negative coliforms, such as *E. coli*, *Klebsiella* species and *Proteus mirabilis*, as well as anaerobes, such as *Bacteroides fragilis*. They are all commensals of the gastrointestinal tract. In many cases more than one organism is involved.

Risk groups

The risk of developing cholecystitis and cholangitis increases with age, and women are more often affected than men.

Clinical features

Biliary tract infections present with right upper quadrant pain, jaundice and fevers. The patients usually look sick and complain of malaise. Typically, patients with cholangitis are more likely to be bacteraemic and hence have higher temperature spikes and these are more commonly accompanied by rigors. The jaundice with acute cholecystitis tends to be milder than that occurring with cholangitis.

Charcot's triad of symptoms consists of fever, rigors and jaundice.

Patients with acute cholecystitis tend to be nauseous and vomit. The right upper quadrant pain may radiate to the shoulder blade tip. On examination, the right upper quadrant tenderness resulting from acute cholecystitis can give rise to a positive Murphy's sign (see Ch. 6). If gallstones are present and are causing an obstruction to the biliary tract, then the jaundice will be accompanied by dark urine and pale stools.

Investigations

Right upper quadrant pain and/or jaundice should be investigated with an ultrasound scan. This can demonstrate the thickened gall bladder wall, gallstones within the gall bladder and fluid around it suggesting acute cholecystitis; or the dilated biliary tracts of cholangitis. An abdominal CT scan will also show these changes. A more detailed view of the biliary tree can be obtained from an ERCP or non-invasively with an MRCP (magnetic resonance cholangiopancreatography). Blood cultures are more likely to be positive with cholangitis than with cholecystitis. The liver function tests will show a raised bilirubin when jaundice is present and usually an obstructive picture with cholangitis, i.e. ALP and GGT more raised than the ALT and AST. There is a neutrophilia on the full blood count and raised inflammatory markers, CRP and ESR.

Treatment

The antibiotics of choice for biliary tract infections are the second-generation cephalosporin, cefuroxime, combined with metronidazole. An obstructed biliary system may require decompression, which can be achieved endoscopically with ERCP, involving a sphincterotomy for gallstones or stenting for strictures; or with surgery. In general, cholecystectomy operations for gallstones are delayed until the infection has settled if the clinical condition allows.

Complications

Cholecystitis can be complicated by gangrene and perforation of the gallbladder, empyema of the gallbladder or pancreatitis due to gallstones. Cholangitis may result in Gram-negative septicaemia and shock; and abscess formation in the liver.

FEVER AND ABNORMAL LIVER FUNCTION TESTS

Patients may present with a PUO and on routine blood tests be found to have mildly deranged LFTs. This presentation can reflect a systemic infection that involves granuloma formation in the liver. Examples would include brucellosis, Q fever (*Coxiella burnetii*), tuberculosis and syphilis.

Liver and biliary tract infections are summarized in Figure 19.7.

Further reading

Lauer GM, Walker BD. Hepatitis C virus infection. New Engl J Med 2001; 345(1):41–52.
NICE. Guidelines for the treatment of chronic hepatitis C in adults. Website: www.nice.org.uk/.

Fig. 19.7 Summary of liver and biliary tract infections

Hepatitis – see Figure 19.1
Non-hepatitis liver infections

Infection	Risk groups	Clinical features	Investigations	Treatment	Other
Leptospirosis/Weil's disease (*Leptospira interrogans icterohaemorrhagiae*)	Those with jobs or hobbies leading to contact with water contaminated by rat urine	First phase: severe headache, malaise, fever, myalgia, anorexia, arthralgia, skin rashes. Conjunctival suffusion, hepatosplenomegaly, lymphadenopathy. Second phase: meningitis, jaundice, renal impairment	Blood, urine and CSF for cultures. PCR and serology. Haemolytic anaemia; abnormal renal and liver function tests	Penicillin or tetracycline. Supportive care for complications	*Complications*: renal impairment, cardiac dysrhythmias, congestive cardiac failure. Mortality up to 20% in elderly. *Prevention*: avoid high-risk water exposure; doxycycline
Pyogenic abscesses (commonest *E. coli*; can have mixed growth of coliforms with anaerobes)	Those with GI tract infections, e.g. diverticulitis or biliary tract infections	Acute: swinging fevers, rigors, sweating, vomiting, anorexia, right upper quadrant pain, jaundice. Chronic: malaise, prolonged fever, right-sided reactive pleural effusion	Ultrasound scan ± aspiration; CT scan. Culture of aspirated contents and blood. Abnormal liver function tests	Second-generation cephalosporin, e.g. cefuroxime with metronidazole. Aspiration of abscess contents	More likely to have multiple abscesses. *Complications*: acute cases may be complicated by Gram-negative septicaemia and shock
Amoebic abscesses (*Entamoeba histolytica*)	Those exposed to contaminated food and water. Those practising oral-anal sex	Asymptomatic or acutely with right upper quadrant pain, fever, malaise, anorexia. Preceding bloody diarrhoea	Ultrasound scan ± aspiration; CT scan. Culture of aspirated contents and stool. Serology. Abnormal liver function tests	Metronidazole and aspiration of abscess contents	Usually single abscess
Hydatid disease (*Echinococcus granulosus*)	Those involved in sheep farming; contact with infected dogs	Asymptomatic or chronically with jaundice, right upper quadrant pain, fever. Dyspnoea, chest pain, haemoptysis. Seizures	Liver ultrasound or CT scan. Chest radiograph or CT scan. CT or MRI scan of brain. Serology. Microscopy of cysts. Eosinophilia	Albendazole and praziquantel. 'PAIR'. Surgical resection. Nil if asymptomatic and calcified	*Complications*: anaphylaxis from released cyst contents
Liver flukes (*Clonorchis sinensis* and *Fasciola hepatica*)	Those eating raw fish or watercress	Asymptomatic or fevers, malaise, right upper quadrant pain, urticaria. Jaundice and cholangitis	Liver ultrasound, CT or MRI scans. Ova from faeces or duodenal aspirate. Serology. Eosinophilia	Praziquantel for clonorchiasis; triclabendazole for fascioliasis	*Complications*: secondary liver abscesses, cholangiocarcinoma, ectopic locations for flukes
Schistosomiasis (*Schistosoma mansoni* and *Schistosoma japonicum*)	See Chapter 24				

(Continued)

Fig. 19.7 Summary of liver and biliary tract infections —continued

			Biliary tract infections			
Infection	Involvement	Risk groups	Clinical features	Investigations	Treatment	Other
Cholecystitis (Gram-negative coliforms and anaerobes)	Gall bladder	Older age, women; those with gallstones	Right upper quadrant pain, milder jaundice, fevers, malaise, nausea, vomiting. Positive Murphy's sign	Ultrasound or CT scan. ERCP or MRCP. Blood cultures less useful. Abnormal liver function tests	Second-generation cephalosporin, e.g. cefuroxime with metronidazole. Cholecystectomy	*Complications:* gangrene and perforation or empyema of gallbladder; pancreatitis from gallstones
Cholangitis (Gram-negative coliforms and anaerobes)	Hepatic and common bile ducts	Older age, women; those with gallstones, strictures, tumours. After pancreatitis or ERCP	Right upper quadrant pain, deeper jaundice, higher fevers, rigors, malaise	Ultrasound or CT scan. ERCP or MRCP. Blood cultures more useful. Abnormal liver function tests.	Second-generation cephalosporin, e.g. cefuroxime with metronidazole. ERCP ± stenting/sphinc-terotomy	*Complications:* Gram-negative septicaemia and shock; liver abscess formation

Urinary tract infections

Objectives

In this chapter you will learn:

- What influences the risk of acquiring a UTI
- How you distinguish clinically between a simple UTI and pyelonephritis
- The investigation results that confirm the diagnosis of a UTI
- What imaging is appropriate for urinary infections.

A urinary tract infection (UTI) is a common infection affecting the urethra and bladder. It usually arises from bacteria commensal to the gastrointestinal tract or perineum. The vast majority of community-acquired UTIs are caused by *Escherichia coli* (up to 95%), whereas nosocomial infections have a higher proportion caused by the other Gram-negative bacteria from the gastrointestinal tract (Fig. 20.1). UTIs are the second most common group of hospital-acquired infections after those resulting from intravenous devices, e.g. peripheral cannulas and central lines.

The infection can extend proximally to involve the ureters and kidneys, at which point it is called pyelonephritis. This involvement of the kidneys means the infection is classified as a complicated UTI. Other factors which constitute a complicated UTI are those infections associated with renal calculi, urinary tract malformations or related to prostheses, e.g. urinary catheters. An infection solely affecting the urethra and bladder is a simple or uncomplicated UTI. The importance of distinguishing between an uncomplicated UTI and a complicated UTI is that it determines the length of antibiotic treatment that will be required.

The organisms responsible for both upper and lower urinary tract infections are detailed in Figure 20.2.

LOWER URINARY TRACT INFECTIONS

Risk factors

There are a number of factors which predispose someone to contracting a UTI:

- Female sex – most probably because females have a shorter urethra than males and so contamination from the gastrointestinal tract and perineum is easier. Also prostatic fluid has bactericidal properties.
- Sexual intercourse – since this can introduce bacteria from the perineum internally.
- Diabetes mellitus – these patients are more susceptible to all infections than the non-diabetic population. Diabetic patients on average have higher levels of glucose in the blood on which bacteria can feed and this is thought to be a contributing factor.
- Immunocompromise – from whatever cause, e.g. haematological, drug related or HIV-related, renders the patient vulnerable to infection. The causative organisms can be the same as in immunocompetent patients but also include less virulent bacteria and fungi.
- Elderly patient – the increased likelihood of immobility, incontinence and urinary catheterization in the elderly accounts for their increased risk of UTIs.
- Structural abnormalities of the urinary tract, e.g. benign prostatic hypertrophy (BPH), a horseshoe kidney (see Fig. 20.3) and a neuropathic bladder – these are significant because they result in incomplete emptying of the bladder and the residual urine is more liable to become infected.
- Instrumentation of the urinary tract, e.g. a urinary catheter, a cystoscopy procedure – these allow the introduction of bacteria into the urinary tract if strict aseptic techniques are not used.

Fig. 20.1 Causative organisms for a UTI in decreasing order of frequency

Community-acquired causes	Hospital-acquired causes
Escherichia coli	Escherichia coli
Staphylococcus saprophyticus	Coliforms (e.g. klebsiella, enterobacter,
Enterococcus faecalis	serratia)
Coliforms (e.g. klebsiella,	Proteus mirabilis
enterobacter, serratia)	Enterococcus faecalis
Candida albicans	Candida albicans
Proteus mirabilis	Pseudomonas aeruginosa
Staphylococcus epidermidis	Staphylococcus epidermidis
Pseudomonas aeruginosa	Staphylococcus saprophyticus

Fig. 20.2 Details of organisms causing UTIs

Organism	Type	Site as commensal	Resistance	Acquired	Other infections caused
Bacterial causes					
Escherichia coli	Gram-negative bacilli (has endotoxin)	GI tract	Commonly to penicillin (produces beta-lactamases)	Both in community and in hospital	GI tract, biliary tree, respiratory tract, neonatal meningitis
Klebsiella	Gram-negative bacilli	GI tract	Commonly to penicillin (produces beta-lactamases)	Most while in hospital	Wound, respiratory tract, neonatal meningitis
Enterobacter and serratia	Gram-negative bacilli	GI tract	May be problems with antibiotic-resistant strains	Most while in hospital	Respiratory tract
Proteus mirabilis	Gram-negative bacilli	GI tract		Most while in hospital	Wound
Enterococcus faecalis*	Gram-positive cocci	GI tract	Resistance to penicillin increasing; vancomycin resistance	Most while in hospital	Endocarditis, wounds and abscesses
Staphylococcus epidermidis	Gram-positive cocci (coagulase-negative)	Skin		Most while in hospital	With prosthetic materials, e.g. catheters, i.v. cannulas
Staphylococcus saprophyticus	Gram-positive cocci (coagulase-negative)	Perineum		Sexually active young women	
Pseudomonas aeruginosa	Gram-negative bacilli	GI tract	Resistance to many antibiotics common	Both in the community and in hospital	Respiratory tract, urinary tract, skin, eye, otitis externa
Fungal causes					
Candida albicans	Yeast	Mouth and GI tract		Most while in hospital	Oral, skin, nail, respiratory, GI and GU tracts, endocarditis, prosthetic materials

Enterococci are a reclassification of group D beta-haemolytic streptococci

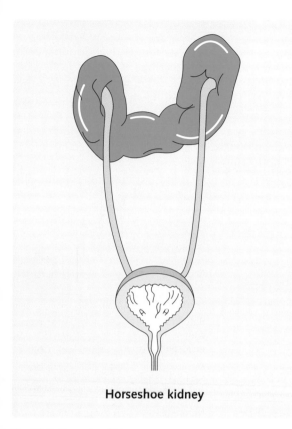

Horseshoe kidney

Fig. 20.3 Horseshoe kidney.

Good practice for women is to pass urine directly after sexual intercourse to reduce the risk of acquiring a UTI.

Clinical features

A patient suffering with a UTI classically complains of:

- dysuria (pain or burning sensation on passing urine)
- frequency (needing to pass urine an increased number of times per day)
- nocturia (getting up at night to urinate)
- urgency (short time period between feeling the sensation to urinate and actually passing urine) and if the patient is unable to resist the urge before finding a suitable place to pass urine then urge incontinence.

Sometimes patients also experience haematuria (blood in the urine). The urine can smell offensive when it is infected, and in elderly patients smelling of urine may also reflect new urinary incontinence that has resulted from the UTI. Elderly patients often have minimal urinary tract symptoms and present with just confusion or a deterioration of their usual mental state. Younger patients usually only present with local symptoms relating to the UTI but older patients and those with many comorbidities are more likely to be systemically unwell with a UTI. They can suffer with fever and malaise as well as confusion.

Investigations

The principal bedside investigation to confirm the clinical suspicion of a UTI is a urine dipstick. Positive results for leucocytes and nitrites support the diagnosis of a UTI. The patient will sometimes test positive for blood and less commonly protein. If a patient not known to be diabetic has a dipstick positive for glucose then a formal fasting glucose should be checked to exclude a new diagnosis of diabetes mellitus. It is equally important in the elderly, especially if they are catheterized, to test the urine after a course of antibiotic therapy because they may test positive for leucocytes all the time even when not actually infected.

In order to confirm the diagnosis of a UTI and identify the organism responsible for causing the infection, the urine needs to be sent for microscopy and culture. Antibiotic sensitivities can be checked if the organism is cultured. This is particularly important in hospital-acquired UTIs, because there is an increased risk the bacteria will be antibiotic-resistant. If the patient is systemically unwell then blood cultures may be positive in addition to urinary cultures.

On blood testing, the full blood count (FBC) shows a leucocytosis, which is typically a neutrophilia with a bacterial infection. The biochemistry results demonstrate a raised C-reactive protein (CRP) reflecting the presence of an infection. The renal function should be checked, as there may be deterioration with

Treatment with trimethoprim can cause a rise in plasma creatinine in patients with already moderately impaired renal function, since trimethoprim competes with the creatinine for excretion into the urine in the distal convoluted tubule. It does not reflect a decrease in overall renal function as the glomerular filtration rate of creatinine is unchanged.

a UTI. A fasting glucose sample should be tested to look for diabetes mellitus.

The indications for imaging the renal tract with an ultrasound scan (USS) when only a simple UTI is suspected are different depending on the sex of the patient. The first UTI in males warrants a USS as a UTI is more unusual and therefore there is a higher likelihood of finding a structural abnormality as the predisposition. In females, if there are repeated UTIs then a USS should be requested to exclude an underlying abnormality.

Treatment

An uncomplicated UTI is readily treatable with nitrofurantoin, trimethoprim, ciprofloxacin or amoxi-cillin as a short oral course: 3 days of antibiotics is usually sufficient to resolve the infection. If, however, the patient is systemically unwell or the infection is catheter-related or hospital-acquired then the initial empirical treatment should be with an intravenous second-generation cephalosporin, e.g. cefuroxime. This therapy can be tailored more specifically once the organism and sensitivities are known. The antibiotic course is typically prescribed for a week. In cases where there is a suspicion that a *Pseudomonas aeruginosa* infection may be responsible for the UTI, particularly to be considered in those with a long-term indwelling urinary catheter, then the antibiotic of choice is ciprofloxacin or a third-generation cephalosporin, e.g. ceftazidime.

In addition to antibiotics some simple measures are recommended: drinking plenty of fluid is important to help flush out the bacteria from the urinary tract and double micturition to ensure an empty bladder. In catheterized patients the urinary catheter should be changed once antibiotics are started, as bacteria can adhere to the prosthetic material and remain a reservoir of infection. The episode of infection should also prompt the clinicians to reassess the indications for urinary catheterization in the patient and if possible take the opportunity for a trial without a catheter.

PYELONEPHRITIS

Pyelonephritis is a more serious infection involving the kidneys and ureters. It can arise as a consequence of a lower UTI, a urinary malformation or related to renal calculi, i.e. is a complicated UTI. The causative organisms of pyelonephritis are the same as for lower UTIs.

Clinical features

The patient typically presents with abdominal pain, which is classically described as loin to groin pain, although some patients suffer with back pain rather than more anterior pain. The pain is usually colicky and sharp in nature. Patients can appear restless as they are unable to find a position in which to get comfortable. Many cases will be preceded by dysuria and other lower urinary tract symptoms, as detailed above. Haematuria is more commonly present with pyelonephritis than with a simple UTI. The patient is also systemically unwell with high fevers, rigors and drenching sweats.

Renal calculi causing obstruction in the renal pelvis or ureters can act as a nidus for infection. Haematuria and loin pain occur with both renal calculi and pyelonephritis. A plain kidneys, ureters and bladder (KUB) radiograph (90% of renal calculi are radio-opaque) followed by an intravenous urogram (IVU) should be performed to exclude renal calculi (see Fig. 20.4). Calculi < 5 mm in diameter are able to pass through the urinary tract but for larger calculi a urological opinion should be sought.

Investigation

The infection is confirmed initially by the bedside using a urine dipstick. As with a simple UTI, positive results for leucocytes and nitrites indicate the presence of urinary infection; blood and protein may also be present. In cases of pyelonephritis, the blood cultures are more likely to be positive in addition to the urine cultures than in an uncomplicated UTI, especially if the patient is systemically unwell. Cultures are useful not only for identifying the causative organism but also for elucidating the antibiotic resistance patterns. Proteus infections can predispose to renal calculi formation, particularly staghorn calculi (see Fig. 20.5).

The haematology results in pyelonephritis are the same as for a simple UTI: showing a neutrophilia with bacterial infection. The renal function impairment can be more significant with pyelonephritis since any obstruction by renal calculi can result in back pressure on the kidney. The other biochemistry results are similar with a raised CRP and the need to check the

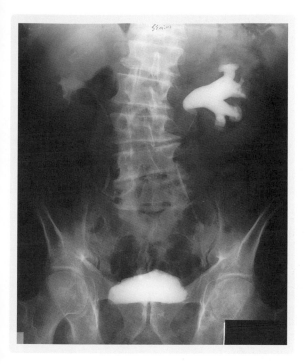

Fig. 20.4 A renal calculus seen in an intravenous urogram. *Source:* Conlon CP, Snydman DR. Mosby's Colour Atlas and Text of Infectious Diseases. Edinburgh: Mosby; 2000: Fig. 10.4.

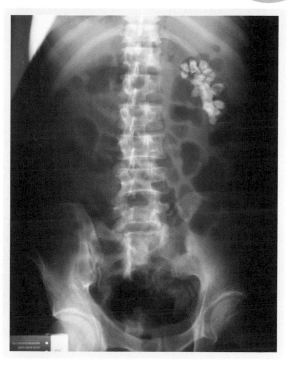

Fig. 20.5 Staghorn calculus.

fasting glucose level. Since most renal calculi contain calcium, if they are found to be present then the calcium levels in both blood and urine need to be ascertained. Hypercalcaemia can cause multiple problems beyond renal calculi, and therefore investigations to elucidate the underlying cause are essential, so that it can be treated.

Unlike with a simple UTI, all cases of pyelonephritis should undergo imaging with an ultrasound scan of the renal tract. It is essential not to miss the development of hydronephrosis secondary to obstruction by renal calculi, because if left uncorrected this can result in chronic renal failure. It also offers the opportunity to look for any anatomical abnormalities that may be predisposing the patient to infection. A KUB radiograph and IVU are used to detect renal calculi.

Treatment

The patient requires intravenous therapy initially, usually with a second-generation cephalosporin, e.g. cefuroxime, or the aminoglycoside, gentamicin. Once the temperature has settled, oral antibiotics chosen according to the bacterial sensitivities, e.g.

co-amoxiclav, ciprofloxacin, can be used to complete the course of treatment. A total of 7–10 days of antibiotics is usually given to treat pyelonephritis.

Pyelonephritis and renal calculi can both be very painful and good analgesia is crucial. Drinking large volumes of water is helpful in that it creates an increased urine output to flush through any bacteria, calculi (< 5 mm) and debris. Renal calculi larger than 5 mm are unlikely to pass through the renal tract and require lithotripsy treatment (shattering with extracorporeal shock waves) or surgical removal. The urology team should be involved for these management decisions.

Complications

The principal concerns with pyelonephritis are the potential to develop Gram-negative septicaemia and chronic renal failure. An obstruction of the renal tract, if not relieved promptly, can result in a dilatation of the ureters and renal pelvis known as hydronephrosis (see Fig. 20.6). Renal scarring can result from repeated infections or from trauma by renal calculi. Repeated infections do not cause renal impairment unless there is an anatomical abnormality of the renal tract or a

Fig. 20.6 Changes seen in hydronephrosis.

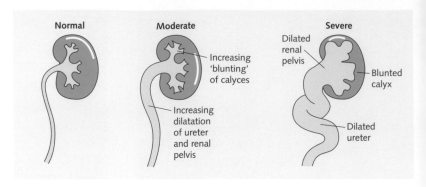

Fig. 20.7 Summary of urinary tract infections

	Lower urinary tract infection (urethra and bladder)	Upper urinary tract infection (ureters and kidneys, i.e. pyelonephritis)
Risk factors	Females, sexual intercourse, diabetes mellitus, immunocompromise, elderly patients, structural abnormalities, e.g. neuropathic bladder; instrumentation of the urinary tract, e.g. catheterization	Structural abnormalities, e.g. ureteric strictures; renal calculi, and all risk factors for a lower UTI
Clinical features	Dysuria, frequency, nocturia, urgency and urge incontinence. Haematuria less common. Confusion or deterioration in mental state. Systemically unwell with fever and malaise	Abdominal 'loin to groin' pain or back pain; dysuria and lower UTI symptoms. Haematuria more common. Systemically unwell with high fevers, rigors and sweats
Investigations	Urine dipstick. Urine for microscopy and culture. Blood cultures if systemically unwell. Renal function. Fasting glucose. Renal tract USS depending on sex of patient	Urine dipstick. Blood and urine cultures. Renal function. Calcium and fasting glucose. Renal tract USS essential. KUB radiograph and IVU for renal calculi
Treatment	Simple UTI: nitrofurantoin, trimethoprim, ciprofloxacin or amoxicillin as an oral course. Complicated or nosocomial UTI: intravenous cefuroxime. Plentiful fluids and double micturition. Catheter change	Initial: intravenous cefuroxime or gentamicin. Completion: oral antibiotic, e.g. co-amoxiclav, ciprofloxacin. Good analgesia. Plentiful fluids. Urological advice for calculi (> 5 mm)
Complications	Bacteraemia, pyelonephritis	Gram-negative septicaemia, hydronephrosis, renal scarring and chronic renal failure

complicating factor such as obstruction or diabetes mellitus. Chronic pyelonephritis results from childhood infections and urinary reflux from the bladder into the ureters on voiding.

Urinary tract infections are summarized in Figure 20.7.

Further reading

Fihn SD. Acute uncomplicated urinary tract infection in women. NEJM 2003; 349:259–266.

Health Protection Agency. Primary care guidance for the diagnosis of UTI. Website: www.hpa.org.uk/infections/topics_az/primary_care_guidance/uti_guide_290404.rtf.

Hooten TM, Stamm WE. Diagnosis and treatment of uncomplicated urinary tract infection. Infect Dis Clin North Am 1997; 11:551–581

MedlinePlus Medical Encyclopedia. Extracorporeal shock wave lithotripsy. Website: www.nlm.nih.gov/medlineplus/ency/article/007113.htm.

Objectives

In this chapter you will learn:

- The differential diagnosis for urethral/vaginal discharge
- The meaning of VDRL, TPHA and FTA serology results
- What predisposes someone to a candida infection
- How to differentiate between the ulcers of syphilis and HSV-1 and -2
- The prevention advice that should be given to patients presenting with a potential STI.

Sexually transmitted infections (STIs) are most common in those aged between 16 and 30 years old. Higher rates of infection are predictably correlated with an increased number of sexual partners. Worldwide there has been a marked increase in the number of infections acquired within the last decade and that is mirrored in the UK, which has witnessed a steady increase in the rates of all STIs. An important landmark in the epidemiology of STIs was the discovery of HIV in the early 1980s, which heralded the beginning of the 'Safe sex' campaign to promote condom use to prevent the transmission of STIs. The important STIs to be familiar with are detailed below:

BACTERIAL CAUSES

Gonorrhoea

Gonorrhoea is caused by *Neisseria gonorrhoeae*, Gram-negative diplococci.

Transmission

Gonorrhoea is acquired either sexually or vertically at birth.

Epidemiology

Gonorrhoea is the second most common STI in the UK. The highest rates of infection are found in males aged 20–24 years and females aged 16–19 years. Gonorrhoea was the only bacterial STI not to show an increase in cases during 2003 and 2004, although the rate of infection had risen sharply between 1998 and 2002. There are approximately between 22 000 and 25 000 cases per year in the UK. In contrast to chlamydia and viral STIs, gonorrhoea tends to occur in concentrated areas, especially affecting urban and deprived populations. In the UK the highest infection rates for gonorrhoea in 2004 were seen in London.

Clinical features

Male patients present with urethritis and a purulent discharge from the penis, 2 days after sexual intercourse. Other symptoms will depend on sexual practice, e.g. pharyngitis with oral–genital sex, proctitis with anal sex. Female patients are often asymptomatic but if not, will complain of dysuria and purulent vaginal discharge. The patient can become systemically unwell with fever and sweats.

Complications

Men may suffer with prostatitis and epididymo-orchitis, whereas women can develop pelvic inflammatory disease (PID) and bartholinitis (inflammation of the Bartholin glands). Pustular skin lesions can develop, particularly on the medial aspect of the upper thighs and area local to the genitalia. In more severe cases, arthritis and septicaemia can result from haematogenous spread; in these cases pustules may be seen on the digits and elsewhere. Neonates can develop gonococcal conjunctivitis with periorbital inflammation.

Investigations

Microscopy and culture of urethral or vaginal discharge identifies the organism. If arthritis is present then microscopy and culture of aspirated joint fluid can reveal the gonococcus. If the patient is

Fitz-Hugh–Curtis syndrome is a rare complication of gonorrhoea infection. It is a perihepatitis that results from direct spread of the infection to the liver capsule and peritoneum from the Fallopian tube. Adhesions can develop (see Fig. 21.1).

The major concern of PID is that 60% of cases are asymptomatic and yet it can lead to infertility in women and ectopic pregnancies. Most cases of PID are sexually transmitted with chlamydia causing the greatest proportion. Other sources of infection are during childbirth and instrumentation.

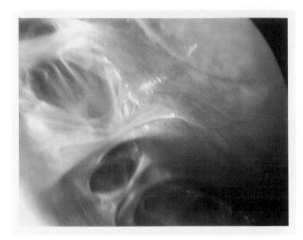

Fig. 21.1 Perihepatitis as a complication of gonorrhoea. *Source:* Conlon CP, Snydman DR. Mosby's Colour Atlas and Text of Infectious Diseases. Edinburgh: Mosby; 2000: Fig. 10.22.

systemically unwell, blood cultures may also be positive.

Treatment

Many gonococci now produce penicillinase (PPNG – penicillinase-producing *Neisseria gonorrhoeae*) so penicillin or ampicillin is no longer seen as first-line therapy. More commonly, drugs like the third-generation cephalosporin, ceftriaxone, or quinolones, e.g. ciprofloxacin, are used, although the prevalence of ciprofloxacin resistance is currently 9% in the UK. It is crucially important that patients abstain from sexual activity until their treatment is completed and their partner has been assessed and treated if necessary, otherwise reinfection is likely to occur.

Prevention

Prevention strategies involve condom usage for sexual intercourse and contact tracing from known cases of gonorrhoea, with investigation and treatment as appropriate. Antenatal screening is important for preventing vertical transmission.

Non-gonococcal urethritis (NGU)

NGU, also known as non-specific urethritis (NSU), can be caused (in order of decreasing frequency) by:

* *Chlamydia trachomatis* (majority of cases, > 50%)
* *Ureaplasma urealyticum*
* Bacteroides
* Mycoplasma.

Transmission

NGU is contracted through sexual intercourse.

Clinical features

Male patients suffer with urethral discharge, dysuria and penile discomfort, although 10–15% are asymptomatic. The majority of female patients are in fact asymptomatic but those who do have symptoms will complain of urethritis and cervicitis. Conjunctivitis and a reactive arthritis are present if the urethritis forms part of Reiter's syndrome.

Reiter's syndrome consists of the triad of urethritis, arthritis and conjunctivitis. Other bacteria not causing urethritis can also be a trigger such as salmonella, shigella and yersinia, which all cause gastroenteritis (see Ch. 18).

Investigations

Microscopy of urethral or cervical discharge will show pus cells. *Chlamydia trachomatis* may be detected by immunofluorescence or by ligase chain reaction.

Treatment

Tetracyclines, e.g. doxycycline, or macrolides, e.g. erythromycin, are the antibiotics used to treat NGU. Sexual abstinence should be emphasized until treatment has been completed and the sexual partner assessed for infection and treated as necessary.

Prevention

Condom usage decreases transmission of infections. Contact tracing, investigation and treatment of sexual partners aims to reduce reinfection and lower the population rate of infection.

Syphilis

Syphilis is caused by *Treponema pallidum*, a spirochaete.

Transmission

Syphilis can be acquired either sexually or vertically via the placenta.

Epidemiology

Since 1997 there has been a substantial rise in the number of cases of syphilis, with the greatest increase seen amongst men who have sex with men. Infection rates are currently the highest they have been since 1984; there were over 2250 new diagnoses of primary and secondary syphilis in 2004 in the UK. The increase in syphilis cases has been associated with outbreaks across the UK: in Bristol, Brighton, Manchester, Newcastle-upon-Tyne, central Scotland and the largest in London. Unlike other bacterial STIs, the highest rates of syphilis infection are seen in older age groups, 25- to 44-year-olds.

Clinical features

There are four stages to syphilis as detailed below:

- Primary – this involves a painless chancre (hard ulcerating papule) on the genitalia and painless regional lymphadenopathy, which resolve spontaneously over weeks to months. The incubation period is on average 21 days but can be up to 3 months.
- Secondary – occurs about 2 months after the primary stage. It consists of a flu-like illness of pyrexia, malaise, pharyngitis, lymphadenopathy and arthralgia. A maculopapular non-itchy rash may also be present. Condylomata lata (wart-like lesions) on the perineum (see Fig. 21.2) and 'snail track' ulcers in the oropharnyx and on the genitalia are classical features of secondary syphilis. Some cases may also suffer with aseptic meningitis.
- Latent – this phase may last for many years.

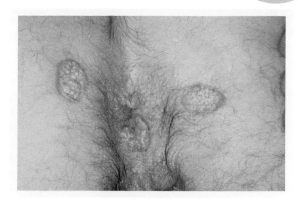

Fig. 21.2 Condylomata lata.
Source: Conlon & Snydman, 2000: Fig. 10.31b.

- Tertiary – involves many body systems. The classic granulomatous lesions known as gummas can occur in the skin, particularly at sites of trauma; in bones with a predilection for the skull, tibia, fibula and clavicle bones; and in viscera especially the liver. The cardiovascular aspects involve aortitis, aortic regurgitation and aortic aneurysms. Neurosyphilis can present as aseptic meningitis, meningitis with cranial nerve palsies, tabes dorsalis (demyelination of dorsal roots leading to lower motor neuron (LMN) signs) and general paralysis of the insane, which is dementia combined with upper motor neuron (UMN) signs. The cardiovascular and neurological features are sometimes referred to as quaternary syphilis.

The differential diagnosis of secondary syphilis includes HIV seroconversion, EBV (Epstein–Barr virus) infection, i.e. glandular fever, and CMV (cytomegalovirus) infection.

Investigations

In vitro culture of *Treponema pallidum* is not possible, so diagnosis relies on clinical signs and serology. Dark-ground microscopy of tissue from chancres, condylomata lata or oropharyngeal ulcers may reveal the organism but it is difficult and not always available. There are a number of serological tests for syphilis, including VDRL (Venereal Disease Research Laboratory), TPHA (*Treponema pallidum* haemagglutination assay) and FTA (fluorescent treponema antibodies). A useful screening test now is the syphilis

Fig. 21.3 Syphilis serology results at each stage of the disease

	VDRL	TPHA	FTA
Primary syphilis	– early, + later (after 3–4 weeks)	±	±
Secondary syphilis	+	+	+
Latent syphilis	–	+	+
Tertiary syphilis	±	+	+
Treated syphilis	–	+	+

ELISA (enzyme-linked immunosorbent assay) to look for IgG and IgM; positive samples are then subjected to the tests shown in Figure 21.3.

False-positive VDRL results occur with EBV, VZV (varicella zoster virus, i.e. chickenpox), measles, mycoplasma infections, pneumococcal pneumonia, tuberculosis, leprosy, malaria, hepatitis, cirrhosis, subacute bacterial endocarditis (SBE), SLE (systemic lupus erythematosus) and pregnancy.

Treatment

Penicillin is given for all stages of syphilis, with the length of course and the preparation of penicillin chosen depending on the stage. Third-generation cephalosporins, such as ceftriaxone, are increasingly used. Tetracyclines, usually doxycycline, are used if the patient is allergic to penicillin. Sexual abstinence until the treatment is completed and the partner is assessed for infection and treated if necessary helps to prevent immediate reinfection.

Prevention

Condom usage reduces sexual transmission rates. Contact tracing, investigation and treatment of partners decrease the disease burden in the population and reinfection between partners. Antenatal screening is used to reduce vertical transmission.

Chlamydia

Chlamydia trachomatis of serotypes D–K are the causative organisms. It is of note that serotypes L1–3 cause lymphogranuloma venereum (see Ch. 8).

Transmission

Chlamydia is acquired sexually or vertically at birth.

Epidemiology

Chlamydia is the most common STI in the UK. There were over 103 000 cases diagnosed in 2004. There has been a steady rise in the number of cases of chlamydia since 1990 with the greatest proportion of infections occurring in London and the North-west of England. Young adults less than 25 years of age are at the highest risk of contracting chlamydia.

Clinical features

Many chlamydial infections are asymptomatic in both males (up to 50%) and females (up to 70%). Both sexes suffer with urethritis if there are symptoms, with cervicitis in addition in females, and proctitis can occur after anal intercourse.

Complications

In men the infection can lead to prostatitis and epididymitis, whereas women can get PID and bartholinitis. PID may result in infertility. Both sexes can suffer with Reiter's syndrome following a chlamydia infection.

Investigations

Direct detection of chlamydia from swabs of the urethra, and cervix in women, is the usual method of confirming the diagnosis. Growth from cell culture is not routinely available.

Treatment

Tetracycline or erythromycin is used for the treatment of chlamydia. Sexual abstinence is advised until treatment is completed and the sexual partner is assessed and treated as necessary.

Prevention

Condom usage is recommended as prophylaxis. Contact tracing, investigation and treatment of partners lessen the spread of chlamydia. Antenatal screening is used to reduce vertical transmission. The National Chlamydia Screening Programme in England began in September 2002.

Chancroid

Chancroid is caused by *Haemophilus ducreyii*, Gram-negative bacilli.

Transmission

Chancroid is acquired sexually.

Epidemiology

Chancroid is more commonly found in tropical regions but cases are seen in temperature climes. In general there are fewer than 100 cases reported annually in the UK, but recently there has been an outbreak of chancroid.

Clinical features

Initially a pustule forms that erodes to reveal an ulcer with a ragged margin. These genital ulcers can appear necrotic. There tend to be multiple ulcers, but single ulcers can occur. The ulcers are deep and very painful and there is associated tender lymphadenopathy.

Chancroid does not give rise to oral ulceration as can occur with genital herpes or secondary syphilis (see Fig. 8.1).

Investigations

The diagnosis is often made as a matter of exclusion, when other causes of genital ulceration have been ruled out. *Haemophilus ducreyii* can be isolated from culture of ulcer tissue or swabs. PCR, where available, is used for diagnosis.

Treatment

Macrolides, e.g. erythromycin or azithromycin; the third-generation cephalosporin, ceftriaxone; ciprofloxacin, co-trimoxazole and co-amoxiclav are all effective in the treatment of chancroid. Sexual abstinence until the sexual partner is assessed and treated, as necessary, is recommended as part of the treatment strategy.

Prevention

Barrier contraception, e.g. condoms, is important in reducing transmission of the infection. Contact tracing, investigation and treatment of partners helps to prevent further spread of infection.

FUNGAL CAUSES

Candida

Candida albicans is a yeast.

Transmission

Candida can be acquired sexually but may result from an alteration of the usual flora of the genital tract. The flora is altered by antibiotic therapy, the oral contraceptive pill (OCP), pregnancy and steroid therapy.

Epidemiology

The number of confirmed genital candida infections has increased over the decade 1990–2000. The highest rates of candida infection are reported in London and the eastern regions. There are now more than 65 000 cases per year in the UK.

Clinical features

Candida presents with pruritus and a curdy discharge in females known as vaginal candidiasis, but may be asymptomatic. Males may develop balanitis.

Investigations

Microscopy and culture of any discharge can identify *Candida albicans*.

Treatment

Most infections resolve with clotrimoxazole cream or pessary in females; more severe infections may require oral fluconazole. It is advised to abstain from sexual intercourse until the treatment is completed and the sexual partner has been assessed to prevent immediate reinfection.

Prevention

Condom usage protects against infection. Contact tracing, investigation and treatment of partners are important to reduce population infection rates.

VIRAL CAUSES

Genital herpes

Genital herpes is most commonly caused by herpes simplex virus 2 (HSV-2), although genital contact with oral lesions due to herpes simplex virus 1 (HSV-1) can lead to genital herpes.

Transmission

Most transmission of HSV-2 is sexual but vertical transfer occurs at birth as a result of asymptomatic viral shedding. The risk of the neonate contracting HSV is greatly increased if the mother has an active infection at the time of delivery.

Epidemiology

The highest rates of HSV infection occur in 20- to 24-year-olds, with females affected more than males. The number of genital HSV infections had been rising annually from 1998 but there has been a reversal of this trend in 2003 and 2004, when just over 19 000 cases were reported. The oral–genital route is becoming increasingly important in the transmission of HSV, as the proportion of new cases of genital herpes due to HSV-1, typically associated with oral herpes, is on the increase.

Clinical features

Genital herpes presents with shallow painful ulcers on the genitalia (see Fig. 21.4), which may coalesce, and associated painful regional lymphadenopathy. The ulcers heal over 10–14 days but the virus remains latent in the dorsal ganglia and can reactivate. Patients describe a tingling sensation that precedes the ulcer lesions. When reactivation occurs it leads to recurrent lesions: genital cold sores. Women may present with urinary retention with a primary attack. Infection can be associated with fever, headache and myalgia.

Neonatal HSV infection can result in encephalitis, meningoencephalitis, conjunctivitis and widespread visceral disease. Although treatment with aciclovir reduces the mortality, this remains significant and hence mothers known to have active genital herpes should have a caesarean section.

Investigations

Vesicular fluid or ulcer swabs can be taken for virus identification by culture or PCR.

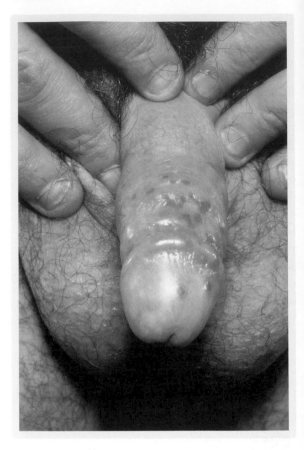

Fig. 21.4 Genital herpes.
Source: Conlon & Snydman, 2000: Fig. 10.35.

Treatment

Genital herpes is treated with aciclovir. Symptomatic relief for the ulcers comes from soaking in warm, salty water. Sexual abstinence is imperative whenever lesions are present, or the tingling sensation indicating imminent presentation, as condoms may not cover all areas affected with ulcers.

Prevention

This involves condom usage for sexual intercourse and contact tracing from known cases with investigation and treatment as appropriate. Antenatal screening is important for preventing vertical transmission.

Genital warts

Genital warts are caused by the human papillomavirus, particularly types 6 and 11.

Transmission

Genital warts can be acquired either sexually or vertically at birth.

Epidemiology

Genital warts are the most prevalent viral STI in the UK. Cases are concentrated amongst those aged less than 24 years, and the highest rates are seen in London. There has been a steady rise in the number of infections since 1995, with nearly 80 000 cases diagnosed in 2004.

Clinical features

The female patient presents with warts on her external genitalia and on the cervix. Males have warts on the urethra, at the meatus and along the penile shaft (see Fig. 21.5). Both sexes may have anal and perineal warts.

Investigations

Usually the warts can be identified clinically but if the diagnosis is in doubt then a biopsy can be taken and cultured.

Treatment

The warts are treated with topical podophyllin, or topical imiquimod, but if they are extensive may require cryotherapy or laser treatment.

Complications

There is an increased risk of cervical carcinoma, and anal tract cancers in those practising anal intercourse.

Prevention

Condom usage is necessary for up to 8 months after treatment to prevent spread. Contact tracing, investigation and treatment of partners are also important for reducing infection rates.

HIV

See Chapter 25.

Hepatitis B and C

See Chapter 19.

PROTOZOAL CAUSES

Trichomoniasis

The causative organism is *Trichomonas vaginalis*.

Transmission

Trichomonas is acquired sexually.

Epidemiology

Trichomonas vaginalis is one of the most common STIs worldwide, with an estimated 167 million cases per year. There have been relatively constant rates of infection in males and females over the last 10 years.

Clinical features

In females, trichomonas infection presents with vaginitis and a foul-smelling discharge. In males it is

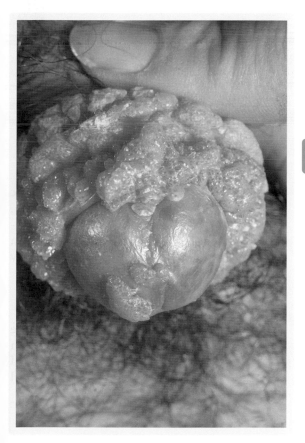

Fig. 21.5 Genital warts.
Source: Conlon & Snydman, 2000: Fig. 10.37.

usually asymptomatic, otherwise they complain of urethritis.

Investigations

Microscopy of a wet film of the discharge to look for motile trichomonads is diagnostic. The discharge can also be cultured to identify the organism.

Treatment

Metronidazole is the treatment of choice. Abstaining from sexual intercourse is recommended until treatment is completed and the sexual partner has been assessed and treated if necessary.

Prevention

Condom usage helps prevent transmission. Contact tracing, investigation and treatment of partners aims to reduce reinfection and population infection rates. This is particularly important given that the majority of infections in males are asymptomatic.

Sexually transmitted infections are summarized in Figure 21.6.

Further reading

Donovan B. Sexually transmissible infections other than HIV. Lancet 2004; 363:545–556.

Health Protection Agency. HIV and STI annual report 2004. Website: www.hpa.org.uk/infections/topics_az/hiv_and_sti/publications/annual2004/annual2004.htm.

LaMontagne DS, Fenton KA, Randall S, et al. on behalf of the National Chlamydia Screening Steering Group. Establishing the National Chlamydia Screening Programme in England: results from the first full year of screening. Sex Transm Infect 2004; 80:335–341.

Kimberlin DW, Rouse DJ. Genital herpes. N Engl J Med 2004; 350:1970–1977.

Fig. 21.6 Summary of sexually transmitted infections

	Symptoms in males	Symptoms in females	Diagnosis	Treatment	Complications
Gonorrhoea (*Neisseria gonorrhoeae*)	Urethritis, urethral discharge. Pharyngitis, proctitis. May have fevers and sweats	Dysuria, vaginal discharge. Pharyngitis, proctitis. May have fevers and sweats	Microscopy and culture of discharge. Blood and aspirated joint fluid for microscopy and culture	Third-generation cephalosporin ceftriaxone, or quinolones, e.g. ciprofloxacin	Prostatitis, epididymo-orchitis, PID, infertility, bartholinitis, septicaemia, septic arthritis, pustular skin rash, neonatal conjunctivitis, Reiter's syndrome
Non-gonococcal urethritis (e.g. *Chlamydia trachomatis, Ureaplasma urealyticum*, bacteroides, mycoplasma)	Dysuria, urethral discharge, penile discomfort	Urethritis, cervicitis	Microscopy and culture of discharge. High vaginal swabs	Tetracyclines, e.g. doxycycline, or macrolides, e.g. erythromycin	Reiter's syndrome
Syphilis (*Treponema pallidum*)	First – chancre; second – flu-like illness with lymphadenopathy, maculopapular rash, condylomata lata, 'snail track' ulcers, aseptic meningitis; latent phase; third – gummas, aortic complications, neurosyphilis, tabes dorsalis, general paralysis of the insane		Serology, syphilis ELISA. Dark-ground microscopy of tissue, e.g. from condylomata lata	All stages – penicillin (or doxycycline if penicillin allergic), third-generation cephalosporins, e.g. ceftriaxone	Aortic complications: aortitis, aortic valve incompetence, aortic aneurysms. Neurosyphilis: meningitis ± cranial nerve palsies
Chlamydia (*Chlamydia trachomatis*, serotypes D–K)	Urethritis. Proctitis	Urethritis and cervicitis. Proctitis	Urethral and cervical swabs for microscopy and culture	Tetracycline or erythromycin	Prostatitis, epididymitis, PID, infertility, bartholinitis, Reiter's syndrome
Candida (*Candida albicans*)	Balanitis	Pruritus and curdy vaginal discharge	Microscopy and culture of discharge	Clotrimoxazole cream ± pessary. Oral fluconazole	
Genital warts (human papillomavirus, usually types 6 and 11)	Warts on urethra, at meatus and along penile shaft	Warts on external genitalia and cervix	Clinical diagnosis usually; if in doubt biopsy for culture	Topical podophyllin. Cryotherapy or laser treatment	Cervical carcinoma and anal tract cancers (if anal intercourse practised)
Trichomoniasis (*Trichomonas vaginalis*)	Urethritis	Vaginitis, foul-smelling discharge	Microscopy of wet film of discharge. Culture of discharge	Metronidazole	
Genital ulcers	See Figure 8.1				

Skin, joint and bone infections

SKIN

Although skin infections are generally noted for their aesthetic insult, some infections such as necrotizing fasciitis are in fact life-threatening. The appearance of a skin infection is the mainstay of diagnosing its aetiology. Rashes are also often due to systemic infections manifesting on the skin, and these are covered in Chapter 14.

Bacterial infections

Cellulitis

Cellulitis is an infection of the dermis and sub-cutaneous tissues.

Organisms

The most common causes are *Streptococcus pyogenes* (group A beta-haemolytic streptococcus) and *Staphylococcus aureus*, including methicillin-resistant *Staph. aureus* (MRSA).

Aetiology

Strep. pyogenes and *Staph. aureus* are frequent commensals on the skin and only cause infection once the skin barrier has been breached. The portal of entry can result from trauma, ulceration of the skin, an insect or animal bite, intravenous drug abuse or an athlete's foot infection which creates cracks between the toes. Certain patients are particularly at risk of developing cellulitis, such as those with diabetes mellitus. Not only does a raised blood glucose level contribute to an increased risk of infection but the complications of diabetes such as peripheral neuro-

pathy, peripheral vascular disease and an increased body mass index (BMI) also render the patient more liable to cellulitis. Any disorder which results in these complications predisposes the patient to cellulitis. A peripheral neuropathy means that the patient has an impaired ability to feel any trauma that could lead to a skin abrasion or ulceration and then underestimates the damage. Peripheral vascular disease indicates a diminished blood flow to the peripheries which can result in ulceration and hinders the healing process. An obese person, as determined by a BMI over 30, can develop pressure ulcers on weight-bearing areas and may have skin folds that can rub against each other to rawness and are moist, which helps the growth of bacteria. These people are also typically unable to view the under surface of their feet to check for damage. Chronic lymphoedema is another risk factor.

> BMI (body mass index) is calculated by the weight in kilograms divided by the height in metres squared, e.g. someone who weighs 56 kg and is 1.6 m tall has a BMI of 22. There are four categories for BMI: 15–20 is underweight; 20–25 is normal; 25–30 is overweight; and > 30 indicates morbid obesity.

Clinical features

Cellulitis presents with an erythematous, hot, swollen, tender area of skin (see Fig. 9.1). The affected area is usually in close proximity to or surrounding the site where the skin integrity was breached. In cases of lower leg cellulitis the web spaces between the toes should be specifically inspected to look for athlete's foot (tinea pedis, see below). Note that cellulitis has a less clear border to the erythema than erysipelas (see below). In some cases an abscess may be present at the site of cellulitis. This is more common where the cellulitis is secondary to a puncture wound, e.g. trauma or from injecting illicit drugs. The regional draining lymph nodes become enlarged in reaction to the infection. The lymphadenopathy is typically mildly tender. Some patients feel systemically unwell with cellulitis, experiencing a fever, sweats and rigors, probably due to bacterial toxins.

Investigations

It is difficult to make an aetiological diagnosis in most cases of cellulites. Skin swabs do not predict the cause of deeper infection and are confounded by the fact that most skin is colonized with a variety of bacteria. For this reason skin biopsies (really only performed for research studies) and purulent material discharging or aspirated from an abscess are preferable samples because of their higher yield of positive results and the relevance of organisms isolated. Blood cultures are sometimes positive in those who are systemically unwell. As with any bacterial infection there will be a neutrophilia and raised CRP on routine blood testing.

Treatment

An oral course of antibiotics is often appropriate for a limited area of cellulitis. However, if the patient is diabetic, systemically unwell or there is an ulcer present, then intravenous antibiotics should be administered. Flucloxacillin provides good cover for both streptococci and methicillin-sensitive *Staph. aureus* and is the treatment of choice for community-acquired cellulitis. Clindamycin or clarithromycin can be used in patients allergic to penicillin. Diabetic patients and those with an ulcer have an increased likelihood of anaerobic organisms and Gram-negative bacilli being present, so the addition of metronidazole may be considered, along with a broadening of antibiotic cover. If the patient is known to have MRSA or is at high risk, e.g. previous prolonged hospital admission, then vancomycin would be more appropriate than flucloxacillin.

In addition to antibiotics there are practical measures to assist in the management of cellulitis. Any limb affected with cellulitis should be elevated. Ulcerated areas require specialist dressings and tissue viability specialist nurses should be involved. If the ulcers weep a significant amount of serous fluid, then daily soaking in permanganate solution can help in drying out the area. Abscesses may require surgical incision and drainage if they are too large for aspiration and do not discharge spontaneously. A surgical opinion should be sought if this is considered appropriate and necessary. Patients with cellulites are at increased risk of venous thrombosis, so prophylactic heparin should be used.

> An ulcer with a significant amount of necrotic tissue will often heal more rapidly once the necrotic tissue is removed. One effective method of achieving this is using maggots to eat away the dead flesh; this is known as 'biotherapy'. NB: maggots do not eat viable tissue!

Erysipelas

Erysipelas is a more superficial infection than cellulitis, affecting the epidermis and dermis.

Organism

Streptococcus pyogenes (group A beta-haemolytic streptococcus) is almost always responsible for causing erysipelas.

Aetiology

Erysipelas predominantly occurs in children, the elderly and immunocompromised patients.

Clinical features

Erysipelas typically affects the face, occurring particularly across the cheeks and periorbitally (see Fig. 22.1). The erythema is clearly demarcated with a slightly raised edge and there may be some blistering. It is more rapidly progressive than cellulitis. There is associated regional lymphadenopathy. Often patients feel unwell with a fever and develop a headache and vomiting secondary to circulating streptococcal toxins.

Investigations

The causative *Strep. pyogenes* may be isolated from blood cultures but the infection is more likely to be confirmed serologically with an ASOT (antistreptolysin O titre). Skin swabs of erysipelas are generally unhelpful.

Treatment

Erysipelas is treated with penicillin or, if the patient is allergic to penicillin, clindamycin or a macrolide such

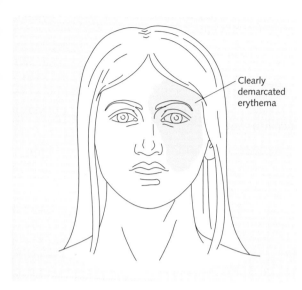

Fig. 22.1 Erysipelas.

Clearly demarcated erythema

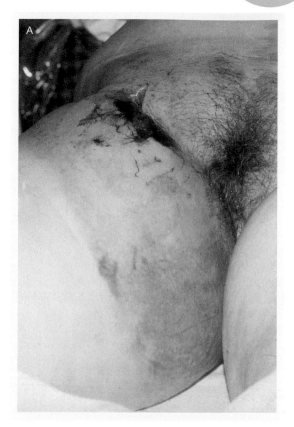

as clarithromycin. Usually an oral course of antibiotics is adequate.

Necrotizing fasciitis

Necrotizing fasciitis is a life-threatening progressive infection in which the organisms penetrate from the skin through the subcutaneous tissues into the deep fascia, and may include muscle.

Organism

Necrotizing fasciitis is most commonly due to *Streptococcus pyogenes*, group A beta-haemolytic streptococcus, but other groups of beta-haemolytic streptococcus can rarely be responsible, e.g. groups C and G. There is often synergistic anaerobic infection.

Pathogenesis

Some streptococci are able to produce enzyme exotoxins such as streptokinase and hyaluronidase. These enzymes are capable of breaking down fibrin and hyaluronic acid in connective tissue respectively, which facilitates the dispersion of the streptococci through the deep tissues. Necrotizing fasciitis may follow a surgical procedure, when the organisms have already gained access to the deeper structures during surgery.

Clinical features

Necrotizing fasciitis manifests as a rapidly progressing cellulitis with necrosis and, unlike cellulitis, severe pain. The affected area can develop blisters and have a

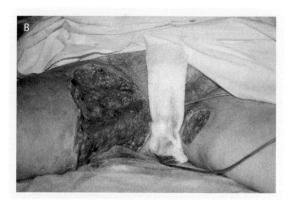

Fig. 22.2 Necrotizing fasciitis: (A) necrotic wound following coronary angiography with subcutaneous necrosis in thigh appearing as bruising; (B) same patient showing extent of debridement of necrotic tissue at operation.
Source: Conlon CP, Snydman DR. Mosby's Colour Atlas and Text of Infectious Diseases. Edinburgh: Mosby; 2000: Fig. 11.12.

dusky appearance (see Fig. 22.2). The patient is usually systemically unwell and suffers with high fevers and rigors but may appear relatively well initially.

Investigations

Plain radiographs of the affected area may show gas in the tissues, while CT or MRI scanning may be more definitive. Microscopy and culture of purulent material and biopsies of involved tissue can isolate the responsible group of beta-haemolytic streptococci. Frozen sections taken at surgery or by biopsy may help. Blood cultures may be positive.

Treatment

The essential management is urgent surgical debridement, possibly with amputation, as antibiotics alone will be ineffectual. Postoperatively it is important to monitor the proximal wound to check for signs of continued infection in case the debridement was not extensive enough and further surgery is required. Antibiotic therapy should be broad spectrum to cover the streptococci and anaerobes; there are theoretical reasons for using clindamycin as it inhibits protein synthesis and may limit the production of streptococcal toxins.

Complications

The major concern with necrotizing fasciitis is the high mortality rate.

Extreme pain associated with cellulitis raises the differential diagnoses of necrotizing fasciitis or clostridial gas gangrene. Both cases require urgent surgical debridement, possibly including an amputation, as antibiotics alone will be insufficient.

Clostridial gas gangrene

Clostridial gas gangrene is a severe infection involving the muscles.

Organism

Clostridial gas gangrene is usually caused by *Clostridium perfringens*, Gram-positive bacilli. Occasionally other clostridial species may be responsible.

Aetiology

Clostridial gas gangrene typically occurs in open fracture wounds or surgical wounds where there is residual dead tissue, especially if there is foreign material present. Since *C. perfringens* is a strict anaerobe, patients with peripheral vascular disease and diabetes mellitus are at an increased risk

because these conditions impair blood flow to the peripheries, hence creating more anaerobic conditions. Nowadays it is rarely seen outside of developing countries.

Pathogenesis

C. perfringens produces an alpha-toxin, which is a phospholipase, and other enzymes that cause the tissue destruction as well as haemolysis and shock. Gas production by the bacteria results in crepitus of the tissues.

Clinical features

Clostridial gas gangrene should be suspected if there is extreme pain experienced over the affected wound. The skin becomes thickened and oedematous with watery blebs, which discharge fluid and later become haemorrhagic. The muscles around the wound go through a step-wise transformation from pale and oedematous through beefy red to dark and black. If a limb is involved then the part distal to the infection becomes cold and pulseless as blood flow is lost. Crepitus, evocatively described as 'cornflakes under cling film', is a late feature. The patient is systemically septic with fever, tachycardia, hypotension and subsequently reduced urine output.

Investigations

C. perfringens can be isolated from tissue and blood cultures. However, the diagnosis of clostridial gas gangrene is essentially made clinically because identifying *C. perfringens* in the wound does not necessarily indicate gas gangrene since the organism could just be a wound contaminant. Detection of the alpha-toxin, by the Naegler reaction, would confirm the diagnosis. A plain radiograph of the affected area might reveal free gas in the tissues.

Treatment

Surgical debridement of the affected tissue, and possibly amputation depending on the severity and extent, is the crucial management. This should not be delayed unnecessarily. In addition, antibiotic therapy with penicillin and metronidazole, to cover other anaerobic organisms, should be administered. The role of antitoxin is not clear cut.

Complications

The septic shock which results from a clostridium gas gangrene infection may cause the development of renal failure and hepatic failure. Without rapid surgery to remove the infected tissue, there is a significant risk of death.

Prevention

All amputation procedures, especially if being performed for peripheral vascular disease, should be covered with prophylactic penicillin antibiotics to prevent the development of clostridium gas gangrene.

Fungal infections

Tinea infections

Tinea infections are superficial, affecting the keratinized epithelium. They can affect any area of skin as well as hair and nails.

Organisms

Tinea infections are caused by the filamentous fungi dermatophytes, which include *Epidermophyton floccosum*, *Trichophyton* species and *Microsporum* species.

Transmission

The dermatophytes are spread either by direct contact or via fomites, e.g. sharing hairbrushes and towels. The infections occur worldwide, although different age groups are more prone to different types of tinea infections. For example, tinea capitis is most common in children, whereas older people are more likely to have tinea unguium.

Clinical features

The common name for tinea infections is ringworm. The pattern that makes this name apt is most apparent when the infection occurs on the body. The different sites affected and their presentations are detailed below:

- Tinea corporis – occurs on the body. It manifests with an irregular circle of erythema which clears from the centre, hence giving the 'ringworm' name (see Fig. 22.3). The lesions are itchy and the erythema is raised and scaling. Pustules may occasionally be seen at the periphery of the lesion.
- Tinea capitis – occurs on the scalp. A spectrum of disease can arise: from a mild diffuse scaling with minimal hair loss through to circular scaling lesions with associated alopecia (hair loss) and broken hairs (see Fig. 22.4), and then the most severe form, a 'kerion', which is a raised lesion that discharges purulent material associated with severe alopecia.
- Tinea cruris – occurs in the groins. The lesions are similar to those seen with tinea corporis but the erythema appears more like plaques, although there may be some central clearing. As with tinea corporis a few pustules may be seen.

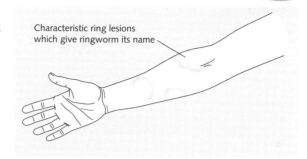

Characteristic ring lesions which give ringworm its name

Fig. 22.3 Tinea corporis.

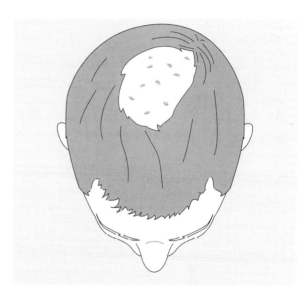

Fig. 22.4 Tinea capitis.

- Tinea pedis – occurs between the toes, and is known as athlete's foot. There is a scaly erythema with fissuring of the skin. Note that rings of erythema are rare.
- Tinea unguium – occurs in the nails. There is usually an asymmetrical distribution of nails affected. The nails have a white or yellow discoloration and become thickened. Loose material may collect under the nails.

The current level of tinea capitis in children, especially those with an Afro-Caribbean hair type, has been reported to be close to reaching epidemic proportions in the London area.

Investigations

The particular species causing the tinea infection can be identified from microscopy and culture of skin scrapings, nail clippings or the loose material, or hair roots. The samples taken depend on which areas are affected.

Treatment

Most tinea infections affecting the skin will resolve with topical clotrimoxazole or terbinafine. Oral preparations of terbinafine or itraconazole may be required for more extensive infections or for nail infections, since the nails are a much more difficult site for the antifungal drugs to penetrate. Terbinafine has proved best in clinical trials.

Candidiasis

Candidiasis is a common infection of the keratinized epidermis of the skin and may involve the nails.

Organism

Candidiasis is usually caused by the yeast *Candida albicans*, although other *Candida* species may be implicated in some settings.

Aetiology

Candida albicans is part of the body's normal flora, particularly found as a commensal of the gastrointestinal tract. As a superficial skin infection, *Candida albicans* tends to occur opportunistically in moist areas such as the groins, especially with nappy-wearing babies, and between skin folds in obese individuals. Diabetes mellitus is a risk factor for candidiasis.

Clinical features

Candidiasis presents as erythematous lesions in moist skin areas, e.g. axillae, groins, and as intertrigo. Vesicles and pustules may be seen at the edges of the erythema. *C. albicans* can affect nails, mimicking tinea unguium.

Investigations

Candidal skin infections are usually diagnosed clinically and this is confirmed with microscopy and culture of skin scrapings.

Treatment

Candidiasis usually responds to topical treatment with clotrimoxazole cream. Very extensive skin involvement or nail infections may require oral itraconazole.

Pityriasis versicolor

Pityriasis versicolor is an infection of the epithelium that has a varying appearance depending on the natural colouring of the patient's skin.

Organism

Pityriasis versicolor is caused by *Malassezia furfur*, a dimorphic fungus.

Aetiology

Pityriasis versicolor usually affects young adults. It is found worldwide but is more common in the tropics. The causative organism is a part of the normal human flora.

Clinical features

In pale-skinned people the infection appears as red/brown scaly macules, whereas dark-skinned people develop hypopigmented areas. Pityriasis versicolor particularly tends to affect the upper part of the trunk.

Investigations

Skin scrapings from the lesions viewed under Wood's light fluoresce yellow and this is characteristic for Pityriasis versicolor.

Treatment

Pityriasis versicolor is treated by washing the area with selenium shampoo and leaving it on for 30 minutes as well as using topical imidazole cream. If the infection persists, then oral itraconazole can be used. Note that a return to normal pigmentation takes months to occur, even with successful treatment.

JOINTS

Septic arthritis

Septic arthritis describes an infection of the joint and synovial fluid.

Organisms

Septic arthritis can be caused by a number of different bacteria, and certain individuals are more susceptible to particular infections, as shown in Figure 22.5.

Pathophysiology

Septic arthritis results from either direct bacterial invasion from overlying cellulitis or osteomyelitis locally; or from haematological spread from bacteraemia. It can occasionally occur following surgery performed on the joint e.g. total hip replacement.

Clinical features

Septic arthritis presents with a hot, swollen, tender joint. There is usually an associated reduced range of movement, both active and passive, due to the pain. Note that a tuberculous septic arthritis presents as a

Fig. 22.5 Bacterial causes of septic arthritis and high-risk groups for each infection

Bacteria	High-risk groups
Staphylococcus aureus	Vast majority of cases, since commensal of the skin and common cause of cellulitis
Streptococcus pyogenes	Patients vulnerable to cellulitis
Haemophilus influenzae type b	Children less than 5 years old; patients without a normally functioning spleen, e.g. after surgical removal, sickle cell anaemia. Now rare
Streptococcus pneumoniae	Splenectomized patients or hyposplenism
Salmonella enteritidis	Sickle cell disease
Mycobacterium tuberculosis	Immunosuppressed patients; TB elsewhere in the body
Neisseria gonorrhoea	Sexually active individuals

cold joint not a hot one (see Ch. 26). Some patients will have a fever and may feel systemically unwell; this is more likely with a septic arthritis due to haematogenous spread.

Investigation

Confirmation of a clinical suspicion of septic arthritis is by joint aspiration. If the synovial fluid is purulent then there is little doubt of the diagnosis. Microscopy and culture are required for isolation of the causative organism, and are important for determining the diagnosis if the synovial fluid appears clear. Blood cultures may be positive for the organism responsible; this is more likely when the septic arthritis results from haematogenous seeding.

Treatment

Broad-spectrum antibiotics are required until the causative organism is identified and antibiotic sensitivities are known. The empirical therapy recommended for septic arthritis is flucloxacillin, or if the patient is allergic to penicillin, clindamycin. If the patient is known to have MRSA or is at high risk, e.g. recent prolonged hospital admission, then vancomycin should be used. Severe infections with synovial articular fluid may also require a surgical washout procedure in addition to antibiotics for resolution. In the case of a prosthetic joint infection, this usually needs removal. Prosthetic surfaces enable bacteria to persist despite antibiotics. These infections are complicated and require specialist input.

Complications

It is crucially important to diagnose a case of septic arthritis promptly because synovium and cartilage can be rapidly damaged, leading to the risk of osteomyelitis and arthritis.

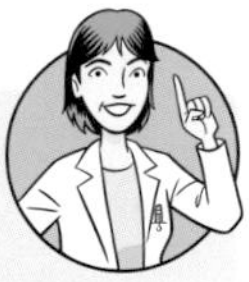

Because of the importance of the hand and the anatomy of the tendon sheaths, hand infections should be promptly referred to a hand surgeon to ensure a good functional result.

BONE

Osteomyelitis

Osteomyelitis is an infection of the bone itself rather than just a joint. It can occur as an acute infection secondary to cellulitis or bacteraemia; or as a chronic infection due to a deep-seated infection local to the bone involved, particularly if there is a prosthetic joint involved.

Organisms

The organisms that are responsible for causing osteomyelitis are slightly different, depending on whether the infection is acute or chronic, as detailed in Figure 22.6.

Aetiology

The high-risk groups identified for particular organisms causing septic arthritis are the same for osteomyelitis. Again *Staph. aureus* causes the vast majority of acute cases of osteomyelitis and to a lesser extent the chronic cases. Open wounds following trauma that involve fractures or penetrate down to bone, are liable to lead to bony infection, which in the short-term may be due to *Clostridium perfringens* or in the longer-term *Pseudomonas aeruginosa* or coliforms. Ear infections,

Fig. 22.6 Bacterial causes of acute and chronic osteomyelitis

Acute osteomyelitis	Chronic osteomyelitis
Staphylococcus aureus	*Staphylococcus aureus*
Streptococcus species	*Streptococcus* species
Clostridium perfringens	*Pseudomonas aeruginosa*
Haemophilus influenzae type b	Coliforms
Salmonella enteritidis	*Salmonella enteritidis*
	Mycobacterium tuberculosis
	Bacteroides

such as chronic otitis media, and chronic sinusitis can lead to chronic osteomyelitis, usually due to one of the species of streptococci or bacteroides.

Broadly speaking, haematogenous spread of organisms to bone is more common in children, when the growing ends of long bones tend to be affected, whereas direct spread into bone from skin ulceration is more likely in older patients. Those who are prone to ulceration of the feet and lower limbs, e.g. due to diabetes mellitus or any other cause of peripheral vascular disease or peripheral sensory neuropathy, are at high risk of osteomyelitis. This occurs because the ulcers are slow to heal and can extend down to bone allowing direct infection with the organisms causing the superficial cellulitis and infecting the ulcers.

Clinical features

Osteomyelitis is often not apparent initially from clinical inspection (see Fig. 22.7A). The suspicion should be raised if ulceration associated with cellulitis is found to extend deeply down to bone, or the skin infection is slow to resolve on appropriate antibiotic therapy. However, the affected bone may be painful and, if it is in the lower limbs, the patient may be reluctant to weight-bear. In diabetics with foot ulcers, studies have shown that if a sterile probe is inserted through the base of the ulcer and hits bone, this is highly predictive of underlying osteomyelitis. Fever may be present.

Investigations

Plain radiographs of the affected area can demonstrate osteomyelitis: loss of integrity of the periosteum and vacuolation of the bone are features (see Fig. 22.7B). It is important to appreciate, however, that the changes

seen on radiographs may lag 1–2 weeks behind the clinical picture. MRI (magnetic resonance imaging) is useful in the further assessment of possible cases of osteomyelitis. In order to identify the organism causing the osteomyelitis, blood cultures are required and cultures of bone biopsies taken during any operative procedures.

Treatment

A more prolonged course of intravenous antibiotics is required for osteomyelitis than for other soft tissue infections, often up to 6 weeks, and some cases require further periods of oral antibiotics. Flucloxacillin is the first-line empirical treatment for osteomyelitis until cultures are available, with vancomycin used if there is a risk of MRSA. Clindamycin is used for penicillin-allergic patients. Once a causative organism has been identified and the antibiotic sensitivities elucidated, the therapy should be adjusted accordingly. Surgical debridement of the affected bone is more commonly required with chronic osteomyelitis than with acute cases.

Skin, joint and bone infections are summarized in Figure 22.8.

Further reading

Cavanagh PR, Lipsky BA, Bradbury AW, Botek G. Treatment for diabetic foot ulcers. Lancet 2005; 366:1725–1735.

Lew DP, Waldvogel FA. Current concepts: osteomyelitis. N Engl J Med 1997; 336:999–1007.

Torok E, Conlon CP. Skin and soft tissue infections. Medicine 2005; 33:84–88.

Zimmerli W, Trampuz A, Ochsner PE. Current concepts: prosthetic-joint infections. N Engl J Med 2004; 351:1645–1654.

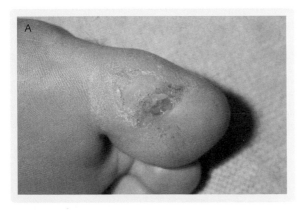
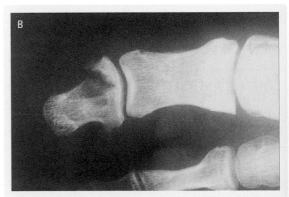

Fig. 22.7 Osteomyelitis: (A) ulcer on toe; (B) plain radiograph. *Source:* Conlon & Snydman, 2000: Fig. 12.17.

Fig. 22.8 Summary of skin, joint and bone infections

Skin infections					
Infection	**Site**	**Clinical features**	**Diagnosis**	**Treatment**	**Complications**
Cellulitis (*Streptococcus pyogenes*; *Staphylococcus aureus*)	Dermis, subcutaneous tissues	Erythematous, hot, swollen, tender area of skin ± abscess. Less clear border of erythema. Tender lymphadenopathy. Fever, rigors, sweats	Discharge, abscess aspirate or skin biopsy for microscopy and culture. Blood cultures	Flucloxacillin (clarithromycin or clindamycin if penicillin allergic). Vancomycin for MRSA	Venous thrombosis
Erysipelas (*Streptococcus pyogenes*)	Epidermis, dermis	Clearly demarcated erythema ± blistering, usually affecting the face. Tender lymphadenopathy. Fever, nausea, vomiting	ASOT. Blood cultures	Penicillin (clindamycin or macrolide, e.g. erythromycin if penicillin allergic)	
Necrotizing fasciitis (*Streptococcus pyogenes*)	Subcutaneous tissues, deep fascia and muscle	Rapidly progressive cellulitis with blisters and necrosis, severe pain. High fevers and rigors	Pus, tissue biopsies and blood for culture. Plain radiographs, MRI and CT scans of limbs	Urgent surgical debridement ± amputation. Clindamycin	Death
Clostridial gas gangrene (*Clostridium perfringens*)	Open fracture wounds or surgical wounds	Extreme pain over wound. Blistering of skin, necrosis of muscles. Crepitus. Septic shock	Tissue and blood cultures with alpha toxin detection. Plain radiographs	Urgent surgical debridement ± amputation. Penicillin with metronidazole. Antitoxin	Septic shock, renal failure, hepatic failure and death
Tinea infections (*Epidermophyton floccosum*, *Trichophyton* species and *Microsporum* species)	Keratinized epithelium, i.e. skin, hair and nails	Tinea corporis: 'ringworm' erythema, pustules. Tinea capitis: scaling lesions, alopecia, 'kerion'. Tinea cruris: erythema plaques, pustules. Tinea pedis: scaling erythema, fissuring. Tinea unguium: thickened, yellow nails	Microscopy and culture of skin scrapings, nail clippings or hair roots	Topical clotrimoxazole or terbinafine. Oral terbinafine or itraconazole	
Candidiasis (*Candida albicans*)	Keratinized epidermis of skin, nails	Erythematous lesions in moist skin areas. Vesicles and pustules. Thickened, yellow nails	Microscopy and culture of skin scrapings	Topical clotrimoxazole. Oral itraconazole	
Pityriasis versicolor (*Malassezia furfur*)	Epidermis	Red/brown scaly macules on pale skin and hypopigmented areas on dark skin	Skin scrapings fluoresce yellow in Wood's light	Selenium shampoo and topical imidazole cream. Oral itraconazole	Delayed return to normal pigmentation

(continued)

Fig. 22.8 Summary of skin, joint and bone infections—*continued*

		Joint and bone infections			
Infection	Site	Clinical features	Diagnosis	Treatment	Complications
Septic arthritis	Joint and synovial fluid	Hot, swollen, tender joint with reduced range of movement. Fever	Joint aspiration for microscopy and culture. Blood cultures	Empirical flucloxacillin (clindamycin if penicillin allergic). Surgical washout of joint	Osteoarthritis, osteomyelitis
Osteomyelitis	Bone	Suspect if deep ulceration penetrating to bone or slow to resolve. Pain, inability to weight-bear. Fever	Plain radiographs and MRI scan. Bone biopsies and blood for cultures	Empirical flucloxacillin (clindamycin if penicillin allergic) for prolonged intravenous course. Surgical debridement	Non-resolution

Endocarditis and pericarditis

Objectives

In this chapter you will learn:

- Which groups of patients are susceptible to develop infective endocarditis
- How to investigate a suspected case of infective endocarditis
- The issues for the management of infective endocarditis
- How to investigate a suspected case of pericarditis.

ENDOCARDITIS

Endocarditis is an infection of the heart valves or endocardial surfaces. Of the three layers of tissue that form the heart, the endocardium is the innermost one and is continuous with the heart valves. Infective endocarditis is a significant infection with approximately 3.3 cases per 100 000 population in the UK.

Aetiology

Endocarditis predominantly affects congenitally abnormal valves or damaged valves. The most common cause for the latter used to be rheumatic valvular disease. As described in Chapter 14, the mitral valve is involved in rheumatic valvular disease far more frequently than any other, followed by the aortic valve. Now infection is more likely to occur on degenerative valves: 60–80% of all cases of infective endocarditis occur in middle-aged to elderly patients with a cardiac lesion, most commonly affecting the mitral valve. Endocarditis more commonly affects the valves on the left side of the heart, except in intravenous drug users (IVDUs) when the tricuspid valve is usually affected. This occurs because bacteria showering into the bloodstream from an infection at a venepuncture site will arrive via the inferior vena cava at the right atrium and the first valve they encounter is the tricuspid valve.

Endocarditis may affect native valves or prosthetic valves. Prosthetic valve endocarditis may be early (in the first 60 days after surgery) or late. Prosthetic valves are particularly susceptible to infection, as bacteria are difficult to remove once adherent to the surface. 2% of patients who have a prosthetic valve will develop infective endocarditis at some stage, and prosthetic valve endocarditis accounts for 20% of all cases, with the aortic valve most commonly affected.

In general, less virulent bacteria are needed to cause endocarditis on rheumatic valves, prosthetic valves or congenitally abnormal valves, e.g. bicuspid aortic valve, whereas more virulent bacteria, such as Staph. aureus, are able to infect normal valves. Endocarditis arises on the heart valve following a bacteraemia. Although endocarditis may follow dental procedures, most cases do not follow a recognized initiating event. The bacteria tend to adhere to any fibrin or thrombus on the heart valves and create a 'vegetation'. Further fibrin and platelets are deposited so that the bacteria are protected from the immune system and antibiotics, and are able to reproduce further.

Organisms

Numerous organisms can cause endocarditis, both bacteria and fungi, as shown in Figure 23.1. Some of the bacteria are notoriously difficult to isolate from blood cultures and the diagnosis is only made from serology.

In the UK the three most common causes of endocarditis are Streptococcus viridans (an alpha-haemolytic streptococcus), Enterococcus faecalis and Staphylococcus aureus. Strep. viridans is responsible for approximately 50% of cases. Very rarely the oral Gram-negative bacteria, known collectively as the 'HACEK' bacteria, can cause endocarditis.

The usual sites for these organisms to be part of the normal body flora indicate which procedures are liable to result in them causing endocarditis, as shown in Figure 23.2.

Fig. 23.1 Causative organisms for endocarditis

Culture positive	Culture negative	Rare causes
Streptococcus viridans	Coxiella burnetii	**H**aemophilus aphrophilus
Enterococci, e.g.	Chlamydia psittaci	**A**ctinobacillus
Enterococcus faecalis	Chlamydia trachomatis	actinomycetemcomitans
Staphylococcus aureus	Brucella species	**C**ardiobacterium hominis
Staphylococcus epidermidis	Bartonella henselae	**E**ikenella corrodens
Candida albicans		**K**ingella kingae

Fig. 23.2 Sites of origin for organisms causing endocarditis and procedures likely to initiate the bacteraemia

Organism	Site as commensal	Precipitant procedure
Streptococcus viridans	Oral cavity and upper respiratory tract	Dental work/cleaning
Streptococcus faecalis	Perineum, gastrointestinal tract	Gastrointestinal or genitourinary tract instrumentation, surgery or infections
Staphylococcus aureus	Skin	Cellulitis, abscesses, secondary to intravenous cannulas and in IVDUs
Staphylococcus epidermidis	Skin	Secondary to intravenous cannulas and in IVDUs; post-prosthetic valve surgery
Candida albicans	Skin, oral cavity and gastrointestinal tract	IVDU
Chlamydia trachomatis	Perineum	Genitourinary tract instrumentation or surgery

Brucella species are acquired mostly from ingestion of unpasteurized dairy produce. *Coxiella burnetii* and *Chlamydia psittaci* are zoonoses that may infect humans through contact with animal excreta. *Bartonella henselae* is another, more recently identified cause of endocarditis. These last three organisms are not easily cultured and should be considered if a patient has clinical features suggesting endocarditis but negative blood cultures.

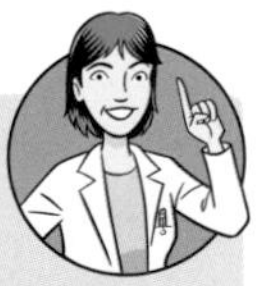

Non-infective causes of endocarditis are marantic endocarditis (metastatic-related); SLE (systemic lupus erythematosus)-related, known as Libman–Sacks syndrome; and Loeffler's endocarditis (endocardial fibrosis associated with eosinophilia).

Clinical features

Endocarditis can present acutely or as a more insidious infection, seen typically when the infection is caused by less virulent organisms. The patient initially tends to present with non-specific symptoms such as fever, malaise, anorexia, weight loss and night sweats. If the vegetations impede the normal functioning of the valve or destroy part of the valve, then a valvular incompetence murmur will develop or the character of an existing murmur will change, which should be detectable clinically. Cases of endocarditis with a more insidious presentation are more likely to develop vasculitic features. These include splinter haemorrhages in the nails, Roth spots on the retina (retinal vasculitis), Janeway lesions (erythematous macules) on the palms, Osler's nodes (tender nodules in the finger pulps and on toes) and microscopic haematuria. Fragments of the vegetations can break off causing emboli to lodge in the capillaries of the systemic circulation from left-sided valvular involvement, e.g. causing a stroke, renal or splenic abscess (see Fig. 23.3), or lodge in the pulmonary circulation from right-sided valvular lesions, e.g. causing lung abscesses. Sometimes the embolic sequelae are in fact the presenting feature. Clubbing can develop after a prolonged infection, so is usually only seen late in subacute cases. Mild splenomegaly is often a feature of endocarditis.

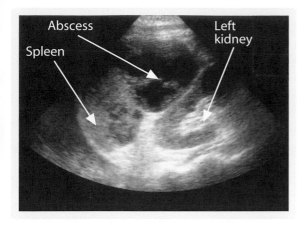

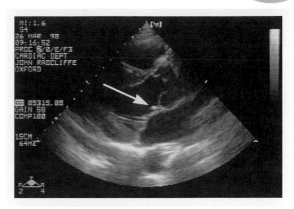

Fig. 23.4 Vegetation on echocardiogram.
Source: Conlon & Snydman, 2000: Fig. 5.10.

Fig. 23.3 Ultrasound of splenic abscess.
Source: Conlon CP, Snydman DR. Mosby's Colour Atlas and
Text of Infectious Diseases. Edinburgh: Mosby; 2000: Fig. 5.8.

> Any patient who presents with a fever and a new murmur has infective endocarditis until proved otherwise. In those cases it is imperative to take multiple sets of blood cultures (minimally three sets), separated either in time or place, before any antibiotic therapy is started.

Investigations

Positive blood cultures and echocardiography findings consistent with endocarditis are the mainstay of the diagnosis of endocarditis. Ideally there should be at least three sets of blood cultures taken from different locations and taken at different times before any antibiotic therapy is started. This maximizes the chances of isolating the causative organism. As mentioned above, some organisms are difficult to grow from blood cultures, and serology for these should be sent if initial blood cultures are negative. It is also important to check the antibiotic sensitivities of the causative organism isolated to ensure the appropriate therapy is given. Initially, a transthoracic echocardiogram (TTE) should be performed looking for vegetations (see Fig. 23.4), abscesses, valvular incompetence or paravalvular leak and dehiscence of a heart valve. The quality of the images from the TTE may not allow the operator to exclude a diagnosis of endocarditis, particularly in obese patients. A transoesophageal echocardiogram (TOE) should be considered, as this is much more sensitive for diagnosis.

On routine blood testing, patients with endocarditis will have raised inflammatory markers, CRP (C-reactive protein) and ESR (erythrocyte sedimentation rate), in addition to a leucocytosis, usually a neutrophilia. The other changes seen on the full blood count are a normochromic-normocytic anaemia, either secondary to splenomegaly or anaemia of chronic disease, and thrombocytopenia. The renal function of the patient may deteriorate, with vasculitic involvement or septic emboli to the kidneys. Mild liver function impairment is not uncommon. Microscopy of the urine will reveal haematuria if there is a renal vasculitis.

The Duke criteria

The diagnosis of infective endocarditis is facilitated by using the Duke criteria. A definitive diagnosis of endocarditis requires two major criteria, or one major and three minor criteria, or five minor criteria to be met.

Major criteria:
- Echocardiography findings of vegetations, abscesses, dehiscence of a heart valve or new valvular regurgitation
- Typical organism in two separate sets of blood cultures, or persistently positive blood cultures taken more than 12 hours apart in three or the majority of four or more sets.

Minor criteria:
- Predisposing cardiac condition, e.g. prosthetic heart valve, congenital valve abnormality
- Temperature > 38 °C
- Vasculitic features, e.g. major emboli or mycotic aneurysm
- Immunological criteria, e.g. glomerulonephritis

- Blood culture results not meeting the major criteria
- Echocardiography findings not meeting the major criteria.

Treatment

The initial empirical treatment of infective endocarditis should cover the three most common organisms: ampicillin for streptococci (*Strep. viridans, Enterococcus faecalis*) and flucloxacillin for *Staph. aureus* (also covers *Staph. epidermidis*) in addition to gentamicin, which has a synergistic action against the Gram-positive organisms and will hold the Gram-negative ones until culture results are available. Vancomycin is used in patients who are allergic to penicillin or who are at high risk of MRSA (methicillin-resistant *Staph. aureus*). Amphotericin or fluconazole is used for endocarditis due to *Candida albicans*. The *Chlamydia* species and *Coxiella burnetii* are best treated with tetracycline. Once the specific organism has been isolated and the sensitivities checked, the antibiotic therapy can be tailored appropriately. Intravenous antibiotic therapy is usually given for four weeks at least.

Valvular repair surgery or valve replacement may be necessary if there is a failure of medical management with appropriate antibiotic therapy or destruction of the affected valve. Prosthetic valves usually need to be replaced, as the infection is difficult to eradicate from the artificial surfaces. Ideally the blood cultures should be sterile before a new prosthetic valve is placed but the clinical condition of the patient must be taken into account with regards to the timing of surgery.

Complications

Septic emboli arising from the vegetations can lodge anywhere in the relevant circulation, i.e. left-sided valvular lesions dispersing emboli into the systemic circulation and right-sided lesions into the pulmonary circulation. The effects of the emboli, such as a stroke, partial loss of vision or lung abscesses, can be apparent before the endocarditis is diagnosed, or subsequently. The major concerns with infective endocarditis are destruction of the affected valve, valvular incompetence leading to heart failure and death. The mortality from endocarditis is greatest in those with a prosthetic valve, when it can reach 35%. An abscess in the aortic root associated with aortic valve endocarditis can result in destruction of the conductive tissue and hence lead to first-degree heart block. For this reason, patients with aortic valve endocarditis should have daily electrocardiograms (ECGs) to monitor the PR interval.

Prophylaxis

Prophylactic antibiotics to cover risky procedures, such as dental work, are recommended for those patients known to have an increased susceptibility to developing endocarditis. The patients at highest risk are:

- Those with:
  - prosthetic valves
  - left-sided valvular disease
  - congenital cyanotic heart disease
  - ventricular septal defect
  - coarctation of the aorta
  - patent ductus arteriosus
- Those who have previously had endocarditis.

Patients with right-sided valvular disease, bicuspid aortic valve and mitral valve prolapse are deemed to be at intermediate risk of developing endocarditis. Patients are advised to inform their dentist and any other health professional who is to undertake a procedure so that a decision on whether antibiotic prophylaxis is required can be made. The antibiotics used are ampicillin or clindamycin, if the patient is allergic to penicillin. However, the role of antibiotic prophylaxis in this setting is increasingly controversial.

PERICARDITIS

Pericarditis is an inflammation of the outermost layer of the heart. This can arise secondary to infection, myocardial infarction, which may be part of Dressler's syndrome, uraemia or malignancy, such as Hodgkin's lymphoma, lung or breast carcinoma. In the UK the most common causes are Coxsackie viral pericarditis and pericarditis following a myocardial infarction. Autoimmune pericarditis also occurs relatively commonly. Only the infective aetiologies will be considered below.

Organisms

Pericarditis can be due to viral, bacterial and fungal infections.

- Viral infections:
  - Coxsackie A and B viruses (enterovirus family, RNA virus)
  - Echoviruses (enterovirus family, RNA virus)
  - Cytomegalovirus (CMV) (herpesvirus family, DNA virus)
  - Epstein Barr virus (EBV) (herpesvirus family, DNA virus).
- Bacterial infections:
  - *Staphylococcus aureus* (Gram-positive cocci)
  - *Streptococcus pneumoniae* (Gram-positive cocci)
  - *Mycobacterium tuberculosis* (acid-fast bacilli)
  - *Haemophilus influenzae* type b (Gram-negative bacilli)
  - Group A, B, C and G beta-haemolytic streptococci (Gram-positive cocci).
- Fungal infections (all rare):
  - *Histoplasma capsulatum* (dimorphic fungi)
  - *Aspergillus fumigatus* (filamentous fungi)
  - *Candida albicans* (yeast).

> The viral causes of pericarditis are also able to give rise to myocarditis, infection of the muscle of the heart. Myocarditis and pericarditis can coexist. Bacteria very rarely infect the myocardium.

Aetiology

Viral pericarditis tends to occur in young adults and is usually a self-limiting infection. Bacterial pericarditis can result from septicaemia, septic emboli from another source of infection or directly from pneumonia affecting the surrounding lung. Tuberculous pericarditis occurs as a post-primary infection, usually from haematogenous spread. Typically only immunocompromised patients develop fungal pericarditis.

Clinical features

Patients with acute pericarditis present with fevers and sharp pleuritic chest pain. Classically any movement, deep breathing and lying down make the pain worse, with some relief obtained from sitting forward. The patient may also become dyspnoeic. On examination there is a pericardial rub, which sounds like someone crunching up a crisp packet, and is best heard with the patient sitting forward. Once the patient develops a reactive pericardial effusion the rub is lost. A peri-cardial effusion makes the heart sounds quieter as they are muffled by the fluid. The pericardial fluid can restrict the heart pump function resulting in cardiac failure and hence a raised jugular venous pressure (JVP), pulmonary and peripheral oedema. In general patients with bacterial pericarditis are more systemically unwell than those with viral pericarditis and have a greater risk of cardiac tamponade. Tuberculous pericarditis is associated with other typical tuberculous symptoms, such as weight loss, night sweats and malaise, and may lead to constrictive pericarditis.

Investigations

The investigation of a suspected case of pericarditis involves confirming the diagnosis and elucidating the causative organism. The ECG has a specific pattern in pericarditis: there is widespread concave ST elevation, involving anterior, lateral and inferior leads (see Fig. 23.5). Subsequently T wave inversion develops in the same leads. The QRS complexes reduce in amplitude with a pericardial effusion. A chest radiograph may show an enlarged cardiac silhouette if there is a pericardial effusion present. Cardiac enzymes may be raised if there is a concomitant myocarditis.

In order to isolate the organism responsible a number of samples need to be sent to the microbiology laboratory. Blood cultures are taken to isolate bacterial and fungal causes; faecal samples and serology are used for viral identification. Ideally a pericardial tap will be performed to obtain pericardial fluid for microscopy and culture, including Ziehl–Neelsen and auramine staining for *M. tuberculosis* and viral culture. Any pericardial tissue obtained can also be cultured for *M. tuberculosis* to help confirm the diagnosis.

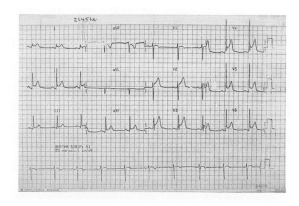

Fig. 23.5 Electrocardiogram showing changes of pericarditis. *Source:* Conlon & Snydman, 2000: Fig. 5.21.

Treatment

Antimicrobial therapy and non-steroidal anti-inflammatory drugs, e.g. aspirin, indometacin or naproxen, are required for pericarditis. Most viral infections do not require specific antiviral therapy, but immunocompromised patients at risk of CMV may benefit from treatment with ganciclovir. The antibiotic cover in case of a bacterial aetiology should be broad spectrum till the organism is identified. Tuberculous pericarditis requires quadruple antituberculous therapy, i.e. rifampicin, isoniazid, pyrazinamide and ethambutol. Steroids are given in combination with antibiotics instead of merely NSAIDs in severe or recurrent cases of bacterial and tuberculous pericarditis. Antifungal therapy is achieved using amphotericin.

Bacterial pericarditis usually requires pericardial drainage (pericardiocentesis) in addition to antibiotic therapy for resolution, whereas viral and fungal cases are less likely to need this. There is a high risk with tuberculous pericarditis of developing constrictive pericarditis, and hence a pericardectomy may need to be performed as a combined procedure with pericardial drainage. Steroids given with antituberculous therapy have been shown to reduce the risk of constriction. In cases of bacterial pericarditis where the pericardial fluid is purulent, then a pericardectomy is recommended.

Complications

A pericardial effusion can increase in size until it causes cardiac tamponade. It is essential this is recognized promptly and the pericardial fluid drained before the heart arrests. Cardiac tamponade is a cause of a pulseless electrical activity (PEA) arrest. Bacterial and tuberculous pericarditis can heal with fibrous tissue and calcification (see Fig. 23.6), thereby resulting in constrictive pericarditis and subsequently heart failure. There is also a significant mortality associated with pericarditis: even with antibiotic therapy and pericardial drainage the mortality of bacterial pericarditis, including tuberculous, is 2–20% and is almost 100% with no treatment at all.

Figure 23.7 summarizes endocarditis and pericarditis.

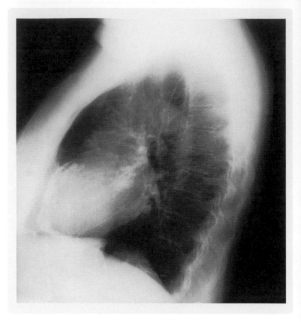

Fig. 23.6 Pericardial calcification in tuberculous pericarditis. *Source:* Conlon & Snydman, 2000: Fig. 5.23.

Cardiac tamponade is a medical emergency. The classical signs are a JVP that rises on inspiration as opposed to the normal fall, and a drop in the systolic blood pressure of > 10 mmHg on inspiration. A significant drop can be felt as the loss of a palpable pulse in inspiration, which returns on expiration. The treatment is urgent pericardiocentesis.

Further reading

British Cardiac Society. Updated guidelines produced in May 2004. Website: www.bcs.com.

British National Formulary. Current recommendations and dosing schedules. Website: www.bnf.com.

Prendergast BD. Diagnostic criteria and problems in infective endocarditis. Heart 2004; 90(6):611–613.

Simmons NA. Recommendations from the Working Party of the British Society of Antimicrobial Chemotherapy. J Antimicrob Chemother 1993; 31:437–438.

Fig. 23.7 Summary of endocarditis and pericarditis

	Organisms	Clinical features	Diagnosis	Treatment	Complications	Prophylaxis
Endocarditis	Bacteria, and rarely fungi	Fever, malaise, anorexia, weight loss, night sweats. New or changed cardiac murmur. Vasculitic features. Clubbing, mild splenomegaly	Multiple blood cultures, echocardiography. Duke criteria	Empirical: ampicillin, flucloxacillin and gentamicin. Prolonged intravenous course	From septic emboli, e.g. causing a stroke, renal or lung abscess. Heart failure, first-degree heart block. Mortality up to 35%	Prophylactic ampicillin (or clindamycin if penicillin allergic) for risky procedures, e.g. dental work in high-risk patients
Pericarditis	Viruses, bacteria, and rarely fungi	Fever, sharp pleuritic chest pain, dyspnoea. Pericardial rub	ECG. Blood and pericardial fluid for microscopy and culture. Faecal samples and serology for viral identification	Viral: NSAIDs, ganciclovir for some cases. Bacterial including TB: broad-spectrum antibiotics and steroids. Pericardiocentesis ± pericardectomy. Fungal: amphotericin and NSAIDs	Cardiac tamponade, constrictive pericarditis, heart failure. Significant mortality	None

Malaria and tropical infections

Objectives

In this chapter you will learn:

- The management of a suspected case of malaria
- The types of leishmaniasis
- The signs that are seen with a case of typhoid
- Who is at risk of brucellosis
- The clinical difference between the types of leprosy
- How a patient with dengue fever may present
- The areas of the body that are affected by schistosomiasis
- Which infections can give rise to elephantiasis.

Malaria

Malaria is responsible for a huge disease burden worldwide. The WHO (World Health Organization) states there are more than 300 million acute illnesses from malaria every year and at least 1 million deaths, of which 90% are in sub-Saharan Africa. Forty percent of the world's population live at risk from malaria, mostly within the poorest countries in tropical and subtropical regions. The WHO have made malaria one of their key targets, launching their Roll Back Malaria programme in October 1998 with the objective of halving the malaria burden in participating countries.

In returning travellers, the infection not to be missed is malaria, as it is life-threatening. It should always be top of the list of differential diagnoses in anyone returning from travelling outside Europe. Malaria is found in Africa, the Middle East, Asia, Central and South America. In the UK malaria is a notifiable disease so all cases must be reported to the Consultant in Communicable Disease Control (CCDC). Although malaria is not endemic in the UK, there are approximately 2000 cases per year from travellers returning from malaria-endemic regions.

Pathogenesis

Malaria is caused by the protozoan *Plasmodium*, of which there are four species: *P. falciparum*, *P. ovale*, *P. vivax* and *P. malariae*. The protozoan infects humans via the female *Anopheles* mosquito and must pass through both hosts to complete the life cycle. Sexual reproduction, known as gametogony, occurs in the mosquito, whereas asexual reproduction, known as schizogony, occurs in humans (Fig. 24.1).

- When the female *Anopheles* mosquito bites a human the sporozoites pass into the bloodstream and are carried to the liver.
- In the hepatocytes asexual reproduction occurs, taking up to 1 month, resulting in the release of merozoites into the bloodstream, which produces the first symptoms of fever.
- The merozoites infect red blood cells to further reproduce asexually, and each release of new merozoites creates the cyclical spikes in fever that characterize malaria. Some merozoites develop into gametocytes so that the human host becomes infectious to mosquitoes.
- When a human with gametocytes in the blood is bitten by a mosquito the gametocytes pass into the mosquito. They are carried to the mosquito's gut where sexual reproduction occurs to create sporozoites, which migrate to the salivary glands and are ready to be introduced into the next human bitten. The cycle thus continues.

P. vivax and *P. ovale* are able to produce sporozoites, called hypnozoites, that can remain dormant in the liver. Therefore these types of plasmodia are able to cause a malaria relapse years after the initial infection. *P. malariae* can remain dormant in the bloodstream.

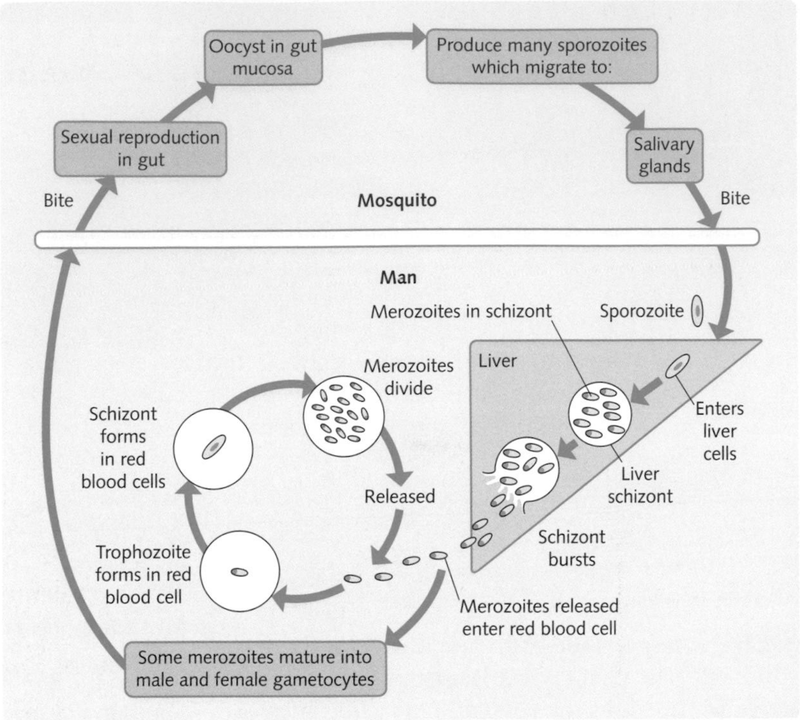

Fig. 24.1 *Plasmodium falciparum* life cycle.
Source: Elliott TS, Hastings M, Desselberger U. Lecture Notes on Medical Microbiology. Oxford: Blackwell Science; 1997: Fig. 21.2.

Fig. 24.2 Table differentiating the four types of plasmodia

	P. falciparum	P. ovale	P. vivax	P. malariae
Incubation	7–14 days	10–18 days	10–17 days	18–42 days
Fever cycle	36–48 hours	36–48 hours	36–48 hours	72 hours
Red cells infected	All, especially the young	Reticulocytes	Reticulocytes	Older cells
Dormancy site	None	Liver	Liver	Blood
Relapses after successful treatment	No	Yes	Yes	Yes
Mortality	20%	Very low	Very low	Very low

The superior ability of *P. falciparum* to infect red blood cells of all ages results in a higher parasitaemia (can be > 20%) than the other plasmodial species (less than 5%), and correlates with a higher morbidity and mortality. The non-falciparum species are collectively known as the benign malarias. Red blood cells infected with *P. falciparum* are more 'sticky' and have a tendency to occlude small blood vessels causing anoxic damage to the vital organs. In the brain this results in 'cerebral malaria'.

The features differentiating the four types of plasmodia are shown in Figure 24.2.

Clinical history

A comprehensive travel history is important for malaria, as the presentation can be up to 1 year after return, for example with *P. malariae*, or malaria due to *P. vivax* or *P. ovale* may have been acquired many years previously and relapse. Equally important is whether any malarial prophylaxis was taken and if so what drugs were used and how good was the compliance. Falciparum malaria is resistant to chloroquine in many parts of the world now, so chloroquine is no longer deemed adequate protection in those places. Some travellers suffer with side-effects from their malarial prophylaxis and might stop taking the drug during their visit. Symptoms of malaria may be suppressed if the person is still taking prophylaxis on their return.

It is not uncommon for adults from endemic areas to lose their immunity to malaria after living in non-endemic areas of the world for a few years. They may then return to their native country to visit friends and relatives and often assume they are still immune and, thus, not take antimalarial prophylaxis. They usually recognize the symptoms of malaria and are typically less ill than those who have never been immune.

Sickle cell anaemia, like other haemoglobinopathies such as thalassaemia, confers some protection against *P. falciparum* malaria, as the protozoa are unable to reproduce as effectively in these red blood cells, hence limiting the potential severity of the disease. Immunity to *P. vivax* also occurs in those who are blood group Duffy-negative, since their erythrocytes lack a receptor required for the binding of merozoites to red blood cells.

Patients describe periodic chills with rigors followed by high fevers associated with drenching sweats and vomiting. There may be a prodrome of headache, malaise, myalgia and anorexia before the fevers develop. Cerebral malaria can present with a variety of neurological symptoms including confusion, reduced consciousness, fits and abnormal movement of the eyes and limbs.

Examination

Although there are classically described fever patterns: tertian (every third day or 48 hours), e.g. with *P. vivax* or *P. ovale*; subtertian (every 36 hours), e.g. with *P. falciparum*; quartan (every fourth day), e.g. with *P. malariae*; these are in fact rare. Most patients have daily (quotidian) or irregular paroxysms of fever. Fevers up to 41°C may be recorded.

The patients are often anaemic because the infected red blood cells are destroyed as the merozoites are released, and this is most profound with *P. falciparum*. Patients may also be jaundiced as a result of the high rate of haemolysis. On abdominal examination it may be possible to palpate hepatosplenomegaly. Splenomegaly is a late sign in *P. falciparum* malaria but

can be massive with *P. malariae* because of the chronicity of the infection.

Cerebral malaria occurs sometimes with falciparum infections and is defined as unrousable coma in the absence of any other cause than malaria. Affected patients decline rapidly from a reduced conscious level to coma and death if untreated. Many patients suffer with fits. The neurological examination can elicit an upper motor neuron pattern with increased tone, hyperreflexia and up-going plantars but there may be other neurological signs, such as nystagmus or flaccid tone.

Investigations

Thin and thick films of blood examined under the microscope can detect the plasmodial parasites (see Fig. 11.3). With an experienced eye the different species can be determined. The vital aspect of seeing *P. falciparum* parasites on the film is to estimate the percentage parasitaemia: this correlates with the severity of the infection. It requires three sets of blood films from consecutive days to all be negative for malaria parasites before the patient would be confirmed as not having malaria.

A parasitaemia of greater than 2% with *P. falciparum* denotes severe malaria. The presence of a schizont on the blood film automatically means the malaria should be classed as severe because imminently the schizonts in the patient will release multiple merozoites and produce a high parasitaemia.

The full blood count will demonstrate the anaemia and thrombocytopenia; a leucocytosis is not a feature. The biochemistry results can show renal impairment and lactic acidosis with *P. falciparum*, and a raised bilirubin level and lactate dehydrogenase from the intravascular haemolysis. It is important to check the glucose level because not only does hypoglycaemia complicate *P. falciparum* malaria but it can also result from treatment with quinine. The urine should be dipsticked for blood, as haemoglobinuria can occur with *P. falciparum* malaria. An electrocardiogram is recommended before treatment with quinine, as it can induce conduction defects and arrhythmias. A lumbar puncture should be performed in cases of cerebral malaria to rule out bacterial meningitis.

Treatment

Quinine, orally or intravenously, is the gold standard treatment for *P. falciparum* malaria, or if the species is unknown or mixed. Quinine should be given for 7 days. However, quinine is poorly tolerated and is less effective in the Far East now. More recently, artemisinin derivatives combined with a second drug (artemisinin combination therapy: ACT) has been shown to be very effective and is being adopted by the WHO as the standard of care for falciparum malaria. If the patient is able to take medication orally then Riamet (artemether with lumefantrine) or Malarone (proguanil with atovaquone) are useful alternatives and usually better tolerated than quinine. Chloroquine is the drug of choice for the benign malarias as long as chloroquine has not been used for prophylaxis. Only a 3-day course is necessary. Malaria due to *P. vivax* or *P. ovale*, should be treated with a 2-week course of primaquine, after the chloroquine, to destroy the hypnozoites (dormant parasites) in the liver and thereby prevent subsequent relapses. It is important to check whether the patient is glucose-6-phosphate dehydrogenase (G6PD) deficient before use because primaquine can cause haemolysis in those patients.

Supportive care is essential in malaria, especially those cases due to *P. falciparum*. Paracetamol is a useful adjunct as an antipyretic agent. Fluid resuscitation is required for the dehydration that can result from insensible losses, such as fever and sweating, as well as vomiting. Severe anaemia may necessitate blood transfusions, and platelet replacement with pools may be required for profound thrombocytopenia. Cardiac monitoring should be undertaken and regular measuring of the blood glucose levels if the patient is receiving quinine therapy, especially if it is given intravenously. Patients with falciparum malaria, particularly cerebral malaria, may require looking after in the intensive care unit. If the renal impairment is severe, then renal replacement therapy, such as haemofiltration, may be essential. The role of exchange transfusion for severe malaria is controversial but it is often used if the parasitaemia is more than 25%.

Complications

P. falciparum malaria can be complicated by:

- CNS: cerebral malaria, including seizures
- Cardiovascular: septic shock; pulmonary oedema
- Respiratory: adult respiratory distress syndrome (ARDS)
- Renal: acute renal failure; blackwater fever (haemoglobinuria)
- Haematological: disseminated intravascular coagulation (DIC); severe anaemia and thrombocytopenia
- Metabolic: hypoglycaemia; lactic acidosis
- Hyperpyrexia.

P. malariae malaria can result in nephrotic syndrome due to chronic glomerulonephritis which can be fatal in young children.

Prophylaxis

The most effective way to prevent infection with malaria is to avoid getting bitten by mosquitoes. Anopheline mosquitoes particularly bite in the early evening, so this is an important time to keep well covered up and use insect repellent liberally. On a worldwide scale the use of bed nets to prevent bites whilst asleep is a highly effective measure. Funding has been directed to attempt to provide bed nets for everyone living in sub-Saharan Africa.

Traditionally chloroquine and proguanil in combination was the mainstay of malarial chemoprophylaxis but currently the levels of chloroquine resistance mean this is no longer adequate in most endemic areas. The drugs currently recommended are mefloquine, doxycycline or Malarone (proguanil with atovaquone). Anyone travelling to a malaria-endemic area should seek advice on the preferred drug for the region to which they are travelling, any potential side-effects and the correct regimen for taking the drug before departure. Important side-effects to be aware of related to these medications are neuropsychiatric reactions with mefloquine and sun sensitivity with doxycycline. Detailed information can be obtained from various websites, e.g. Centers for Disease Control and Prevention: www.cdc.gov/travel.

OTHER PROTOZOAN INFECTIONS

Leishmaniasis

Leishmaniasis is a devastating disease to contract as it can be disfiguring or life-threatening. Given the stigma associated with the disfigurement, leishmaniasis is vastly under-reported worldwide. The WHO estimates there are 12 million people infected worldwide, whilst 350 million people are threatened by the disease.

Organism

Leishmaniasis is caused by the protozoan *Leishmania*, of which there are numerous species, such as *L. donovani*, *L. aethiopica* and *L. braziliensis*.

Epidemiology

Leishmaniasis occurs in Africa, Central and South America, India, the Middle East and coastal regions in the Mediterranean, although the different species of *Leishmania* are only responsible for disease in certain areas, for example *L. aethiopica* is only found in east Africa and *L. braziliensis* in Central and South America.

Pathogenesis

The *Leishmania* protozoa are carried by female sandflies (Fig. 24.3).

Clinical features

The clinical manifestations of leishmaniasis depend on the species of *Leishmania* causing the infection and the host immune system.

Visceral leishmaniasis (also known as kala-azar) – usually due to *L. donovani* or *L. aethiopica*; it is not caused by 'New World' species.

Visceral leishmanias results from the lymphatic spread of the protozoa around the body with minimal if any skin lesions. Immunocompromised patients are most at risk of developing visceral

leishmaniasis. The skin is not totally unaffected, though, as it becomes hyperpigmented on the face, hands, feet and abdomen, hence the name kala-azar, which means black sickness. The patient tends to present with episodic fevers and associated rigors and sweats, substantial weight loss, malaise, anorexia and hepatosplenomegaly. The other features are more variable and are shown in Figure 24.4.

Visceral leishmaniasis can be transmitted via blood transfusions and, rarely, dirty needles.

Cutaneous leishmaniasis (localized or diffuse) – caused by most species of *Leishmania* but not *L. donovani*, *L. aethiopica* or *L. infantum*.

In the cutaneous form of the disease, lesions arise from the site of the sandfly bite. A papule develops at the bite site, which is itchy and progressively increases

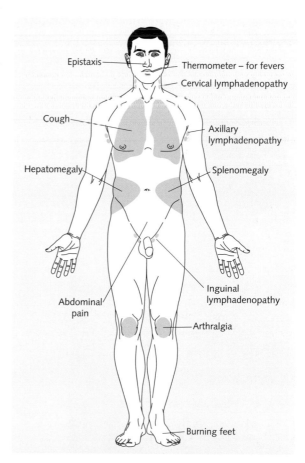

Fig. 24.3 *Leishmania* life cycle.

Fig. 24.4 Body map for features of visceral leishmaniasis.

in size. A crust subsequently develops and then falls off to reveal an ulcer with a raised border. The lesions heal with scarring and, depending on the site and extent of the affected area, are variably disfiguring. The healing process is slow, usually taking months to years, with some lesions healing spontaneously without treatment.

Mucocutaneous leishmaniasis (also known as espundia) – usually due to *L. braziliensis* (rarely to *L. panamensis* or *L. guyanensis*).

In mucocutaneous disease the initial skin lesions are generally on the lower limbs and heal in a similar pattern to the cutaneous form over a 6-month period. Years later the person then develops lesions involving the mucous membranes of the nose, mouth and throat and the surrounding tissue (Fig. 24.5). The affected areas ulcerate and are destroyed. As a result it is seriously disfiguring and renders the patient vulnerable to respiratory tract infections.

Investigations

The diagnosis can be confirmed by identifying the *Leishmania* protozoa with microscopy, histology (Wright's and Giemsa stains) or culture (specialized media required). In cutaneous disease the appropriate specimens are cutaneous scrapings of the margins of any ulcers, a punch biopsy along an active border of an ulcer or needle-aspirated material from nodular/papular lesions. In visceral leishmaniasis, lymph nodes, spleen or bone marrow can be examined to isolate the *Leishmania* protozoa. Serology can be used to confirm the diagnosis in mucocutaneous and visceral disease. PCR is now the best method to differentiate between species. The leishmanin skin test, a delayed hypersensitivity skin test, is of limited use since it is not positive in early cutaneous disease or at any stage in visceral leishmaniasis.

The full blood count in visceral leishmaniasis usually shows anaemia, neutropenia and thrombocytopenia, usually secondary to the hypersplenism.

Treatment

Cutaneous lesions can be surgically removed, or treated with local cryotherapy or topical paromomycin, especially when occurring in cosmetically sensitive areas. Those patients with a risk of mucosal disease (i.e. infected with *L. braziliensis*) should receive systemic treatment. Visceral leishmaniasis always requires systemic treatment. Intravenous stibogluconate remains the treatment of choice, although intravenous amphotericin B and pentamidine are used as alternatives or in resistant cases. Liposomal amphotericin B is very effective but also very expensive, and thus unaffordable in developing countries.

Prognosis

Untreated visceral leishmaniasis in developing countries is fatal within 2 years, often from secondary infections. There is a variable response of all types of leishmaniasis to treatment, and relapses are not uncommon.

Prevention

Since there is no vaccination or chemoprophylaxis available for leishmaniasis, the mainstay of prevention is to avoid sandfly bites. The sandflies tend to be most active in the evening and at night. Avoiding bites can be achieved by using insect repellent liberally and covering up with clothing as well as sleeping under impregnated bed nets.

Trypanosomiasis

Trypanosomiasis covers a number of diseases: the two forms of African sleeping sickness and Chagas' disease. The features of African sleeping sickness are shown in Figure 24.6.

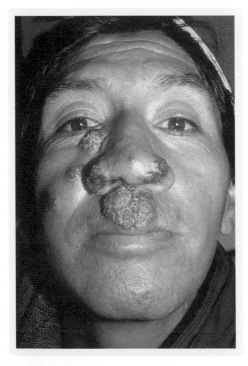

Fig. 24.5 Mucocutaneous leishmaniasis.

Fig. 24.6 Comparison of the types of African trypanosomiasis

Organism	*Trypanosoma brucei gambiense*	*Trypanosoma brucei rhodesiense*
Geography	West coast Africa	East coast Africa
Transmission	Tsetse fly (bite during the day)	
Clinical course	More indolent, over several years	Acute, over a few months
Clinical features:		
Stage 1 (time of bite)	Infrequent feature	Commonly have a 'trypanosoma chancre' at site of bite, which heals over a month
Stage 2 (weeks to months later)	Marked lymphadenopathy, especially of posterior cervical chain, known as 'Winterbottom's sign' (see Fig. 24.7). Hepatosplenomegaly present but other organs less commonly affected. Low-grade fever	Acute, swinging fever; myocarditis, purpura, haemolysis, hepatitis, hepatosplenomegaly, oedema, pleural and pericardial effusions and nephritis more common. Lymphadenopathy less marked
Stage 3 (later)	Prominent CNS features: meningoencephalitis, personality changes, focal neurological signs, especially extrapyramidal; progression from daytime somnolence to coma and death	CNS features not as severe or common
Severity	Mild	Severe, death within 1 year
Investigations	Organisms isolated from blood (thick and thin films), bone marrow and lymph node aspirates, CSF. Serology may be helpful	
Treatment	Most effective if started before CNS involvement Pre-CNS (since neither penetrates blood–brain barrier): suramin, pentamidine – *T. b. gambiense* only Post-CNS: melarsoprol, nitrofurazone, difluoromethylornithine	
Prevention	Insect repellents, clothing covering limbs, bed nets. Pentamidine has been used as prophylaxis but breeds resistant organisms	

Rhodesia was the former name for Zimbabwe, hence the organism responsible for the East African disease being named *Trypanosoma brucei rhodesiense*.

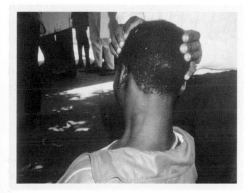

Fig. 24.7 Winterbottom's sign.

Chagas' disease (American trypanosomiasis)

Chagas' disease is the form of trypanosomiasis that occurs in Central and South America.

Organism

Chagas' disease is caused by *Trypanosoma cruzi*.

Transmission

Trypanosoma cruzi is transmitted via reduviid insects, which tend to bite at night-time. Chagas' disease can also be acquired from blood transfusions or transplacentally.

Clinical features

Initially a 'chagoma' develops at the site of the insect bite. This is an erythematous papule and there is often associated local lymphadenopathy. The chagoma and lymphadenopathy are self-limiting. If the bite happens to be to the eye, then orbital swelling and unilateral conjunctivitis occur; this is known as 'Romaña's sign'.

There are two patterns of presentation: acute, with an incubation period of 1–2 weeks, or chronic, which occurs many years later. The acute form of the disease is more common in children. The acute illness may be asymptomatic but the patient more usually has a fever, macular rash, truncal and facial oedema, lymphadenopathy and hepatosplenomegaly. Typically the illness is self-limiting, although patients can die as a result of myocarditis and fatal meningoencephalitis.

The chronic disease is usually asymptomatic. If not, there are cardiac features and may be gastrointestinal complications. The cardiac aspects include cardiomyopathies, arrhythmias, emboli, cardiac failure and sudden death. The gastrointestinal problems are megaoesophagus, dilated stomach and megacolon and their subsequent complications.

Diagnosis

The diagnosis can be made during the acute phase of the illness by isolating the organism from blood and biopsied tissue or by xenodiagnosis. In the chronic phase, serology is used to confirm a diagnosis of Chagas' disease.

Treatment

The current treatment for Chagas' disease is benzimidazole. Nifurtimox has been used previously.

Prevention

There is no vaccine or chemoprophylaxis for Chagas' disease. The best approach is preventing insect bites by using insect repellents and sleeping under a bed net. Vector control is important in avoiding outbreaks. All blood products should be screened to prevent transmission by this route.

Amoebiasis

See Chapters 18 and 19.

Giardiasis

Giardiasis is caused by the protozoan *Giardia lamblia*.

Epidemiology

Although giardiasis is found worldwide, it is more prevalent in the tropics and an important cause of diarrhoea in returning travellers. In Europe and North America there have been outbreaks associated with contaminated water supplies.

Transmission

Giardia is transmitted via the faecal–oral route. Cysts can also be ingested from contaminated water. Person-to-person transmission can occur within institutions.

Pathogenesis

The pathogenesis of *Giardia* is detailed in Figure 24.8.

Clinical features

Giardiasis presents with watery diarrhoea which can be explosive. There is associated mild abdominal pain and bloating. Some patients develop steatorrhoea and malabsorption. A more chronic diarrhoea can occur in HIV-positive patients.

Investigations

The *G. lamblia* protozoa can be identified from stool and duodenal aspirate cultures. The stool can also be inspected under the microscope for cysts and trophozoites.

Treatment

Metronidazole or tinidazole are effective treatments for giardiasis.

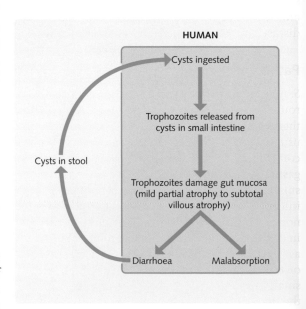

Fig. 24.8 *Giardia* life cycle and pathogenesis.

Prevention

Giardiasis can be prevented with good hygiene practices and ensuring clean water supplies.

BACTERIAL INFECTIONS

Typhoid and paratyphoid

Typhoid and paratyphoid are endemic in poorer regions of the world where sanitation is inadequate and clean drinking water supplies unreliable, especially in Asia, sub-Saharan Africa and South America. The WHO estimates there are 21.7 million cases of typhoid and 5.4 million cases of paratyphoid every year worldwide. Typhoid and paratyphoid are notifiable diseases which should be reported to the CCDC. They are not uncommon as a cause of fever in a returning traveller. There are approximately 150 cases of each reported in the UK; of the paratyphoid isolates, most are serotype A.

Organisms

Typhoid and paratyphoid are enteric fevers caused by the Gram-negative bacilli *Salmonella typhi* and *Salmonella paratyphi* (serotypes A, B and C – rare) respectively. The two organisms give rise to clinically indistinguishable illnesses, although paratyphoid is usually milder. Unlike *Salmonella enteritidis*, these salmonella species do not cause gastroenteritis, although diarrhoea can be a feature later in the disease.

Pathogenesis

S. typhi and *S. paratyphi* are spread via the faecal–oral route, with an infective dose that is proportional to the attack rate. Contaminated food and water are the usual sources although poor personal hygiene can contribute to infection. The bacilli can resist the gastric acid in the stomach and are absorbed via the small intestine. The resultant breaches in intestinal integrity can lead to secondary bacteraemias with non-typhi organisms. The bacilli reside and reproduce in the lymphatic tissue of the small intestine, known as Peyer's patches, and may be responsible for some of the abdominal signs and symptoms. From the small intestine the bacilli disseminate around the body via the bloodstream and lymphatics. The incubation period is 5–21 days.

Clinical features

Typhoid and paratyphoid have an insidious onset with headache being the prominent feature. There is then a classical weekly pattern:

- First:
  - step-wise rising fever with a relative bradycardia
  - associated dry cough, myalgia, arthralgia, anorexia, nausea and constipation (sometimes diarrhoea later on)
- Second (week of signs):
  - rose spots (erythematous maculopapular rash on trunk)
  - hepatosplenomegaly or splenomegaly
  - cervical lymphadenopathy
  - abdominal tenderness
- Third (week of complications):
  - lobar pneumonia
  - pericarditis
  - meningitis, cognitive impairment, polyneuropathy
  - acute cholecystitis
  - visceral abscesses
  - intestinal haemorrhage and perforation
  - urinary tract infection
  - osteomyelitis
    haemolytic anaemia
- Fourth (week of convalescence):
  - gradual recuperation over next weeks to months.

In general, paratyphoid results in a milder illness than typhoid.

Investigations

The diagnosis of either typhoid or paratyphoid is confirmed by isolating *S. typhi* or *S. paratyphi* respectively from cultures. The most appropriate cultures to take depend on the week of the illness and the symptoms experienced: blood cultures are most likely to be positive in the first to third weeks; urine cultures in the second week; stool cultures in the second to fourth weeks. Cultures of duodenal aspirates can sometimes identify the salmonella bacilli. Cultures of bone marrow can be extremely useful in diagnosing typhoid and paratyphoid because of their sensitivity and because the organism can be isolated for a prolonged period even after starting antibiotics, for example 98% of bone marrow cultures will be positive prior to antibiotics and 50%

will be positive after 5 days of a course of treatment. Since obtaining bone marrow specimens is an invasive procedure, this is usually reserved for cases where other cultures have been negative but there remains a significant clinical suspicion. The serological Widal test is no longer performed as the results are unreliable.

The full blood count shows a leucopenia (although a leucocytosis is more common in children) and anaemia. The liver function tests (LFTs) may be deranged with a hepatitic picture.

A 'typhoid hepatitis' can be distinguished from a 'viral hepatitis' by the presence of:

- Bradycardia
- Fever > 40°C
- Serum transaminases much lower than in a viral hepatitis.

Treatment

Traditionally typhoid and paratyphoid were treated with chloramphenicol, trimethoprim, co-trimoxazole or amoxicillin but resistance to these antibiotics has risen. In 1999 the UK Reference Laboratory found that 26% of strains were multidrug resistant. The first-line antibiotics are now the quinolones, such as ciprofloxacin and ofloxacin. However, there is an increase in quinolone-resistant typhoid now being imported to the UK. Third-generation cephalosporins, such as ceftriaxone, and the macrolide, azithromycin, are alternative treatments. A 2-week course of antibiotics is given. Steroid therapy given in addition to antibiotics can significantly reduce the mortality in severe cases. Relapse rates are lower with the newer drug regimens, only 1–6% of cases.

Chronic carriage

Following an infection of typhoid or paratyphoid the patient will excrete the salmonella bacilli in stool or urine for several weeks but some patients continue to have the bacilli detectable for more than 1 year after infection and are known as chronic carriers. This occurs in 1–3% of infections. Chronic carriage of the salmonella bacilli remains a problem because these patients are infectious to others. Chronic carriage is more common in women and those with biliary or urinary tract abnormalities. Eradication of chronic

carriage requires a prolonged course of quinolones, usually ciprofloxacin. Very rarely chronic carriage in the gall bladder necessitates a cholecystectomy.

Prognosis

The mortality of typhoid is 15–20% in untreated cases, which is reduced to 1% with appropriate antibiotic therapy.

Prevention

Typhoid and paratyphoid infection rates can be reduced by ensuring good basic hygiene practices, proper sewage disposal and access to clean drinking water. There is a vaccine available against the polysaccharide Vi (virulence) antigen of typhoid, which gives protection for 3 years. It is recommended for travellers to affected countries. A better conjugate vaccine is in clinical trials.

Brucellosis

Brucellosis is caused by intracellular Gram-negative coccobacilli of the genus *Brucella*, of which there are three species as shown in Figure 24.9.

Risk factors

Given that the reservoirs for *Brucella* are in domesticated animals, those who work closely with them are at risk, such as farmers and veterinary practitioners. The ingestion of unpasteurized milk from infected animals is also a source of disease.

Clinical features

The incubation period for brucellosis is 1–3 weeks and the disease can affect any organ system. The patient usually presents with the generalized symptoms of fever, malaise, myalgia, night sweats and weight loss. On examination there is hepatomegaly and, in severe infections, splenomegaly. Lymphadenopathy may occur. The patient can additionally have complications

Fig. 24.9 Comparison of *Brucella* species

Species	Animal reservoir	Geography
B. abortus	Cattle	Worldwide
B. melitensis	Goats, sheep	Mediterranean
B. suis	Pigs	Far East, USA

such as arthritis, osteomyelitis, meningoencephalitis, endocarditis and orchitis. Some patients can have a chronic form of the illness with episodes of fever, myalgia, malaise and depression over several months.

Diagnosis

The *Brucella* organisms can be isolated from prolonged incubation of blood cultures or bone marrow cultures. The diagnosis can also be confirmed using acute and convalescent serology.

Treatment

A combination of doxycycline and rifampicin is used for uncomplicated disease. Complicated infections are usually treated with doxycycline and parenteral aminoglycoside (either streptomycin or gentamicin). Co-trimoxazole can be used instead of doxycycline in children. Treatment needs to be for 3–6 weeks.

Prevention

Good personal hygiene is essential when handling animals, to prevent transmission, as is the pasteurization of milk before consumption.

Typhus

Typhus is a rickettsial infection, of which there are many varieties, but the main ones to note are:

- Epidemic typhus – *Rickettsia prowazekii* (louse-borne)
- Rocky Mountain spotted fever – *Rickettsia rickettsii* (tick-borne).

They are zoonoses: the principal hosts for *R. prowazekii* are humans and squirrels, whereas *R. rickettsii* is found in dogs and rodents. Each is transmitted via insects: lice and ticks respectively. Other types of typhus include murine typhus, tick typhus and scrub typhus. Epidemic typhus is found in Africa, Central and South America and Asia, whereas Rocky Mountain spotted fever is acquired only in North and South America. Typhus is a notifiable disease; therefore all cases need to be reported to the CCDC.

Pathogenesis

Rickettsiae are Gram-negative bacilli. They produce their multiorgan effects by invading the endothelial cells of small blood vessels, resulting in widespread vasculitis.

Clinical features

Epidemic typhus

After an incubation period of 2–21 days the patient presents with a sudden onset of high fever (> 39°C), headache, profound malaise and myalgia. Once raised, the temperature usually remains high. Conjunctivitis and orbital pain can accompany the headache. A generalized maculopapular rash develops 4–6 days following the onset of fever; the rash also involves the soles and palms, and progresses to become purpuric in nature. About a week into the illness the patient suffers with photophobia, neck stiffness, vomiting and deafness. The meningoencephalitic symptoms can progress to extrapyramidal symptoms, such as bradykinesia, tremor and chorea; or coma. Any organ can be affected by the vasculitis; see below. Patients may develop splenomegaly at the peak of their disease. By the third week of the illness, the patient begins to improve but the return to normal health is generally slow.

Rocky Mountain spotted fever (RMSF)

An eschar, which is an ulcerated lesion with a black scar, may develop at the site of the tick bite (see Fig. 24.10). Local lymphadenopathy usually occurs with an eschar. The symptoms are otherwise similar to those of epidemic typhus but there may be a shorter incubation period.

African tick typhus

This is the most common form of typhus imported to the UK. It usually presents with fever, headache and a rash, which is usually erythematous and macular but can be vesicular. There is often an eschar. The symptoms are much milder than in epidemic typhus or RMSF.

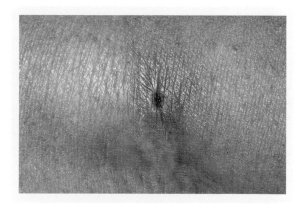

Fig. 24.10 Eschar at site of tick bite.
Source: Conlon CP, Snydman DR. Mosby's Colour Atlas and Text of Infectious Diseases. Edinburgh: Mosby; 2000: Fig. 15.39.

Investigations

The diagnosis is usually confirmed with acute and convalescent serology. The organisms are very difficult to culture. Skin biopsies can be used to diagnose Rocky Mountain spotted fever. Thrombocytopenia occurs in up to 50% of cases.

Complications

The complications of typhus can be severe and mostly result from widespread vasculitis. They include haemolysis, thrombocytopenia, disseminated intravascular coagulation (DIC), shock, respiratory failure, renal failure, myocarditis, stroke, reduced consciousness, coma and death. Thrombotic occlusion of distal extremities can lead to gangrene. The rickettsiae can remain dormant in lymph nodes for years and then cause recurrent illness; this recrudescence is known as Brill–Zinsser disease.

Treatment

All types of typhus are treated similarly with either tetracycline or chloramphenicol. Supportive treatment for the severe multisystem involvement is crucial. Blood products are required for DIC and haemorrhage resulting from thrombocytopenia. Adequate fluid replacement and maintenance for shock can be challenging to achieve and often necessitates invasive cardiac monitoring. Respiratory support with intubation and ventilation may be required for respiratory failure. Renal replacement therapy, e.g. with haemofiltration, may be necessary until the renal function improves.

Prevention

The mainstay of preventing typhus is avoidance of the arthropod vector bites with insect repellent and clothing. Short-term courses of doxycycline prophylactically can be useful for travellers to high-risk areas. An immunization to protect against *Rickettsia prowazekii* is available for high-risk groups.

Tuberculosis

See Chapter 26.

Leprosy (Hansen's disease)

Leprosy can be a very deforming and disabling condition and there is a strong stigma attached to it in endemic countries. Leprosy occurs in Africa, Asia,

India, North and South America and Southern Europe. It is an internationally notifiable disease. The WHO organized the World Health Assembly resolution which aimed to reduce the prevalence of leprosy to less than 1 case per 10 000 population in endemic countries by the year 2000, but by the end of 2005 intensive efforts were still needed to reach the leprosy elimination target in five countries: Brazil, India, Madagascar, Mozambique, and Nepal. The widespread implementation of multidrug therapy (MDT) under this resolution has meant that leprosy is no longer necessarily the devastating disease it once was.

> Since leprosy is spread by close contact, reducing the bacterial burden in a community should reduce the overall prevalence. Leprosy colonies were set up on this principle of isolating affected patients.

Organism

Leprosy is caused by *Mycobacterium leprae*.

Pathogenesis

The incubation for leprosy is long: 2–6 years, since *M. leprae* is very slow growing. The peripheral nerves and the skin of the extremities are most commonly involved because the mycobacterium prefers cooler conditions for growth. The clinical picture is dependent on the host immune response, as shown in Figure 24.11. For an unknown reason males are more susceptible than females to developing leprosy.

Clinical features

The skin lesions are hypopigmented, scaly, hairless, non-sweating and anaesthetic. The affected nerves are thickened and may be tender. The face including the eyes, the gluteal region and the extremities are the most frequently involved sites. The typical pattern is:

* Tuberculoid leprosy – patient usually has a single lesion with clearly demarcated edges, central healing and atrophy. The affected nerves are in the same area and may present as a nerve palsy.
* Lepromatous leprosy – the skin is usually involved first and there are numerous lesions present. These can be macules, papules, nodules or plaques. The nasal tissue is often involved, initially giving rhinitis but further damage can result in collapse

Fig. 24.11 Comparison of tuberculoid and lepromatous leprosy

Tuberculoid leprosy	Lepromatous leprosy
Good cell-mediated immunity	Poor cell-mediated immunity
More limited disease	More generalized disease
Few bacilli in lesions	Many bacilli in lesions
Less infectious	More infectious
Nerve damage occurs early	Nerve damage is a late feature

of the nasal bridge. The skin of the face can become indurated, which gives the classic 'leonine' appearance. The nerve involvement is typically later than with tuberculoid leprosy. Patients also develop a symmetrical 'glove and stocking' sensory neuropathy. This renders them vulnerable to injury and damage to the limbs. The eyes can be affected with an iritis.

There is also an intermediary form:

- Borderline leprosy – the patient has a variable number of skin lesions and nerve involvement is common.

Investigations

The diagnosis can usually be made clinically, which is especially important in low-resource environments. The acid-fast bacilli (AFBs) can be seen in skin or nasal mucosal smears but *M. leprae* does not grow on artificial culture. Culture is only possible on armadillo tail or mouse footpad tissue. Skin and nerve biopsies can histologically confirm a diagnosis of leprosy. PCR can also be used to detect *M. leprae*. Leprosy can give a false-positive result for rheumatoid factor.

Treatment

All cases of leprosy should be treated with MDT, consisting of dapsone and clofazimine daily with rifampicin given monthly. A monthly dose of clofazimine is added for lepromatous leprosy. The treatment course should be at least 2 years or until AFBs are no longer detectable. The drug therapy should be administered from a specialist centre that is additionally able to support the patient with physiotherapy and occupational therapy. Surgical input may be required for damaged limbs or to save sight if there is eye involvement.

If a new case of leprosy is diagnosed, it is important to examine close family contacts for any evidence of skin lesions.

Relapsing fever

Relapsing fever is particularly found in Africa, India, South America, the Middle East and Mediterranean Europe. It is a notifiable disease in the UK and therefore cases should be reported to the CCDC.

Organism

There are two main species of spirochaete that are responsible for causing relapsing fever: *Borrelia recurrentis* and *Borrelia duttoni*. *B. recurrentis* is louse-borne whereas *B. duttoni* is tick-borne.

Clinical features

The incubation period is 7–10 days for relapsing fever. The patient presents with a sudden onset of high fever, rigors, headache and myalgia. There may be a purpuric rash. The patient then tends to deteriorate with a reduced conscious level, haemorrhage and shock. Jaundice and hepatosplenomegaly are also features. Classically the patient starts to recover and then has a relapse of lessening severity. Relapsing fever due to *B. recurrentis* (louse-borne) usually has more frequent relapses with a shorter initial illness than the tick-borne relapsing fevers.

Diagnosis

The diagnosis of relapsing fever can be confirmed by identifying the spirochaetes from blood samples on microscopy.

Treatment

Tetracycline or erythromycin is the treatment of choice for relapsing fever.

The effect of killing large numbers of the spirochaetes following the first dose of antibiotics can precipitate a deterioration of the patient's clinical state to the point of requiring management in an intensive care unit. This is known as a 'Jarisch–Herxheimer reaction'.

Complications

Relapsing fever can be fatal.

Prevention

Louse-borne infections can be reduced by 'de-lousing' the patient; this involves washing the person's body, clothes and bedding with 1% Lysol. Tick-borne infections can be prevented with liberal use of insect repellent, including treating bed nets. Doxycycline can be used as prophylaxis.

Buruli ulcer

Buruli ulcers only occur in tropical regions, comprising Africa, Australasia and Central America.

Organism

A Buruli ulcer is caused by *Mycobacterium ulcerans*, which is an atypical or opportunistic mycobacterium.

Clinical features

M. ulcerans gives rise to superficial skin ulcers. These are self-limiting but heal with scarring.

Diagnosis

Microscopy of the necrotic tissue from the base of an ulcer can reveal the mycobacteria.

Treatment

Local excision of the ulcer is the only effective method for preventing scarring as the ulcer heals and the subsequent morbidity that arises. Usually skin grafting is required following the excision.

Complications

The scarring results in severe contractures and hence deformities and disability.

VIRAL INFECTIONS

Yellow fever

Yellow fever is found in a narrow equatorial area across Africa and South America. It is an internationally notifiable disease, with proof of vaccination required when entering a country from an endemic area.

Organism

Yellow fever is caused by a flavivirus. It is arthropod-borne by mosquitoes; different species are found in different regions, for example *Aedes africanus* in Africa, *Haemagogus* species in South America, and *Aedes aegypti* in urban areas. Mosquitoes remain infectious for life.

Clinical features

The incubation period of yellow fever is 3–6 days. A wide clinical spectrum of disease can occur, ranging from a mild flu-like illness to a severe form. The severe illness has three stages:

- First phase: acute onset of high fever and headache, retrobulbar pain, suffused conjunctivae, myalgia and arthralgia. There can be a relative bradycardia, like with typhoid, after the first day. Vomiting and epigastric pain indicate severe disease.
- Second phase: 'phase of calm'.
- Third phase: high fever, jaundice, hepatomegaly and haemorrhagic features, such as ecchymosis, bleeding gums, haematemesis and melaena.

Diagnosis

The flavivirus can be isolated from blood in the first 3 days of the illness. A liver biopsy can show midzone necrosis and eosinophilic degeneration of hepatocytes.

Treatment

There is no specific antiviral therapy available, but supportive care with fluids, blood products and analgesia is essential.

Complications

Yellow fever can be complicated by haemorrhagic shock, acute renal failure, coma and death. The mortality can be up to 40% in severe cases.

Prevention

There is an effective vaccination against yellow fever. Since it is a live vaccine, it is not suitable for immuno-suppressed patients or those under 9 months. Avoiding mosquito bites is important and can be achieved by using insect repellent, appropriate clothing and sleeping under an impregnated bed net.

Dengue fever

Dengue fever is the most significant arthropod-borne viral disease worldwide according to the WHO. It is endemic in South-east Asia, India, Central and South America and sub-Saharan Africa, with the highest burden of disease in South-east Asia. It is a debilitating viral disease that can result in dengue haemorrhagic fever (DHF) or dengue shock syndrome (DSS). Only DHF is a notifiable disease in the UK, requiring reporting to the CCDC. There are about 100 cases per year in the UK in returned travellers.

Organism

Dengue fever is caused by a flavivirus, of which there are four serotypes: DEN 1 to 4. Both humans and monkeys are reservoirs for the flavivirus, which is transmitted by the *Aedes aegypti* mosquito.

Aedes aegypti is a daytime biting mosquito, whereas the female anopheline mosquito that transmits malaria is most likely to bite during the evening and overnight.

Pathogenesis

The incubation period in humans is 5–8 days. Humans are only infectious to mosquitoes when viraemic, which occurs during the first 3 days of the illness. The incubation period in mosquitoes is 2 weeks and they remain infectious for life, which is why dengue is often endemic in an area. Immunity post-infection is lifelong but is only to the serotype of the infection experienced, not any of the others. There is some evidence to suggest that subsequent infection with a different serotype from the original infection results in the development of DHF or DSS, especially in children.

Clinical features

Dengue fever presents with an abrupt onset of fever, rigors and headache. The fever lasts about 5 days but may recur to give a second peak. This pattern is known as a 'saddleback fever'. There is a severe arthralgia and myalgia often involving the back that has given rise to the nickname for dengue fever as the 'breakbone fever'. A maculopapular rash develops between days 3–5 of the illness, usually starting from the limbs and then spreading over the trunk. Most infections are self-limiting with a rapid improvement in symptoms occurring 3–4 days after the rash appears. Some patients suffer with malaise and depression for a prolonged period after the fever has settled.

Dengue haemorrhagic fever has an onset that mimics the classical presentation described above but then the patient deteriorates between day 2–7 of the illness. The patient abruptly begins to haemorrhage into the skin, resulting in purpura; into the gums and mucous membranes, which can produce epistaxis; into the gastrointestinal tract, giving rise to haematemesis and melaena. The combination of sepsis and blood loss induces shock (dengue shock syndrome).

Investigations

The diagnosis of dengue fever can be confirmed using serology or tissue culture for the flavivirus. The full blood count can show a lymphocytosis and with DHF there will also be an anaemia and thrombocytopenia. In addition there are deranged clotting results and low complement levels in DHF. In cases where renal impairment occurs secondary to shock then the urea and creatinine will be raised accordingly.

Complications

DHF or DSS can lead to respiratory and renal failure in addition. The mortality can be as high as 40–50% but with good supportive care this can be reduced to 1–2%.

Treatment

There is no specific antiviral therapy available. Supportive management on an intensive care unit is required for DHF or DSS. Measures undertaken would include targeted fluid resuscitation, blood products for the coagulopathy and thrombocytopenia; ventilatory support and renal replacement therapy, such as haemofiltration.

Prevention

Since there is no vaccine or chemoprophylaxis available, the mainstay of preventing dengue fever is to avoid being bitten by the *A. aegypti* mosquito. Liberal use of insect repellents and covering up with clothes during the daytime are important measures to achieve this.

Rift Valley fever

Rift Valley fever is found in sub-Saharan Africa and Egypt.

Organism

Rift Valley fever is caused by a phlebovirus, which is transmitted by mosquitoes. There are large reservoirs of infection in endemic areas in domesticated cattle.

Clinical features

In most cases Rift Valley fever is an acute, self-limiting febrile illness from which the patient will make a complete recovery. The incubation period is 3–7 days. The patient then develops fever, headache, photophobia, myalgia and arthralgia. There is usually a biphasic fever pattern with several days of absent fever in the middle.

Complications

Less than 5% of patients will experience the haemorrhagic and neurological complications of the infection. The haemorrhagic features include purpura on the skin, retinal haemorrhages, haematemesis and melaena. The neurological features can consist of meningoencephalitis, retinitis and blindness (resulting from retinitis, retinal haemorrhages and retinal detachment). Some patients may also develop liver failure.

Diagnosis

The diagnosis of Rift Valley fever can be made from serology or viral isolation from blood.

Treatment

Although there is no established drug treatment for Rift Valley fever some success has been achieved using interferon and ribavirin. Convalescent serum (i.e. antibodies from a recovering patient) is recommended for patients with complications.

Prevention

The most effective method of prevention is the vaccination of domesticated cattle to reduce the local reservoir. There is also a human vaccine available for those who are at risk.

Sandfly fever (also known as phlebotomus fever or pappataci fever)

Sandfly fever occurs in the Mediterranean regions, North Africa, the Middle East and India.

Organism

Sandfly fever is caused by a phlebovirus which is transmitted via the sandfly, *Phlebotomus papatasii* (hence the alternative names).

Clinical features

The incubation period is 3–6 days. Sandfly fever presents with a sudden onset of fever, and severe orbital pain with conjunctival suffusion. This can be accompanied by neck and limb stiffness. It is a self-limiting illness, with no complications, lasting just a few days.

Diagnosis

The diagnosis can be confirmed using serology. If a lumbar puncture is performed as a result of the neck stiffness, then the opening pressure of the CSF may be raised, and on further investigation, a pleocytosis with raised protein levels may be seen. Patients may also have a leucopenia in the blood.

Treatment

There is no specific treatment available.

Japanese B encephalitis

Japanese B encephalitis occurs throughout the Far East, not just Japan. It is the most severe of all the viral encephalitides. As an encephalitic infection, Japanese B encephalitis is a notifiable disease in the UK, therefore any case should be reported to the CCDC.

Organism

Japanese B encephalitis is caused by a flavivirus. A *Culex* species of mosquito is its vector and this mosquito breeds in rice paddy areas. Birds and pigs are the reservoirs for this flavivirus.

Clinical features

Most infections are asymptomatic but those that manifest clinically are severe. The incubation period is 4–14 days. There is a sudden onset of high fever, meningitis symptoms (headache, neck stiffness and photophobia), suffused conjunctivae and neurological signs, such as hemiparesis and fits. The patient tends to adopt a particular posture with head extended and flexed limbs. Over the course of several days patients may have a reducing conscious level that deteriorates to coma and their limbs can become rigid.

Diagnosis

The diagnosis is usually confirmed from serology. The CSF may be normal or demonstrate a pleocytosis with a raised protein level.

Treatment

There is no specific antiviral treatment for Japanese B encephalitis, but convalescent serum has been reported as useful if given early.

Complications

The mortality can be as high as 50% in the initial acute phase but deaths can occur spontaneously during the slow recovery phase. Those patients who survive are often left with neurological impairments. These can range from mental deficits, deafness, upper motor neuron lesions and emotional lability.

Prevention

There is an effective vaccine available, given as a course of three immunizations. A booster is required after 5 years for continued protection.

VIRAL HAEMORRHAGIC FEVERS

Whilst yellow fever, dengue fever and Rift Valley fever can all result in haemorrhagic features, the following viruses are the ones known as the viral haemorrhagic fevers (VHF). The viral haemorrhagic fevers are all notifiable diseases in the UK and therefore all cases should be reported to the CCDC.

Lassa fever

Lassa fever occurs in sub-Saharan West Africa. It is named after Lassa in Nigeria, where the illness was first identified.

Organism

Lassa fever is caused by an arenavirus.

Transmission

The virus is contracted following direct contact with affected rats or from food and water contaminated with rat urine. Transmission can occur from contaminated blood in the hospital setting.

Any patient genuinely suspected of having a VHF must be strictly isolated until the diagnosis is ascertained and expert help sought immediately. Such a patient will have returned from an endemic area in Africa within the past 21 days; because of the short incubation period, anyone who has been back more than 21 days cannot have VHF. The isolation requires a negative-pressure room with a chemical toilet, and only essential staff, wearing full protective suits including mask and goggles (see Fig. 24.12), are to attend the patient. These isolation precautions are obviously necessary for confirmed cases. Any equipment used to retrieve bodily fluids from a confirmed case must be disposed of, initially into chemical disinfectant, and the laboratory informed of the infectious risk of these specimens. There are specialized isolation units for patients with a VHF in the UK.

Clinical features

Most infections are asymptomatic – up to 90% of cases. The incubation period is 7–18 days. In the first week the patients present with fever, headache, malaise, myalgia and severe backache. In those who undergo a deterioration of their illness, the haemorrhagic features develop after 1 week. These include epistaxis and gastrointestinal haemorrhage. Diarrhoea and vomiting are also common symptoms. The net result is usually shock, although the patients typically are bradycardic as well as hypotensive. The distinguishing features for Lassa fever are the facial oedema and pharyngeal ulceration. Occasionally patients have a maculopapular rash.

Investigations

The virus can be isolated from samples of blood, urine and pharyngeal secretions. The diagnosis can also be confirmed from serology using an ELISA. The other laboratory findings associated with Lassa fever are leucopenia and acute renal failure.

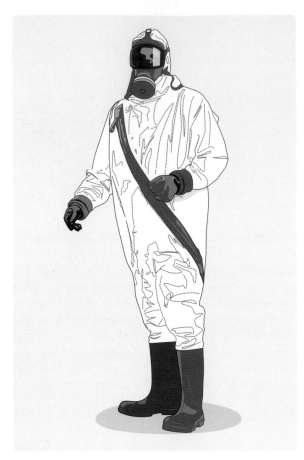

Fig. 24.12 Full protective suit.

Treatment

Ribavirin can be a beneficial treatment if used within the first week of the illness. Convalescent serum is also used as therapy for Lassa fever. The most important element of management, though, is adherence to the strict isolation requirements for a VHF.

Complications

Patients are often profoundly weak and have alopecia for a prolonged period of weeks if they survive the acute illness. The mortality of Lassa fever can be as high as 30% of cases. Many patients suffer with deafness, which does not resolve in all cases.

Prevention

There is no vaccine available against Lassa fever. Rodent control is an important part of preventing human infections.

Ebola virus disease

Ebola virus disease has intermittently caused epidemics in southern Sudan and northern Zaire.

Organism

Ebola virus disease is caused by Ebola virus, which is a filovirus.

Transmission

The virus can be transmitted from person to person and from exposure to contaminated blood but the natural reservoir is unknown.

Clinical features

There is an incubation of 7–14 days for Ebola virus disease. The patient then presents with high fever, severe headache and myalgia, abdominal pain, cough and chest pain. There are often herpetic lesions in the oral cavity and pharynx, and mucosal haemorrhages can be seen in these areas from the onset of bleeding. Patients have diarrhoea the severity of which is the best clinical indicator of the severity of the illness overall. From day 5 the haemorrhagic features become apparent with haemoptysis, haematemesis and bloody diarrhoea. At a similar time to the onset of bleeding, patients develop a measles-like rash, rather than purpura, which tends to start on the face and spread to the rest of the body, but this is extremely difficult to see on African skin. Patients also have hepatosplenomegaly. Neuropsychiatric complications are not unusual.

Investigations

The diagnosis of Ebola virus disease can be confirmed by isolating the virus from blood or by serology. Patients tend to have a leucopenia initially and subsequently develop a lymphocytosis. Dipstick testing the urine reveals a high level of albuminuria.

Treatment

There is no drug treatment available for Ebola virus disease. Convalescent serum is a recommended therapy. Crucially, the management of the patient must include strict compliance with the isolation precautions.

Prognosis

The mortality rate is up to 80% of cases.

Prevention

There is no vaccine available against Ebola virus disease.

Marburg virus disease

Marburg virus has caused small outbreaks in the past but in 2005 the largest outbreak of VHF due to Marburg virus occurred in Angola. The clinical features and epidemiology are similar to that seen with Ebola virus; both are filoviruses. The reservoir remains unknown. Marburg appears to be more virulent than Ebola and is more commonly spread nosocomially.

Congo-Crimean haemorrhagic fever (C-CHF)

Congo-Crimean haemorrhagic fever occurs in Africa and Asia predominantly, but has also been reported from eastern Europe, Russia and the Middle East.

Organism

C-CHF is caused by a bunyavirus, which is transmitted via ixodid ticks of the *Hyalomma* genus. Nosocomial transmission from infected blood also occurs.

Clinical features

Most cases of C-CHF are an acute, self-limiting, mild viral illness. The incubation period is 3–6 days. The patient initially suffers with a flu-like illness involving fever, headache, chills, myalgia and vomiting. On day 4 or 5 of the illness the haemorrhagic complications occur: severe haemorrhage results in shock as well as a petechial rash and haemorrhages visible on the soft palate.

Investigations

The diagnosis can be made from serology and viral isolation from blood. The full blood count may show a leucopenia and thrombocytopenia. The LFTs may also be deranged.

Treatment

There is no specific treatment for C-CHF. The essential aspect of management is adherence to the strict isolation and barrier nursing requirements of VHF.

Prognosis

The mortality can be up to 70% of cases during epidemics.

Prevention

There is no vaccine available against Congo-Crimean haemorrhagic fever.

TREMATODE INFECTIONS

Schistosomiasis (previously known as Bilharzia)

Schistosomiasis has been described by the WHO as the second most important tropical disease in terms of public health importance after malaria. It is endemic in many developing countries with the highest prevalence of disease seen in sub-Saharan Africa, Brazil, southern China and the Philippines. There are more than 200 million people infected worldwide with 20 000 deaths annually.

Organisms

Schistosomiasis is caused by the trematode *Schistosoma*, of which there are three main species: *Schistosoma mansoni*, *S. japonicum* and *S. haematobium*. These are blood flukes.

Pathogenesis

Trematodes undergo both sexual reproduction in humans and asexual reproduction in their mollusc intermediate hosts (Fig. 24.13). The pathology that occurs in humans is as a result of a type IV hypersensitivity reaction to the eggs. The inflammatory reaction leads to healing by fibrosis, and it is the fibrosis that usually leads to clinical problems.

Clinical features

The first symptom noted is a local dermatitis at the site of cercarial invasion, known as 'swimmer's itch'. After an incubation period of 1–3 weeks the patient feels unwell with fever, malaise and myalgia; this is known as 'Katayama fever'. There may be symptoms related to the migration path of the cercariae, such as wheeze and cough. Subsequent symptoms are detailed in Figure 24.14.

Fig. 24.13 Schistosome life cycle.

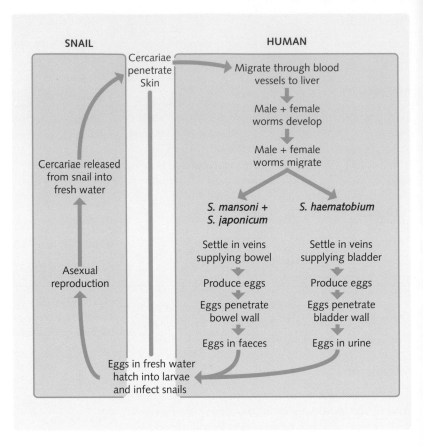

Occasionally, eggs are deposited elsewhere in the body and can become symptomatic, for example in the lungs, brain or spinal cord.

Investigations

The diagnosis can be confirmed by isolating the characteristic eggs in faeces or urine depending on the species. In non-endemic areas, serology may also be helpful. Rectal biopsy samples for eggs can be diagnostic in all species of *Schistosoma*. A liver biopsy can demonstrate the chronic inflammation and fibrosis resulting from the presence of the eggs in *S. mansoni* and *S. japonicum*. An ultrasound scan of the renal tract is important in following up cases of *S. haematobium* to check for related morbidity. There is often an eosinophilia on the full blood count, particularly at the time of the 'Katayama fever'.

Treatment

Praziquantel is the treatment of choice for schisto-somiasis. Just one dose is required for *S. haematobium* and two doses for *S. mansoni* and *S. japonicum*. This is effective when there is no further exposure to the cercariae in freshwater after treatment but in endemic areas repeated reinfection renders attempts at eradication in the local population hopeless.

Complications

The fibrotic complications seen with schistosomiasis are portal hypertension and its sequelae with *S. mansoni* and *S. japonicum*; and hydronephrosis, pyelonephritis and chronic renal failure with *S. haematobium*. *S. mansoni* may also lead to pulmonary hypertension in patients when eggs are shunted to the lungs to bypass a fibrotic liver. In addition, *S. japonicum* and *S. haematobium* have been shown to predispose to colonic and bladder carcinomas respectively in endemic areas.

Prevention

Avoidance of freshwater contact in endemic areas is the only way to avoid contracting schistosomiasis. Any swimming or paddling in freshwater known to contain the snails is high-risk behaviour. Chlorination of water kills schistosomes, so properly chlorinated swimming pools should not be a source of infection.

Fig. 24.14 Table differentiating the three species of *Schistosoma*

	S. mansoni	S. japonicum	S. haematobium
Regions affected	Africa, Middle East, South America	South-east Asia and China	Africa, Middle East, Egypt
Pathology	Eggs from female worms penetrate intestinal wall and pass into faeces. Eggs trapped in intestinal wall can result in inflammation and fibrosis in portal vein leading to portal hypertension		Eggs from female worm penetrate bladder wall and pass into urine. Eggs trapped in bladder wall can cause inflammation and fibrosis resulting in obstruction of ureters, hydronephrosis and renal failure
Veins affected	Inferior mesenteric	Superior and inferior mesenteric	Pelvic and vesical
Clinical features	Abdominal pain and diarrhoea ± blood, can mimic inflammatory bowel disease Wheeze and cough more likely with *S. japonicum* Later hepatosplenomegaly Transverse myelitis with *S. mansoni*		Frequency, dysuria, haematuria, haematospermia and incontinence Later hydronephrosis and renal failure Transverse myelitis with *S. haematobium*
Diagnosis	Faecal microscopy for eggs Liver biopsy shows hepatic fibrosis, granulomatous inflammation and portal hypertension		Urine microscopy for eggs (midday collection) USS renal tract for morbidity Bladder biopsy

Fasciola hepatica

See Chapter 19.

Opisthorcis sinensis

See Chapter 19.

Schistosomiasis is endemic around Lake Malawi, but most travellers, despite their good intentions on leaving home, cannot resist swimming in the beautiful lake. Symptoms in any traveller exposed to Lake Malawi should raise the possibility of schistosomiasis.

Lung flukes

Lung flukes occur in tropical climates around the world.

Organism

Lung flukes are of the *Paragonimus* genus. Different species are prevalent in different areas of the world.

Pathogenesis

The life cycle of lung flukes is shown in Figure 24.15. The worms and eggs induce granuloma formation.

Clinical features

The patient presents with a chronic cough productive of brown purulent sputum. There may be haemoptysis. Night sweats and chest pains can accompany the cough, thereby mimicking tuberculosis or bronchiectasis. A pleural effusion or pneumothorax can complicate this pulmonary infection. Children are more commonly affected.

Complications

Occasionally the flukes can migrate to ectopic sites in the body and these can be symptomatic. For example there can be subcutaneous nodules or space-occupying symptoms from spinal cord or cerebral disease.

Investigations

The diagnosis can be confirmed by isolating the lung fluke from sputum, faeces, gastric washings and tissue

Fig. 24.15 Lung fluke life cycle.

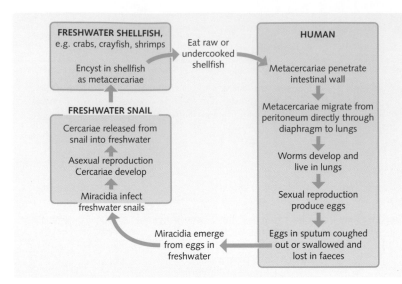

biopsies. Serology is also useful in diagnosis. There is usually a significant eosinophilia seen on the full blood count. A chest radiograph or CT scan can demonstrate the lung lesions.

Treatment

Praziquantel is the treatment of choice for lung flukes. Triclabendazole, bithionol and niclofan have also been used successfully.

Prevention

Lung fluke infections can be prevented by not consuming raw or inadequately cooked crustaceans, in particular crabs, crayfish and shrimps in endemic areas.

NEMATODE INFECTIONS

Nematode infections can be divided into tissue nematodes and intestinal nematodes. The different types of intestinal nematode infections are compared in Figure 24.16.

Filariasis

Filariasis can be caused by the tissue nematodes:

- *Onchocerca volvulus*
- *Wuchereria bancrofti*
- *Loa loa*.

These are all vector-borne infections with similar features. The general life cycle is shown in Figure 24.17.

The details of the different filarial infections are shown in Figure 24.18.

CESTODE INFECTIONS

Cestodes are more commonly known as tapeworms. These infections occur worldwide.

Organisms

The tapeworms acquired from beef are called *Taenia saginata* and those from pork are *Taenia solium*. Tapeworms have a head that is attached to segments, known as proglottids, that form a chain. *T. saginata* can grow up to 10 m in length and has suckers on the head, whereas *T. solium* has hooks and suckers on the head and can reach a maximum length of 6 m.

Transmission

The tapeworms are acquired by ingesting meat contaminated with *Taenia* larvae.

Pathogenesis

The *Taenia* larvae develop into tapeworms in the gastrointestinal tract and reside in the small bowel.

Fig. 24.16 Comparison of intestinal nematode infections

	Strongyloidiasis	Hookworm	Roundworm	Whipworm	Threadworm or pinworm
Organisms	Strongyloides stercoralis	Ancylostoma duodenale; Necator americanus	Ascaris lumbricoides	Trichuris trichiura	Enterobius vermicularis
Size and features	Very small, up to 2.5 mm in length. Two larval forms	Have teeth or cutting plates in buccal capsule to attach to bowel mucosa and cause bleeding. ~ 1 cm in length	Like garden worm, 25 cm in length	Medium length, up to 4.5 cm	Small, up to 12 mm length
Geography	Tropics	Both: Africa, Southeast Asia A. duodenale: Europe, India, Middle East N. americanus: America	Worldwide, especially in poor areas and in Asia	Worldwide, especially in tropical climates	Worldwide but more common in temperate climates
Transmission	Percutaneously	Percutaneously through feet	Faecal–oral route	Faecal–oral route	Faecal–oral route; autoinfection
Pathogenesis	Migrate to upper airways, then coughed up and swallowed into GI tract, then colonize GI tract	Larvae from soil migrate in blood to upper GI tract via lungs and attach to GI tract mucosa to draw blood	Larvae hatch from eggs in jejunum, penetrate bowel wall and migrates through liver and lung back to GI tract	Larvae hatch from eggs in small intestine, develop into adults in caecum	Larvae hatch in small bowel and adults live in caecum. Females lay eggs at anus at night
Site in GI tract	Small bowel	Small bowel	Small bowel	Large bowel	Small and large bowel
Symptoms	Larva currens (Ch. 12) then cough and dyspnoea. Nausea and anorexia with heavy GI infection	Itching at site of larval entry. Ulcer-like abdominal pain	Asymptomatic to abdominal pain and distension, anorexia, nausea, vomiting. Cough, dyspnoea	Asymptomatic to bloody diarrhoea and abdominal pain. Anorexia and tenesmus	Pruritus ani since eggs intensely itchy. Occasionally abdominal pain or diarrhoea
Complications	Intestinal malabsorption, weight loss, death in heavy infection, secondary Gram-negative septicaemia	Anaemia (in heavy infection can lose up to 100 ml blood/day)	Biliary tract and bowel obstruction especially ileocaecal, appendix. Pulmonary eosinophilia. Malnutrition as competes for nutrients	Weight loss. Appendicitis, rectal prolapse in children. Colonic ulceration and anaemia with heavy infections	Scratching can lead to secondary bacterial infections, abscesses and autoinfection
Investigations	Microscopy of faeces or duodenal aspirate. Eosinophilia	Ova in stool (number indicates severity). Eosinophilia	Ova from stool, worms on barium studies. Eosinophilia	Ova from stool. Worms visualized on sigmoidoscopy	Sticky tape to perianal area/perineum to get ova for microscopy. Ova in stool. Eosinophilia
Treatment	Thiabendazole, albendazole. Broad-spectrum antibiotics if secondary Gram-negative septicaemia	Mebendazole. Iron tablets if anaemic	Levamisole, mebendazole, piperazine	Mebendazole, pyrantel pamoate	Mebendazole, piperazine. Treat all family to prevent spread
Prevention	Wearing shoes on feet and good personal hygiene	Wearing shoes on feet	Good personal hygiene and sanitation	Good personal hygiene	Good personal hygiene

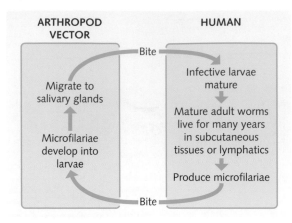

Fig. 24.17 Filiarial life cycle.

Clinical features

The patient presents with mild abdominal pain and diarrhoea. The infection may be discovered by finding proglottids in the faeces or seeing these in underwear or the bed.

Complications

Pancreatitis and appendicitis can occur due to obstruction of the pancreatic duct or appendix respectively, by the tapeworms. Cysticercosis is described below.

Investigations

The diagnosis can be confirmed by visualizing the proglottids or detecting ova in faeces or perianal swabs. On the full blood count there may be an eosinophilia.

Treatment

Taenia infections are treated with niclosamide or praziquantel. With *Taenia solium* it is necessary to flush the stomach through with saline in order to clear the ova and prevent immediate reinfection.

Prevention

Meat needs to be stored and cooked correctly to prevent the transmission of tapeworms. It is also important to check the meat before consumption.

Cysticercosis

Cysticercosis occurs when a patient becomes infected by the intermediate larval forms of *T. solium*. This can occur from undercooked pork, which may contain hatched eggs, or by autoinfection with the ova from stool. It typically occurs in Asia, Africa and South

Fig. 24.18 Comparison of filarial infections

	Onchocerca volvulus	*Wuchereria bancrofti*	*Loa loa*
Vector	Female blackfly (bite during the day)	*Anopheles* and *Aedes* mosquitoes (bite at night)	*Chrysops* fly
Geography	Africa, Central and South America, Saudi Arabia	Asia, Africa, South America and India	Africa
Site of adults	Subcutaneous tissues	Lymphatics	Subcutaneous and periorbital tissues
Incubation	1 year	10–12 months	
Clinical features	Nodule at bite site. Skin: hypopigmentation, lichenification, atrophy. Lymphadenopathy, elephantiasis (see Fig. 24.19). Eyes: uveitis, keratitis, cataract, optic neuritis, atrophy and blindness	Fever. Lymphangitis heals with fibrosis, granuloma formation, secondary lymphoedema and elephantiasis (see Fig. 24.19). Scrotum affected. Chylous ascites and pleural effusions	Skin: urticaria, pruritus, lymphoedema. Joints: arthritis, Calabar swellings. Eyes: chorioretinitis, worms migrate across conjunctiva
Diagnosis	Microscopy of skin/eye snips kept in saline and slit lamp examination of eye show microfilariae	Thick and thin blood films at night (when microfilariae released; coincides with mosquito activity – 9 p.m. to 1 a.m.)	Microscopy of daytime blood film, worm seen in subcutaneous tissues or conjunctiva. Serology
Treatment	Ivermectin now drug of choice for all three; diethylcarbamazine (DEC) can be used as secondary treatment		

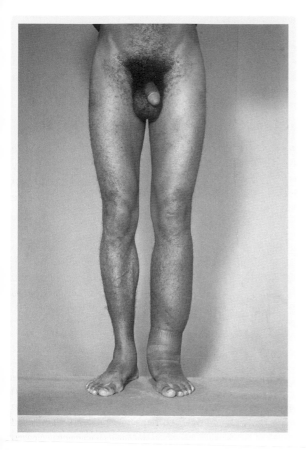

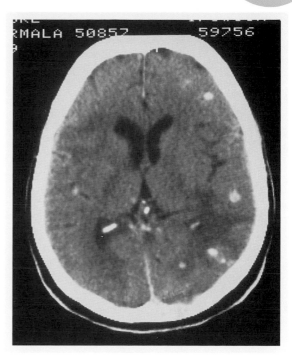

Fig. 24.20 CT scan of head showing calcification in a patient with cerebral cysticercosis.
Source: Conlon & Snydman, 2000: Fig. 7.16.

Fig. 24.19 Elephantiasis seen with filariasis.
Source: Conlon & Snydman, 2000: Fig. 15.16.

Investigations

With cerebral involvement, the CT or MRI scan is helpful as the cysticerci have a classical appearance (Fig. 24.20). The subcutaneous lesions are usually amenable to biopsy, which can demonstrate the organism. Serology can be used to confirm the clinical suspicion. There is an eosinophilia on the full blood count.

Treatment

Praziquantel and albendazole are both effective treatments and may be given together. Since killing the organism can cause a marked inflammatory response, it is recommended that steroids are given with the antimicrobials, especially with cerebral involvement, but it prevents ocular cases being treated with drugs. Antiepileptic therapy may also be required in cerebral cases. Surgery may be appropriate in some cases.

Hydatid disease

See Chapter 19.

Figure 24.21 summarizes the more commonly encountered and important tropical infections.

America. The larvae penetrate the bowel and are disseminated around the body via the bloodstream. Any tissue can be infected and develop the small, fluid-filled cysticerci, but there is a propensity for the brain, eyes and skin to be involved. The cysticerci may not produce symptoms and may be discovered incidentally.

Clinical features

- Cerebral – epilepsy (most common presentation), raised intracranial pressure, focal neurology, e.g. hemiplegia, cognitive deficits.
- Ocular – retinitis, uveitis, conjunctivitis, retinal detachment, blindness.
- Subcutaneous – small nodules under the skin (up to 5 mm diameter).

Further reading

Azad AF, Beard CB. Rickettsial pathogens and their arthropod vectors. Emerg Infect Dis 1998; 4:179–186

Centers for Disease Control and Prevention. Travel information. Website: www.cdc.gov/travel.

Myint HY, Tipmanee P, Nosten F, Day NP, Pukrittayakamee S, Looareesuwan S, White NJ. A systematic overview of published antimalarial drug trials. Trans R Soc Trop Med Hyg 2004; 98:73–81

Olliaro PL, Guerin PJ, Gerstl S, Haaskjold AA, Rottingen JA, Sundar S. Treatment options for visceral leishmaniasis: a systematic review of clinical studies done in India, 1980-2004. Lancet Infect Dis 2005; 5:763–774

Ryan ET, Kain KC. Primary Care: health advice and immunizations for travellers. NEJM 2000; 342:1716–1725

Ryan ET, Wilson ME, Kain KC. Current concepts: illness after international travel. NEJM 2002; 347:505–516

SEAQUAMAT. South East Asian Quinine vs Artesunate Severe Malaria Trial. Website: www.seaquamat.info.

Vennervald BJ, Dunne DW. Morbidity in schistosomiasis: an update. Curr Opin Infect Dis 2004; 17:439–447

WHO (World Health Organization). Website: www.who.int/en. Has excellent information on many of the conditions mentioned in this chapter including: Roll Back Malaria programme; World Health Assembly resolution on leprosy.

Fig. 24.21 Summary of the more commonly encountered and important tropical infections

Infection (organism)	Clinical features	Investigations	Treatment	Complications	Prevention
Malaria (*Plasmodium falciparum*, *P. vivax*, *P. malariae*, *P. ovale*)	High fevers, drenching sweats, chills, rigors, vomiting, confusion, reduced consciousness, seizures. Anaemia, jaundice, hepatosplenomegaly. Abnormal neurological examination	Thin and thick blood films. Anaemia, thrombocytopenia. Abnormal renal function, lactic acidosis, raised bilirubin and lactate dehydrogenase. Hypoglycaemia. Haemoglobinuria. ECG. Lumbar puncture	Artemisinin in combination therapy first line, or over quinine for falciparum malaria. Chloroquine for benign malarias. Primaquine course for hypnozoite eradication. Supportive care	CNS, cardiovascular, respiratory, renal, haematological and metabolic complications occur. Mortality considerable from falciparum malaria. Relapse with *P. vivax*, *P. ovale*	Chemoprophylaxis, drug choice dependent on areas to be visited. Sleeping under impregnated bed nets, liberal insect repellent use and covering clothing especially in evenings
Leishmaniasis (e.g. *Leishmania donovani*, *L. aethiopica*, *L. braziliensis*)	Visceral: fever, rigors, sweats, weight loss, malaise, anorexia, hepatosplenomegaly, hyperpigmentation Cutaneous: papule then crusted ulcer at bite site Mucocutaneous: as cutaneous on lower limbs; later ulceration and destruction of mucous membranes of nose, mouth, throat	Tissue (e.g. skin scraping or punch biopsy of ulcers; lymph node, bone marrow) for microscopy, histology and culture. Serology. PCR. Anaemia, neutropenia, thrombocytopenia in visceral disease	Cutaneous lesions: surgical removal, treatment with local cryotherapy or topical paromomycin Visceral or potential mucocutaneous disease: intravenous stibogluconate first choice; or intravenous amphotericin B, pentamidine	Disfiguring scarring from healing cutaneous lesions. Destruction of nose, mouth, throat; and respiratory infections in mucocutaneous disease. Untreated visceral leishmaniasis fatal within 2 years. Relapse of disease	Avoidance of sandfly bites by liberal insect repellent use and covering clothing in evenings particularly, and sleeping under impregnated bed nets
Giardiasis (*Giardia lamblia*)	Explosive watery diarrhoea. Mild abdominal pain, bloating. Steatorrhoea, malabsorption. Chronic diarrhoea with HIV	Stool, duodenal aspirates for culture. Microscopy of stool for cysts and trophozoites	Metronidazole or tinidazole	Malabsorption	Good personal hygiene and access to clean water supplies
Typhoid and Paratyphoid (*Salmonella typhi* and *Salmonella paratyphi*)	First week: fever, relative bradycardia, dry cough, myalgia, arthralgia, anorexia, nausea, constipation Second week: rose spots, hepatosplenomegaly, cervical lymphadenopathy, abdominal tenderness Third week: complications	Blood, urine, stool, bone marrow, duodenal aspirates for culture. Leucopenia, anaemia. 'Hepatitic' picture with LFTs	Quinolones, e.g. ciprofloxacin and ofloxacin. Third generation cephalosporins, e.g. ceftriaxone, and the macrolide, azithromycin used as alternatives. Steroid therapy with antibiotics for severe cases	Lobar pneumonia, pericarditis, meningitis, cognitive impairment, polyneuropathy, acute cholecystitis, visceral abscesses, intestinal haemorrhage and perforation, urinary tract infection, osteomyelitis, haemolytic anaemia. Mortality up to 15–20% if untreated. Chronic carriage	Immunization. Good basic hygiene practices, proper sewage disposal and access to clean drinking water

(continued)

Fig. 24.21 Summary of the more commonly encountered and important tropical infections—continued

Infection (organism)	Clinical features	Investigations	Treatment	Complications	Prevention
Brucellosis (*Brucella suis*, *B. abortus*, *B. melitensis*)	Fever, malaise, myalgia, night sweats, weight loss. Hepatosp enomegaly, lymphadenopathy	Prolonged incubation of blood or bone marrow cultures. Acute and convalescent serology	Prolonged course of doxycycline and rifampicin or doxycycline and aminoglycoside, e.g. gentamicin	Arthritis, osteomyelitis, meningoencephalitis, endocarditis, orchitis	Good personal hygiene handling animals. Pasteurization of milk
Typhus (e.g. *Rickettsiae prowazekii*, *R. rickettsii*)	Endemic: high fever, headache, profound malaise, myalgia, conjunctivitis, orbital pain. Generalized maculopapular rash, turns purpuric. Vasculitis. Meningoencephalitis, extrapyra-midal signs. Splenomegaly RMSF: eschar with local lymphadenopathy, as endemic African tick typhus: fever, headache, erythematous rash, eschar; milder symptoms	Acute and convalescent serology. Skin biopsies for RMSF. Thrombocytopenia.	Tetracycline or chloramphenicol. Supportive care	Haemolysis, thrombocy-topenia, DIC, shock, gangrene of distal extremities, respiratory failure, renal failure, myocarditis, stroke, reduced consciousness, coma and death. Brill–Zinsser disease	Principally avoidance of insect bites with liberal use of insect repellent and covering clothing. Immunization, chemoprophylaxis with doxycycline
Dengue fever (flavivirus, four serotypes: DEN 1 to 4)	'Saddleback' fever, rigors, headache, severe arthralgia and myalgia. Maculopapular rash	Serology or tissue culture. Lymphocytosis	No specific antiviral therapy. Supportive care	Dengue haemorrhagic fever, dengue shock syndrome. Renal and respiratory failure. Mortality up to 50%	Avoidance of *A. aegypti* mosquito bites, liberal use of insect repellent and covering clothes during the daytime
Schistosomiasis (*Schistosoma mansoni*, *S. japonicum*, *S. haematobium*)	'Swimmer's itch' then 'Katayama fever'. Wheeze, cough. Frequency, dysuria, haematuria, haematospermia, incontinence with *S. haematobium*. Abdominal pain, diarrhoea in other types	Microscopy for eggs from urine or stool. Rectal and bladder or liver biopsy. Renal tract ultrasound scan. Eosinophilia. Serology in non-endemic areas	Praziquantel	Hydronephrosis, pyelonephritis, renal failure with *S. haematobium*. Portal hypertension, hepatosplenomegaly with others. Transverse myelit s with *S. haematobium*, *S. mansoni*. Pulmonary hypertension with *S. mansoni*. Colonic or bladder carcinomas with *S. japonicum* or *S. haematobium*	Avoidance of freshwater contact in endemic areas

Human immunodeficiency virus (HIV) and opportunistic infections

25

Objectives

In this chapter you will learn:

- How HIV can be acquired
- What is meant by the 'window period' relating to HIV testing
- The groups of drugs used to treat HIV
- The AIDS-defining conditions
- The complications of early HIV disease
- How to manage an HIV-positive patient who has reduced visual acuity.

HUMAN IMMUNODEFICIENCY VIRUS (HIV)

HIV is endemic around the world, but the highest rates of morbidity and mortality are in sub-Saharan Africa. The WHO (World Health Organization) reported in their 'Global Summary of the AIDS (acquired immunodeficiency syndrome) Epidemic in December 2004' that the number of people currently living with HIV was 39.4 million and that there had been 4.9 million new infections worldwide in 2004. Although sub-Saharan Africa has 10% of the world's population, more than 60% of all people living with HIV reside there, 25.4 million people according to the WHO.

It is estimated by the Health Protection Agency that there are 53 000 people living with HIV in the UK. The highest rates of transmission in the UK used to be amongst men who have sexual intercourse with men. However, heterosexual acquisitions of HIV have increased markedly, so that since 1999 this has become the most common route of sexual transmission. In 2002/2003 in the UK, 76% of new heterosexual infections were in those from Africa or who had been exposed in Africa.

HIV was identified in 1984, but with access to treatment it is no longer the death sentence it once was. The WHO reported there were 3.1 million deaths worldwide in 2004, with 2.3 million of these in sub-Saharan Africa. Hence, in December 2003 there was a combined WHO/UNAIDS (Joint United Nations Programme on HIV/AIDS) '3 by 5' programme set up which aimed to provide access to treatment to 3 million people in developing countries by the end of 2005.

Virus

HIV is a retrovirus, made up of single-stranded RNA (ribonucleic acid). The significance of this is that the single-stranded RNA (ssRNA) has to transcribe a mirror image of itself to form double-stranded DNA (dsDNA) before it can replicate or translate into proteins (see Fig. 25.1). Since this method of replication involves no 'proof reading', the enzyme is error prone and mutations in the HIV genome are common. Because reverse transcriptase does not occur in human cells, there is no human equivalent of the reverse transcriptase enzyme and this can be a potential target for antiretroviral therapy.

Pathogenesis

HIV is such a successful pathogen because it is able to undermine both the humoral and cellular immune systems. The humoral immune system involves the formation of antibodies by B lymphocytes against foreign antigens. The cellular immune system consists of T lymphocytes, namely helper $CD4^+$ cells and cytotoxic $CD8^+$ cells. HIV primarily infects $CD4^+$ cells and destroys the cells when the new virus particles are released, leading to a progressive reduction in $CD4^+$ cell numbers. B lymphocytes need help from T lymphocytes to produce antibody responses to new antigens, so antibody responses decline as the $CD4^+$ numbers drop. Thus, there is progressive loss of the ability to respond to new and latent pathogens,

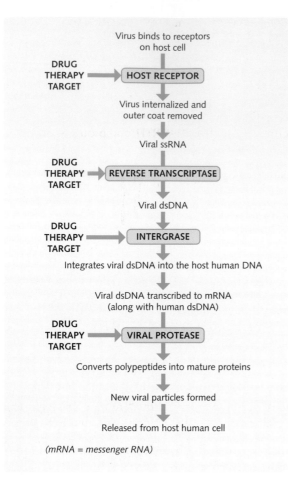

Virus binds to receptors on host cell

DRUG THERAPY TARGET → **HOST RECEPTOR**

Virus internalized and outer coat removed

Viral ssRNA

DRUG THERAPY TARGET → **REVERSE TRANSCRIPTASE**

Viral dsDNA

DRUG THERAPY TARGET → **INTERGRASE**

Integrates viral dsDNA into the host human DNA

Viral dsDNA transcribed to mRNA (along with human dsDNA)

DRUG THERAPY TARGET → **VIRAL PROTEASE**

Converts polypeptides into mature proteins

New viral particles formed

Released from host human cell

(mRNA = messenger RNA)

Fig. 25.1 HIV replication and translation, with targets for drug therapy.

so opportunistic infections become increasingly common.

Transmission

HIV is a typical blood-borne virus and is transmitted sexually, via blood and vertically from mother to child. Sexual transmission is the most common means of spread. There is some evidence to suggest that women are more prone to be infected by a positive partner than the converse. Blood transmission can occur through blood products, although all of these are now screened in the UK. Needle sharing in IVDUs (intravenous drug users) and accidental needle-stick injuries to health professionals are recognized means of transmission. Vertical spread from mother to child can occur whilst in utero but most transmissions occur during labour and via breast-feeding.

Primary HIV infection

Most HIV infections are initially asymptomatic but some may have an overt primary infection, sometimes called a seroconversion illness. After an incubation period of about 6 weeks some patients will experience a flu-like illness during the time of their seroconversion. The patient experiences:

- Fever, malaise, myalgia
- Sore throat, cervical lymphadenopathy
- A generalized maculopapular rash
- Occasionally diarrhoea.

Infrequently there may be a neurological presentation with meningoencephalitis or radiculitis.

The differential diagnosis of an HIV seroconversion illness includes glandular fever, i.e. Epstein–Barr virus (EBV) and cytomegalovirus (CMV).

Diagnosis

All patients should receive pre-test counselling which explains the nature of the test, and explores the implications of a positive result and the availability of treatment. Any doctor should be able to provide this counselling. The current HIV test is an antibody test to the virus. PCR (polymerase chain reaction) tests to detect viral DNA are available but not licensed for testing; they are useful, however, in assessing whether infants born to positive mothers are infected.

Patients and health professionals need to be aware of the 'window period' that occurs with the antibody HIV test. It may take around 6 weeks after infection for the HIV test to become positive (and in some cases up to 3 months). Therefore a negative result should be re-checked after this time interval and only then, if there has been no risk behaviour between the two tests, can patients be confidently told they do not have HIV.

If a patient tests as positive for HIV, then the viral load and CD4+ count also need to be checked as they have implications for treatment and prophylaxis against opportunistic infections. HIV-positive patients frequently have a lymphopenia on the full blood count.

Beware though, a leucopenia is a normal variation for Afro-Caribbean patients; their normal range is lower than for Caucasian patients.

Monitoring

Patients who are HIV positive should be followed up on a regular basis as outpatients to ensure they remain well and to decide when it is appropriate to start antiretroviral therapy. There are two blood test results which are used as a basis for forming the decision on therapy:

- Viral load – whilst on therapy, aim to achieve an undetectable level, i.e. < 50 copies/ml
- CD4+ count:
  - normal > 800×10^6/ml
  - AIDS < 200×10^6/ml.

The levels of both the viral load and the CD4+ cell count vary over the course of a patient's HIV illness as shown in Figure 25.2.

Treatment

The aims with antiretroviral therapy are:

- Restore immune function
- Prevent opportunistic infections
- Maintain health and slow progression of disease
- In pregnant women to prevent vertical transmission.

It has become clear over the years since 1984 of treating HIV that single- or double-agent therapy is not effective as the virus develops resistance and therefore all patients must receive at least three antiretroviral drugs in combination for successful treatment. The groups of drugs used are: nucleotide reverse transcriptase inhibitors (NRTI), non-nucleotide reverse transcriptase inhibitors (NNRTI), and protease inhibitors (PI). Usually the combination therapy, known as 'HAART' (highly active antiretroviral therapy), uses two NRTIs and either a PI or an NNRTI. The groups of antiretroviral drugs and their major side-effects are shown in Figure 25.3.

Given the potentially toxic nature of HAART, patients should be regularly followed with blood tests: full blood count to check for anaemia, neutropenia and thrombocytopenia; liver function tests; and renal function tests for dose adjustments and complications.

There is a new class of drug available for use in HIV that acts to prevent the virus fusing with the host cell: a fusion inhibitor, e.g. enfuvirtide. Enfuvirtide is licensed to be used in combination with other HAART drugs when the patient has failed to respond to or been intolerant of other antiretroviral regimens.

There are increasing concerns about the long-term use of HIV therapies. Lipid metabolism is altered and there may be an increased risk of premature cardiovascular disease. In addition, there may be problems, such as lactic acidosis, that arise because of mitochondrial damage.

Prevention

Measures aimed at preventing HIV infection focus on the three routes of transmission: sexual, blood-borne and vertical. The sexual spread of HIV can be limited

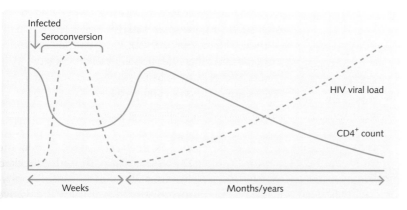

Fig. 25.2 Variations in viral load and CD4+ cell count over time.

Infected
Seroconversion

HIV viral load

CD4+ count

Weeks

Months/years

Fig. 25.3 Groups of antiretroviral drugs and their major side-effects

	NRTI	NNRTI	Protease inhibitors
Examples	Zidovudine (AZT) Stavudine Lamivudine (relatively free of side-effects) Didanosine	Nevirapine Efavirenz	Ritonavir Saquinavir Nelfinavir Lopinavir
Major side-effects	Gastrointestinal (GI) disturbance Pancreatitis Peripheral neuropathy Rashes Lactic acidosis Blood disorders, e.g. anaemia	Interacts with P450 system, so many drug interactions Rashes Neuropsychiatric reactions (efavirenz) Hepatitis (nevirapine)	Interacts with P450 system, so many drug interactions GI disturbance Hepatitis Lipodystrophy Insulin resistance Pancreatitis Blood disorders, e.g. anaemia Rashes

Fig. 25.4 Table of AIDS-defining illnesses

AIDS-defining infections	AIDS-defining tumours (associated viral infections)	Other AIDS-defining conditions (associated viral infections)
Pneumocystis jerovecii pneumonia (PCP) Mycobacteria: disseminated TB, atypical mycobacteria, e.g. *Mycobacterium avium-intracellulare* (MAI) CMV retinitis/colitis/oesophagitis/encephalitis *Toxoplasma gondii* *Cryptococcus neoformans* *Cryptosporidium parvum* *Isospora belli* Microsporidia Oesophageal or disseminated candidiasis Chronic or disseminated herpes simplex infections	Kaposi's sarcoma (human herpes virus 8, HHV-8) Lymphomas, e.g. Burkitt's (EBV); body cavity (HHV-8)	Progressive multifocal leucoencephalopathy (JC virus, a papovavirus) AIDS dementia

by using barrier contraception such as condoms, and limiting high-risk behaviours such as promiscuity. Blood products are now routinely screened in the UK for HIV, which should limit transmission. Sharing needles amongst IVDUs is a high-risk activity, although more for hepatitis C than HIV (see Ch. 19), and needle-exchange programmes are aimed at preventing this potential source of infection. Health professionals may be liable to infection from needle-stick injuries but all hospitals have a policy for post-exposure prophylaxis in order to limit the risk of transmission.

There are a number of measures to limit vertical transmission of HIV and for this reason testing is encouraged in antenatal clinics. HIV-positive mothers who take antiretroviral therapy during their pregnancy, deliver via caesarean section and do not breast-feed their child can reduce the risk of transmission from 25% (up to 40%) to less than 2%.

AIDS-defining illnesses

AIDS-defining illnesses usually occur with a CD4$^+$ count less than 200×10^6/ml. They include infections, tumours and other disorders as detailed in Figure 25.4.

Summary of non-infectious AIDS-defining illnesses

Kaposi's sarcoma

Kaposi's sarcoma (KS) presents with multiple, well-demarcated, purple lesions affecting the buccal mucosa and skin, but can also involve the gastrointestinal tract, lungs and lymph nodes. In general, visceral KS has a worse prognosis than that confined to the skin. It is associated with HHV-8 infection, which is sexually transmitted. KS may be treated with local radiotherapy or with chemotherapy using drugs such as doxorubicin or vincristine and bleomycin. The KS will recur unless immune function is improved with antiretroviral therapy.

Lymphoma

The lymphomas are usually non-Hodgkin's lymphomas (NHLs) of the large B cell type and include Burkitt's lymphoma. These are generally all associated with EBV infection, although some body cavity lymphomas have been shown to be associated with HHV-8. In HIV-positive patients, the NHLs are frequently extranodal, affecting the brain, lungs and gastrointestinal tract and the 'B' symptoms (i.e. fevers > 38°C, drenching night sweats, and > 10% weight loss) are often prominent. The prognosis is often poor with cerebral lymphomas but lymphoma outside the central nervous system (CNS) often responds well to 'CHOP'-type chemotherapy (cyclophosphamide, doxorubicin hydrochloride, Oncovin (vincristine) and prednisolone) in conjunction with HAART.

Progressive multifocal leucoencephalopathy

Progressive multifocal leucoencephalopathy (PML) is characterized by demyelination of the white matter of the brain. This gives rise to a progression of neurological and cognitive losses that occur in an erratic pattern. The demyelination is relentless and inevitably fatal. There is as yet no known cure. PML is associated with JC virus, which is a papovavirus. MRI and CT scans of the brain show multiple lesions in the white matter with no contrast enhancement or mass effect (see Fig. 25.5). The definitive diagnosis is made from a brain biopsy.

AIDS dementia

AIDS dementia is a progressive condition that is usually fatal. It may be associated with a cerebellar syndrome. The only therapy is HAART against the HIV thought to be driving the process.

OPPORTUNISTIC INFECTIONS

The different infections that arise secondary to HIV infection occur at predictable levels of CD4+ cell count, as shown in Figure 25.6.

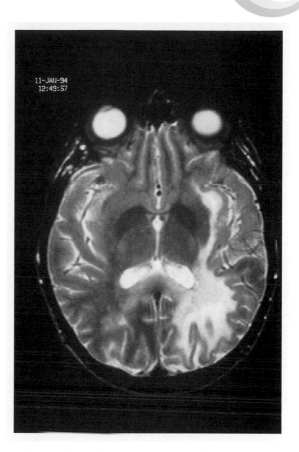

Fig. 25.5 MRI scan showing progressive multifocal leucoencephalopathy (PML).
Source: Conlon CP, Snydman DR. Mosby's Colour Atlas and Text of Infectious Diseases. Edinburgh: Mosby; 2000: Fig. 13.57.

Early HIV

In early HIV disease the infections experienced are:

- Shingles (varicella zoster virus) – see Chapter 14
- Oral candidiasis
- Recurrent herpes simplex infections.

The patients can also suffer with seborrhoeic dermatitis, which has been associated with the yeast *Pityrosporum ovale*. Typically the patient has discrete, erythematous lesions that may develop a yellow crust. The lesions occur in areas with hair follicles including the scalp and in skin folds, such as in the groins. Treatment is with topical steroids combined with an antifungal, such as combined hydrocortisone and clotrimoxazole, and ketoconazole shampoo if the scalp is affected.

Fig. 25.6 Opportunistic infections in relation to the CD4⁺ cell count.
Source: Conlon & Snydman, 2000: Fig. 13.40.

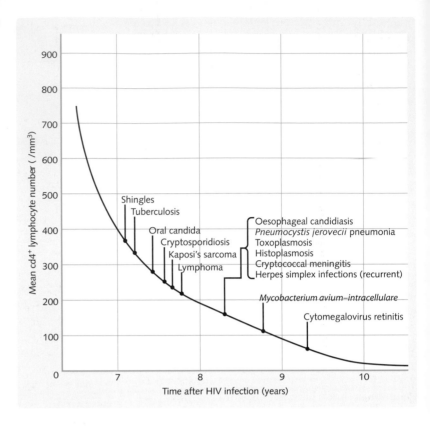

Oral candidiasis

Candidiasis is caused by the yeast *Candida albicans*. The oral lesions appear as white clods on the tongue (superior surface only) and hard palate. They can easily be removed, unlike the lesions of oral hairy leucoplakia. The treatment is with nystatin, either as a liquid to use as a mouthwash or pastilles to suck. Sometimes systemic treatment with oral azoles may be needed.

Herpes simplex virus 1 and 2 (HSV-1 and -2)

Chronic herpes simplex infections occur with a low CD4⁺ cell count and can disseminate around the body. When the infection is herpetic stomatitis, HSV-1 is usually responsible although HSV-2 may be the cause. Recurrent genital ulceration is more commonly due to HSV-2 but can result from HSV-1. The treatment is with aciclovir. Further details are given in Chapter 21.

HSV encephalitis – see Chapter 15.

Late HIV

The infections experienced in late HIV are detailed below in the decreasing order of frequency with which they tend to occur.

Oesophageal candidiasis

As with oral candidiasis, the organism responsible for the infection is *C. albicans*. The patients suffer with dysphagia (difficulty swallowing) and odynophagia (pain on swallowing). The investigation of choice is endoscopy, which shows an ulcerated oesophagus with plaques of *Candida* (see Fig. 25.7). A barium swallow may demonstrate a 'moth-eaten' oesophageal mucosa (see Fig. 12.6). The treatment for this more extensive candidiasis is with an oral azole, such as fluconazole.

Pneumocystis jerovecii **pneumonia (PCP)**

P. carinii has recently been renamed as *P. jerovecii*.

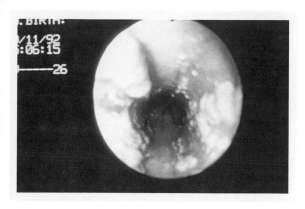

Fig. 25.7 Endoscopic appearance of *Candida*.
Source: Conlon & Snydman, 2000: Fig. 9.1.

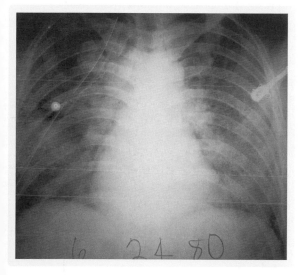

Fig. 25.8 Chest radiograph of Pneumocystis pneumonia in HIV infection.
Source: Conlon & Snydman, 2000: Fig. 13.45.

PCP is the most common infection to occur secondary to HIV infection.

Clinical features

The patient presents with dyspnoea (difficulty breathing), tachypnoea (raised respiratory rate), a dry cough and fever. The classical feature for PCP is that the oxygen saturations decrease on exertion.

Investigations

The chest radiograph may be normal or show a diffuse alveolar shadowing that typically spares the lower zones (see Fig. 25.8). Microscopy of bronchoalveolar (BAL) washings or biopsies of lung tissue can isolate the *P. jerovecii* organism, using a silver stain.

Treatment

The first choice of therapy for PCP is co-trimoxazole, usually given with high-dose steroids. Pentamidine is a second-line agent.

Prophylaxis

Patients who have previously had PCP or those who have a CD4$^+$ cell count less than 200×10^6/ml should receive prophylactic co-trimoxazole to prevent PCP.

Toxoplasmosis

Toxoplasmosis is caused by the protozoan *Toxoplasma gondii*. It can give rise to encephalitis and multiple cerebral abscesses.

Clinical features

The patient tends to present with either seizures or focal neurological deficits, such as a hemiparesis. These are often accompanied by headache and confusion.

Investigations

An MRI or CT scan of the head with contrast will demonstrate the multiple ring-enhancing lesions that are classical for toxoplasmosis. MRI is more sensitive than CT for detection of the lesions. Serology can confirm the diagnosis but the gold standard is to biopsy one of the brain lesions. This, however, is rarely done unless there is no response to treatment.

A single lesion on an MRI scan of the head is unusual in toxoplasmosis and an alternative cause should be sought. The differential diagnoses in an HIV-positive patient would include cerebral lymphoma, tuberculoma or focal cryptococcal infection.

Treatment

The treatment of choice for toxoplasmosis is a combination of pyrimethamine and sulphadiazine. Since pyrimethamine is a folate antagonist, patients usually require folic acid supplementation whilst on treatment. Patients are also given anticonvulsants to prevent seizures until treatment is completed. Alternative therapies are co-trimoxazole or a combination of clindamycin and primaquine.

Prophylaxis

Prophylaxis is required for HIV-positive patients following treatment. Prophylactic co-trimoxazole given to prevent PCP dramatically reduces infection rates for toxoplasmosis.

Cryptococcus neoformans

The typical cryptococcal infection is meningitis, although the fungi can infect other areas such as the lungs or disseminate. It is the most common cause of fungal meningitis.

Cryptococcal meningitis

Clinical features

The patient presents with the meningitis triad of symptoms, i.e. headache, neck stiffness and photophobia. These symptoms are often insidious in onset and may continue for several days before presentation. Seizures and focal neurological signs are uncommon.

Investigations

Those with suspected cryptococcal meningitis should have a lumbar puncture. Indian ink staining of the CSF reveals the fungi. The cryptococcal antigen test on CSF is a very useful rapid test and the fungus is easy to grow in culture. The biochemical results of the CSF are shown in Chapter 2.

Treatment

Cryptococcal meningitis should be treated initially with amphotericin B and flucytosine. Fluconazole can be used to complete therapy and for maintenance.

Mycobacterium tuberculosis

Tuberculosis is common in HIV-positive patients and is more likely to be disseminated (see Ch. 26).

Cryptosporidium parvum

Clinical features

The patient presents with severe chronic watery diarrhoea, which may produce profuse volumes. It tends to be associated with nausea, vomiting, anorexia and abdominal pain.

Investigations

Ziehl–Nielsen staining of a stool sample or tissue biopsy reveals the red cysts which are diagnostic for *C. parvum*.

Treatment

C. parvum has been treated with a variety of drugs, none of which convincingly alter the natural course of disease. However, recent studies have shown that a drug called nitozoxanide has significant beneficial effects.

Isospora belli

Clinical features

Patients present with severe diarrhoea and malabsorption.

Investigations

The *I. belli* oocysts can be identified in stool samples.

Treatment

I. belli responds to co-trimoxazole treatment.

Microsporidia

Clinical features

Microsporidia infection results in diarrhoea.

Investigations

The diagnosis is confirmed by identifying spores in stool samples with a fluorescent stain.

Treatment

Microsporidia are treated effectively with albendazole.

Atypical mycobacterial infections

The most commonly acquired atypical mycobacterium in HIV-positive patients is *M. avium-intracellulare* (MAI) complex.

MAI

Clinical features

The patient presents with the constitutional symptoms also seen in tuberculosis: weight loss, fevers, drenching night sweats and malaise. In addition, there are often an anaemia, abnormal liver function tests and chronic diarrhoea.

Investigations

Unlike *M. tuberculosis* MAI can often be cultured from blood. It can also be isolated from sputum, stool and biopsied tissue.

Treatment

MAI is often resistant to the standard quadruple therapy used to treat tuberculosis. It is usually treated with quinolones, such as ciprofloxacin; macrolides, such as azithromycin and clarithromycin; and the rifamycin: rifabutin.

Prophylaxis

Rifabutin was used for prophylaxis against MAI in those who had a low CD4+ cell count. Nowadays, one would hope to use antiretrovirals to improve the CD4$^+$ count.

Cytomegalovirus (CMV)

CMV can cause a disseminated infection in HIV and this can be life-threatening. CMV infections are more common in transplant patients whose immunocompromise is secondary to the drugs preventing rejection. An important infection not to miss is CMV retinitis because this is sight-threatening.

CMV retinitis

Clinical features
The patient can present with reduced acuity, floaters across the field of vision, visual field loss, orbital pain and in advanced cases blindness.

Diagnosis
The diagnosis is made clinically from the classical description of the retina on fundoscopy. It is referred to as the 'pizza pie' or 'tomato ketchup and cheese' retina, describing the haemorrhages and pale ischaemic areas seen respectively.

Treatment
CMV retinitis is treated initially with ganciclovir or valganciclovir. Maintenance therapy is with valganciclovir. Foscarnet is an alternative treatment and cidofovir is used when ganciclovir and foscarnet are contraindicated. These latter two drugs are nephrotoxic.

Ganciclovir can cause profound myelosuppression when given with zidovudine (AZT) and is therefore not appropriate to be used in combination.

Prophylaxis
Patients require lifelong prophylaxis against CMV retinitis once it has occurred unless the antiretroviral therapy they are taking can markedly improve their immune status.

CMV colitis

Clinical features
CMV colitis presents with abdominal pain that can mimic an acute appendicitis and bloody diarrhoea.

Investigations
A sigmoidoscopy reveals the ulcerated mucosa. Tissue taken from a rectal biopsy can demonstrate the inclusion bodies that are the hallmark of CMV colitis. These inclusion bodies confirm the diagnosis. A plain abdominal radiograph may show dilated loops of large bowel.

Treatment
CMV colitis is treated with ganciclovir.

CMV encephalitis

This is a rare cause of encephalitis.

Clinical features
The patient presents in the typical manner with the triad of meningitis symptoms, headache, neck stiffness and photophobia; and a decreased level of consciousness (see Ch. 15).

Investigations
PCR of the cerebrospinal fluid (CSF) can identify CMV as the causative organism.

Treatment
CMV encephalitis is extremely difficult to treat but may respond to ganciclovir.

CMV pneumonia

Although CMV pneumonitis occurs in immunocompromised hosts, such as bone marrow transplant recipients, it is a very rare cause of pneumonia in people with HIV.

Clinical features
The patient presents with a dry cough and similarly to PCP the oxygen saturations decrease on exertion.

Treatment
CMV pneumonia is treated with ganciclovir.

There are other conditions which occur frequently in HIV-positive patients but are not AIDS-defining:

Oral hairy leucoplakia

Oral hairy leucoplakia presents as white lesions on the tongue, which may be painful. It can be differentiated clinically from *Candida albicans* because it affects the lateral borders of the tongue unlike *C. albicans* and because it is more difficult to scrape from the tongue, whereas *C. albicans* is easily removed. It is associated with EBV infection. The treatment is with aciclovir, although there is a variable response.

Pneumococcal pneumonia

HIV-positive patients have an increased incidence of acquiring pneumonia caused by the encapsulated bacteria *Streptococcus pneumoniae*, see Chapter 17.

Aspergillus fumigatus

Aspergillus fumigatus tends to cause either an aspergilloma in an old lung cavity or invasive aspergillosis that can disseminate in HIV-positive patients. Invasive aspergillosis has a very poor prognosis.

Clinical features
The patient presents with shortness of breath and a dry cough. Haemoptysis can be massive if the *A. fumigatus* erodes into a pulmonary vessel.

Investigations
The diagnosis is suspected if the fungus is seen on microscopy of sputum or BAL specimens. The chest radiograph shows diffuse lung disease with invasive aspergillosis or an aspergilloma, which is a ball of fungus in an old lung cavity (e.g. from previous tuberculosis; see Fig. 12.3). However, the diagnosis is only proven by culturing the fungus from lung tissue or other sterile sites.

Treatment
Aspergillus fumigatus has been treated with amphotericin B or itraconazole in the past but newer drugs such as voriconazole and caspofungin are alternatives.

Giardiasis

Giardiasis is caused by *Giardia lamblia*. Further details are given in Chapter 24.

HIV enteritis

Clinical features
HIV enteritis presents with diarrhoea, malabsorption and marked weight loss.

Diagnosis
This is a diagnosis of exclusion, i.e. there is no other infective cause or pathology identified.

HIV infection and its consequences are continuously changing. New drugs are being brought to the market and there is increasing interest in immunomodulating therapy for this disease. Increasingly, more attention is paid to treating HIV than opportunistic infections as the latter are progressively becoming more rare, at least in developed countries.

Figure 25.9 provides a summary of HIV and opportunistic infections.

Further reading

Hammer SM. Management of newly acquired HIV infection. NEJM 2005; 353:1702–1710.

Kovacs JA, Masur H. Drug therapy: prophylaxis against opportunistic infections in patients with human immunodeficiency virus infection. N Engl J Med 2000; 342:1416–1429.

Fig. 25.9 Summary of HIV and more common, important opportunistic infections

Infection (organism)	Clinical features	Investigations	Treatment	Complications	Prevention
Human immunodeficiency virus, HIV (HIV-1 and -2)	Seroconversion illness: fever, malaise, myalgia, sore throat, lymphadenopathy, generalized maculopapular rash, diarrhoea, meningoencephalitis, radiculitis. Opportunistic infections	HIV testing: antibody and PCR. Viral load and CD4+ count. Lymphopenia	'HAART' involving at least three antiretroviral drugs	AIDS, opportunistic infections, tumours	Barrier contraception, reduced number of sexual partners. Blood product screening, not sharing needles amongst IVDUs. Post-exposure prophylaxis for needle-stick injuries. Antiretroviral therapy during pregnancy, caesarean section delivery, not breast-feeding
Candidiasis (*Candida albicans*)	Oral: white clods on the tongue, hard palate. Oesophageal: dysphagia, odynophagia	Oral: clinical Oesophageal: endoscopy, barium swallow	Oral: nystatin mouthwash or pastilles Oesophageal: oral azole, e.g. fluconazole	Oesophageal: systemic candidiasis	None
Pneumocystis jirovecii pneumonia, PCP (*Pneumocystis jirovecii*)	Dyspnoea, tachypnoea, dry cough, fever, oxygen desaturation with exercise	Microscopy of BAL washings, biopsied lung tissue with silver stain. CXR: diffuse alveolar shadowing	Co-trimoxazole with high-dose steroids. Pentamidine as alternative	Respiratory failure	Prophylactic co-trimoxazole if CD4+ count < 200×10^6/ml or previously infected
Toxoplasmosis (*Toxoplasma gondii*)	Seizures, focal neurological deficits, e.g. hemiparesis, headache, confusion	MRI or CT scan of the head with contrast: multiple ring-enhancing lesions. Serology. Brain biopsy	Pyrimethamine and sulphadiazine. Folic acid supplements, anticonvulsants	Encephalitis, epilepsy, focal neurological deficits, e.g. hemiparesis	Prophylactic co-trimoxazole
Cryptococcal meningitis (*Cryptococcus neoformans*)	Headache, neck stiffness, photophobia. Focal neurology, seizures uncommon	Lumbar puncture for CSF for biochemistry, microscopy (Indian ink), culture. Cryptococcal antigen test on CSF	Amphotericin B and flucytosine initially. Fluconazole for maintenance	Disseminated fungaemia, pneumonia	

(continued)

Fig. 25.9 Summary of HIV and more common, important opportunistic infections—*continued*

Infection (organism)	Clinical features	Investigations	Treatment	Complications	Prevention
Atypical mycobacterial infections (e.g. *M. avium-intracellulare*)	Weight loss, fevers, drenching night sweats, malaise, anaemia, chronic diarrhoea	Blood, sputum, stool and biopsied tissue for culture. LFTs	Quinolones, e.g. ciprofloxacin; macrolides, e.g. azithromycin, clarithromycin; the rifamycin: rifabutin	Disseminated infection	Rifabutin in the past, now aim to increase CD4+ count with HAART
Cytomegalovirus, CMV (cytomegalovirus)	Retinitis: reduced acuity, floaters, visual field loss, orbital pain. Colitis: abdominal pain, bloody diarrhoea	Retinitis: fundoscopy Colitis: sigmoidoscopy, histology of rectal biopsy tissue. AXR	Retinitis: ganciclovir or valganciclovir initially. Maintenance therapy valganciclovir. Foscarnet, cidofovir are alternatives Colitis: ganciclovir	Disseminated infection, death. Loss of sight from CMV retinitis. Rarely, infection causes encephalitis, pneumonia	CMV retinitis: lifelong prophylaxis required once infected, unless significant rise in CD4+ count. Drug choice requires specialist advice
Aspergilloma or invasive aspergillosis (*Aspergillus fumigatus*)	Shortness of breath, dry cough, massive haemoptysis	Microscopy of sputum, BAL washing; culture of lung tissue. CXR: aspergilloma or diffuse lung disease	Amphotericin B, itraconazole, voriconazole or caspofungin	Massive haemoptysis, death from invasive aspergillosis	None

Objectives

In this chapter you will learn:

- How tuberculosis develops
- The factors that may predispose to reactivation of old tuberculosis
- The constitutional symptoms of tuberculosis
- The high-risk groups for developing tuberculosis
- What investigations to order for someone suspected to have pulmonary tuberculosis
- The side-effects associated with the first-line antituberculous drugs.

Tuberculosis is caused by *Mycobacterium tuberculosis*. Worldwide, tuberculosis is the infection with the highest mortality rate: 2 million deaths per year according to the WHO (World Health Organization). In 1993 the WHO declared tuberculosis a global emergency. In order to comprehend the scale of the problem: the WHO estimate that between 2002 and 2020 there will be approximately 1000 million people who will become newly infected, over 150 million people who will fall ill and 36 million who will die. In the UK there are over 7000 cases reported per year.

The *M. tuberculosis* organisms are acid–alcohol-fast bacilli (AAFB) due to the impermeability of their cell wall. This enables the bacilli to resist the host immune system, even reproduce within phagocytic cells, and results in the caseating (cheese-like) granulomas that typify tuberculosis. Diagnostically it means that the bacteria cannot be identified from Gram staining like most others but require different techniques involving either the Ziehl–Nielsen stain or auramine staining.

PATHOGENESIS

M. tuberculosis is usually spread via aerosol droplets; hence the predominance of primary tuberculosis in the lungs. When the bacteria are inhaled they become deposited in the lung alveoli. The alveolar macrophages are the front line of the immune response and phago-cytose the bacteria. As mentioned above, the mycobac-terial cell wall protects the organisms from intracellular digestion and even allows them to multiply within the macrophages. The mycobacteria are carried by the macrophages to the draining hilar lymph nodes, which

enlarge in response to the infection. The local periph-eral lung lesion and the enlarged draining hilar lymph nodes are known as the 'Ghon focus' and constitute primary tuberculosis (see Fig. 26.1). In both these areas the immune reaction results in the classic caseating granulomas, which heal with fibrosis and often calcify. A small number of AAFB remain dormant in the lesions once they have healed and can be reactivated many years later when the host immunity is impaired.

> The causes of reactivation of tuberculosis include steroid therapy and other immunosuppressant drugs, malignancies, diabetes mellitus, malnutrition, HIV infection, chronic ill health and as part of normal ageing.

Those with an impaired immune system are unable to overcome the primary infection and the mycobacteria spread either locally within the lung or via the bloodstream to other sites (Fig. 26.2). The pulmonary sequelae of tuberculosis are:

- A parenchymal infection
- Pleural effusions
- Tuberculous empyema
- Bronchiectasis
- Aspergilloma in an old tuberculous cavity
- Haemoptysis (massive if there is erosion into a blood vessel in the wall of a cavity)
- Collapse of lobes of the lung secondary to bronchial compression by enlarged lymph nodes.

When the right middle lobe collapses due to lymph node enlargement and bronchiectasis develops distally, this is known as Brock's syndrome.

Extrapulmonary tuberculosis can occur independently of pulmonary tuberculosis as both a primary infection or as a result of reactivation. The most common site for extrapulmonary tuberculosis is in the gastrointestinal tract at the ileocaecal region. Other areas involved include lymph nodes, meninges, kidneys, bone, joints, the skin and the peritoneum. Miliary tuberculosis describes the dissemination of tiny foci of mycobacteria throughout the body.

HISTORY

The majority of patients will be unaware of the primary infection as they do not suffer any symptoms. A few will complain of a dry cough or develop erythema nodosum (see Ch. 1). It is the constitutional symptoms of tuberculosis, irrespective of the site of infection, that tend to cause patients to seek medical attention. These are:

- Fevers, with or without rigors
- Drenching night sweats
- Marked weight loss
- General malaise and lethargy

and have usually lasted for several months before presentation. The significant weight loss that occurs with tuberculosis is the reason this disease was known as 'consumption' in the 19th century.

The type of tuberculosis determines the rather more specific symptoms that may accompany the constitutional ones and help the clinician localize the affected areas (see Fig. 26.3).

RISK FACTORS

Once tuberculosis is suspected, the patient should be asked about potential risk factors for acquiring tuberculosis. These include:

- Contacts from a known case of pulmonary tuberculosis
- HIV infection
- Immunosuppression from drug therapy, e.g. steroids, cytotoxic chemotherapy, or from malignancies, e.g. lymphoma
- Immigrants or travellers from countries with a high prevalence of tuberculosis, such as the Indian subcontinent, Eastern Europe, Russia and sub-Saharan Africa

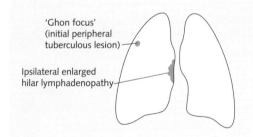

'Ghon focus'
(initial peripheral
tuberculous lesion)

Ipsilateral enlarged
hilar lymphadenopathy

Fig. 26.1 Diagram of Ghon focus on chest radiograph.

Fig. 26.2 The stages and variations of tuberculosis.

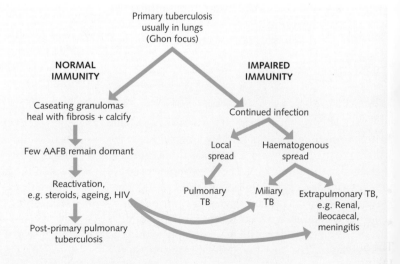

Primary tuberculosis
usually in lungs
(Ghon focus)

NORMAL IMMUNITY

IMPAIRED IMMUNITY

Caseating granulomas
heal with fibrosis + calcify

Continued infection

Few AAFB remain dormant

Local spread

Haematogenous spread

Reactivation,
e.g. steroids, ageing, HIV

Pulmonary TB

Miliary TB

Extrapulmonary TB,
e.g. Renal,
ileocaecal,
meningitis

Post-primary pulmonary
tuberculosis

Fig. 26.3 Signs and symptoms of tuberculosis

	Symptoms	Signs
Pulmonary TB	Cough productive of purulent sputum Haemoptysis Shortness of breath	Often nil to auscultate, but can have coarse crepitations (usually lung apices affected) Pleural effusion
Extrapulmonary TB CNS: meningitis	Neck stiffness Headache Photophobia	Neck stiffness, Kernig's sign
Eyes: choroiditis	Blurred vision Ocular pain unusual Red eyes	Reduced visual acuity Ciliary injection
Skin: lupus vulgaris	Brown lesions, may have ulcers	Brown plaques which may ulcerate; can occur at mucocutaneous junctions
Lymph nodes, including scrofula	Swollen glands in neck or groin which may discharge pus via a sinus to skin	Cervical or inguinal lymphadenopathy with sinuses discharging purulent material (cold abscesses)
CVS: constrictive pericarditis	Chest pain Shortness of breath	Pericardial rub if no effusion Quiet heart sounds with an effusion Signs of heart failure
GI: ileocaecal	Abdominal pain	Mass in right iliac fossa
GI: peritoneal	Distended abdomen	Ascites
Adrenals: Addison's disease	Weakness, collapse Nausea, vomiting, diarrhoea Abdominal pain Myalgia Confusion	Postural hypotension Pigmentation, e.g. buccal, scars, palmar creases Dehydration
GU: renal	Dysuria Haematuria	Sterile pyuria
Skeletal: arthritis and osteomyelitis	Joint/bone pain Inability to weight-bear	Localized swelling (not hot, i.e. cold abscess) Localized pain

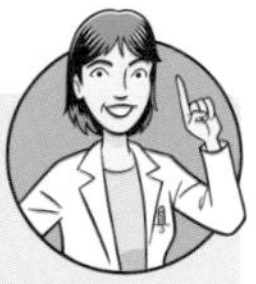

It is highly important to ascertain from the history if there is a risk of multidrug-resistant tuberculosis (MDR TB). Patients who have not completed their full course of antituberculous chemotherapy or had poor compliance with the treatment course; those in contact with a case of MDR TB or from a country with a high prevalence of MDR TB are especially at risk.

- Patients who have spent a significant time in an institution, e.g. prison
- Homeless or malnourished individuals.

The other factor which is important to consider when taking a history is whether the patient has ever received the BCG (bacille Calmette–Guérin) vaccination and at what age, as this can affect the interpretation of some investigations.

GENERAL EXAMINATION

Classically a patient with tuberculosis looks cachectic with a gaunt face, from the marked weight loss. This is, of course, dependent on the premorbid nutritional status and the time period for which the person has had tuberculosis. Some patients develop erythema nodosum in association with the infection. The other signs depend on the site involved by the tuberculosis and are described in Figure 26.3.

INVESTIGATIONS

Tuberculosis can be notoriously difficult to diagnose. The problems arise because there is no gold standard test and the tests available have poor sensitivity and specificity for *M. tuberculosis*. There are numerous environmental mycobacteria which are in general not pathogenic to immunocompetent humans but can contaminate test specimens, although they may be of significance in immunocompromised patients.

The mainstay of diagnosing tuberculosis involves isolating *M. tuberculosis* by microscopy or culture. The specimens used for microscopy and culture depend on the potential source of infection. For microscopy there are two stains used for AAFB:

- Ziehl–Nielsen (ZN) – AAFB are stained red
- Auramine – AAFB fluoresce golden yellow. This is more sensitive than ZN.

In order to culture AAFB there are two types of culture media available:

- Liquid media, e.g. Bactec
- Solid media, e.g. Lowenstein–Jensen.

The significant difference between the two media is the time taken for the *M. tuberculosis* to grow: 10 days for the liquid medium compared with 6 weeks for the solid medium, but the disadvantage of the liquid medium is that the exact mycobacterial species cannot be determined. Testing for the drug sensitivities of the *M. tuberculosis* takes a further 2 weeks from when the culture becomes positive.

For a suspected case of pulmonary TB the AAFB may be obtained from sputum in those who have a productive cough, otherwise induced sputum, bronchoalveolar lavage (BAL) washings from a bronchoscopy or early-morning gastric lavage specimens can be sent for analysis. The gastric lavage is done early in the morning on the basis that overnight lung secretions are brought up and swallowed so the greatest concentration of bacteria should be present in the morning. This can be a useful technique in children who are less able to produce sputum. Given the detection rate is poor, at least three separate sputum specimens, ideally from consecutive days, are required. If on microscopy there are no AAFB seen in all three specimens then the person would be termed 'smear negative' for tuberculosis, and if the cultures are also negative then the person is 'culture negative'. Some patients are 'smear negative' and 'culture positive' but it is unusual to have the opposite combination.

For suspected cases of extrapulmonary tuberculosis, the specimens relevant to the symptoms are used for microscopy and culture, e.g. CSF (cerebrospinal fluid) for tuberculous meningitis, early-morning urine specimens (EMUs) for renal tuberculosis, ascitic fluid for peritoneal tuberculosis (although there is a very poor detection rate), aspirated joint fluid for a tuberculous septic arthritis. In cases of suspected tuberculous meningitis, the CSF should also be examined for protein and glucose levels, as these are characteristic for different organisms causing meningitis (see Ch. 2).

It is of note that *M. tuberculosis* is rarely grown from routine blood cultures but this may occur in the setting of immunosuppression, such as HIV disease.

In some cases a tissue biopsy may be the most appropriate specimen, e.g. peritoneal biopsy for peritoneal TB, a lymph node for scrofula, or bone marrow and lymph node biopsies for miliary tuberculosis. The biopsied tissue should be examined histologically as well as being cultured. The histological examination will show caseating granulomas with giant Langhan's cells in cases of tuberculosis.

Radiological imaging can be an important part of establishing the diagnosis of tuberculosis, most of all in pulmonary tuberculosis. The chest radiograph can demonstrate apical fibrosis with cavitation and paratracheal and hilar lymphadenopathy (see Fig. 26.4).

In some cases the chest radiograph may not be conclusive and a CT scan of the chest may be required. A CT scan of the abdomen and pelvis can be useful in revealing peritoneal thickening, ascites, lymphadenopathy, renal and genital tract involvement. A CT or MRI scan of the head may highlight meningeal thickening in cases of meningitis, in addition to ascertaining that it is safe to perform a lumbar puncture to obtain CSF for microscopy and culture.

Skin testing with either the Heaf or Mantoux test can be done as part of the investigations for diagnosis but is more commonly used in the management of contacts of an index case, see below. The Heaf test involves injecting tuberculin purified protein derivative in a circle of six dots using a stamp into the patient's forearm and 48 hours later looking at the erythematous response and grading this from 0 to 4 (see Fig. 26.5). The Mantoux test entails injecting a set volume of tuberculin purified protein derivative intradermally into the upper arm and measuring the diameter of the swelling at 48 hours. There are three grades of diameter – less than 5 mm, 5–10 mm, and greater than 10 mm – which have a varying significance depending on the local prevalence of tuberculosis and whether the individual has received BCG vaccination.

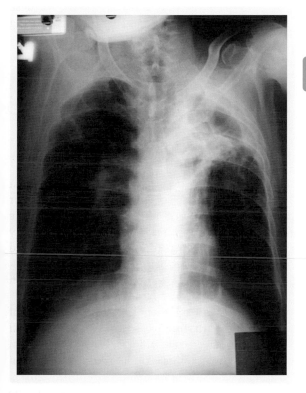

Fig. 26.4 Chest radiograph of tuberculosis.

There is currently research into an ELISA (enzyme-linked immunosorbent assay) technique diagnostic test for tuberculosis, called Elispot, which is not yet available clinically but appears promising. Last of all, in cases where the suspicion for tuberculosis remains high despite an inability to isolate the organism or obtain convincing radiological evidence of tuberculosis, a trial of antituberculous therapy may be warranted as an investigation.

Because tuberculosis is intimately associated with HIV, it is recommended that all patients diagnosed with tuberculosis be offered HIV counselling and testing (see Ch. 25).

TREATMENT

The treatment of tuberculosis involves the use of at least three active drugs to ensure resistance does not develop. Quadruple therapy with rifampicin, isoniazid, pyrazinamide and ethambutol is now recommended by NICE (National Institute for Clinical Excellence) as the standard treatment in the UK. Previously triple therapy was commonly used, with the addition of ethambutol reserved for cases where there was concern about isoniazid resistance. MDR TB requires complex regimens and expert advice.

The main side-effects of the antituberculous drugs are shown in Figure 26.6. The liver function tests can become deranged to five times normal before the drugs have to be stopped, but this needs to be monitored. The orange colouring of all bodily secretions with rifampicin can be used as a way of monitoring whether patients are actually taking their medication. It is a problem for contact lens wearers, though, who have to revert to wearing glasses.

Fig. 26.5 Heaf and Mantoux tests.

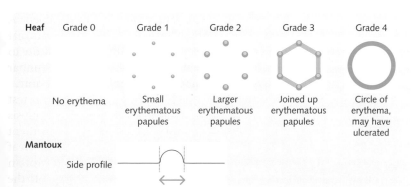

Fig. 26.6 Antituberculous drugs and their main side-effects

Drug	Side-effect	Action required
Rifampicin	Hepatitis Orange bodily fluids Enzyme inducer	Check liver function tests Reassure Contraceptive advice if uses pill
Isoniazid	Hepatitis Interstitial nephritis Peripheral neuropathy Agranulocytosis	Check liver function tests Check renal function Give pyridoxine 10 mg daily Check WCC differential
Pyrazinamide	Hepatitis Arthralgia	Check liver function tests Stop if gout develops
Ethambutol	Retrobulbar optic neuritis	Ophthalmology review

The regimen for taking antituberculous chemotherapy depends on which type of tuberculosis the patient has: pulmonary tuberculosis requires a total of 6 months' therapy with 2 months of all the drugs and then 4 months of just rifampicin and isoniazid. Most types of extrapulmonary tuberculosis, e.g. lymph nodes, joints, abdominal TB, genitourinary TB, are treated with the same regimen as pulmonary tuberculosis. However, spinal tuberculosis with spinal cord involvement and tuberculosis affecting the central nervous system (CNS), e.g. meninges, necessitate a course of 12 months of therapy, again with a reduction of drugs to just rifampicin and isoniazid part way through the course. At the time of going to press, the NICE guidelines for tuberculosis were still in consultation and there were varied opinions on the treatment regimens for extrapulmonary and miliary tuberculosis in particular. As a result, practices will probably vary from hospital to hospital, but local guidelines should be followed. Miliary tuberculosis has classically been treated with a total of 9–12 months of therapy (with tailoring of the number of drugs part way through the course) but the proposed NICE guidelines were suggesting a shorter course of just 6 months, unless there was meningeal involvement, which should be actively searched for.

In proven or suspected cases of MDR TB, each drug for which there is resistance needs to be replaced with at least two of the second-line drugs, such as the aminoglycosides: amikacin or streptomycin; the quinolones: levofloxacin or moxifloxacin; the macrolides: clarithromycin or azithromycin; and other older drugs such as PAS, cycloserine or ethionamide. In these cases a greater number of drugs are continued throughout the course of treatment and treatment usually must be given for 18–24 months.

If patients are poorly compliant with therapy, then DOT (directly observed therapy) may be beneficial both to them for clearing the infection and to the public in preventing further spread. DOT involves the patient swallowing the medication while being observed by a responsible person. The drug dosages are adjusted from the usual daily amount for this thrice-weekly regimen.

PUBLIC HEALTH

Tuberculosis is a notifiable disease and therefore all cases must be notified to the local Public Health Department. Their role is for contact tracing: following up any potential contacts of the index case of tuberculosis. This is usually only important in cases of pulmonary tuberculous, particularly 'smear-positive' cases, when the infection risk to others is greatest. Contacts identified as being at risk of contracting tuberculosis should have a Mantoux skin test and a chest radiograph to assess if they are infected or require prophylactic treatment. All children under the age of 2 years in close contact, e.g. living in the same household as a case of 'smear-positive' or open tuberculosis, should receive a course of treatment.

PROPHYLAXIS

Antituberculous prophylaxis is recommended for those who become positive on skin testing after contact with a case of tuberculosis and those children who are identified as positive with Heaf or Mantoux testing when screened prior to BCG vaccination. Children and adults not vaccinated with BCG, immigrating to the UK with a positive Mantoux test may be recommended a course of prophylaxis. The currently recommended regimen is either isoniazid alone for 6 months or rifampicin and isoniazid combined for 3 months.

In the UK the BCG vaccine was routinely administered to children between the ages of 10 and 14 years if they had a Heaf Grade 0 or 1, but this is under review with the NICE guidelines consultation. Neonates deemed at high risk, e.g. born to immigrant parents, are vaccinated at birth. Vaccination is also recommended for those who are Mantoux-negative contacts of a case of open pulmonary tuberculosis, Mantoux-negative immigrants from high-risk areas, and health workers including students in the clinical setting.

Information on tuberculosis is summarized in Figure 26.7.

Further reading

Frieden TR, Sterling TR, Munsiff SS, et al. Tuberculosis. Lancet 2003; 362:887–899.

Joint Tuberculosis Committee of the British Thoracic Society. Chemotherapy and management of tuberculosis in the United Kingdom: recommendations 1998. Thorax 1998; 53(7):536–548.

Joint Tuberculosis Committee of the British Thoracic Society. Guidelines. Website: www.brit-thoracic.org.uk.

NICE. Guidelines on tuberculosis. Website: www.nice.org.uk.

Thwaites GE, Bang ND, Dung NH, et al. Dexamethasone for the treatment of tuberculous meningitis in adolescents and adults. N Engl J Med 2004; 351:1741–1751.

Fig. 26.7 Summary of tuberculosis

Infection (organism)	Types	Clinical features	Investigations	Treatment	Complications	Prophylaxis
Tuberculosis (*Mycobacterium tuberculosis*)	Pulmonary tuberculosis	Constitutional symptoms: fever ± rigors, drenching night sweats, marked weight loss, malaise, lethargy, erythema nodosum. Productive cough, haemoptysis, dyspnoea	Microscopy and culture of sputum, induced sputum, BAL washings, early-morning gastric lavage specimens. CXR, CT chest. Heaf or Mantoux testing. HIV testing	Quadruple therapy with rifampicin, isoniazid, pyrazinamide and ethambutol for 2 months then 4 months of just rifampicin and isoniazid	Extrapulmonary, miliary tuberculosis. Death	BCG vaccination. Chemoprophylaxis with isoniazid (6 months) or isoniazid and rifampicin (3 months) for contacts becoming skin-test positive, or skin-test positive, non-BCG-vaccinated immigrants to the UK
	Extrapulmonary tuberculosis, e.g. GI tract, lymph nodes	Constitutional symptoms. See Figure 26.3 for specific clinical features	e.g. CSF, early-morning urine specimens, ascitic fluid, synovial fluid, biopsied tissue for microscopy and culture. Histology of tissue. Appropriate radiological imaging, e.g. CT abdomen or CT brain. Heaf or Mantoux testing. HIV testing	As pulmonary TB, except spinal TB with spinal cord affected or TB affecting the meninges when total of 12 months' therapy needed. Reduction from four drugs to just rifampicin and isoniazid part way through course	Miliary tuberculosis. Death	
	Miliary tuberculosis	Constitutional symptoms. Also, e.g. cough, abdominal pain, lymphadenopathy, meningitis depending on sites of involvement	Microscopy and culture of any appropriate specimens, e.g. BAL washings, CSF, biopsied tissue. Appropriate radiological imaging, e.g. CXR, CT chest, USS abdomen. Heaf or Mantoux testing. HIV testing	Total of 6–12 months' therapy needed (opinions vary). Reduction from four drugs to just rifampicin and isoniazid part way through course	Death	

HISTORY, EXAMINATION AND COMMON INVESTIGATIONS

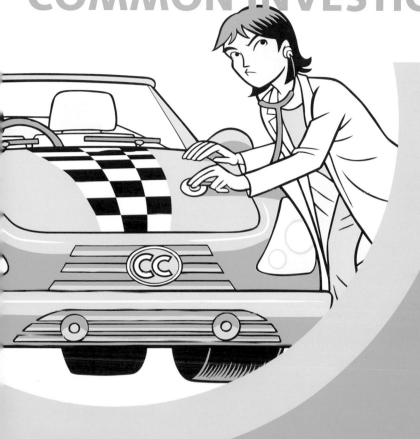

It is a great skill to be able to take a good history and something everyone needs to practise. Each person will develop their own style of eliciting the relevant information. The areas outlined below give a structure to what needs to be covered.

INTRODUCTION

It is vitally important that you introduce yourself to the patient and explain clearly who you are and what you are going to do. The setting for the interview should ideally be private, after all hospital cubicle curtains are not soundproof!

Not all patients presenting with infectious diseases will speak English as their first language. Often a family member will act as a translator, which is very helpful in the acute setting, but may not always be appropriate or facilitate relevant information being divulged. It may therefore be appropriate to organize to have an independent professional translator.

SCENE-SETTING INFORMATION

There are some initial factual pieces of information which help to set the scene for the rest of the history. These include:

- Age of patient
- Sex
- Ethnic origin and country of birth
- Occupation
- Marital status.

If there is a neurological element to the presenting complaint, then whether the patient is left- or right-handed may be important.

PRESENTING COMPLAINT (PC)

This is the main problem precipitating the consultation or admission. It is best to document this as the patient actually describes it rather than your interpretation. For example, a patient may complain of having red eyes, which could be due to haemorrhage from a viral haemorrhagic illness or could be from inflammation that may be infective, such as a bacterial conjunctivitis, or non-infective as part of Reiter's syndrome. Equally important is to clarify any medical terms the patient uses to ensure both patient and clinician understand each other. For example, a rigor describes the vigorous and uncontrollable shaking associated with a fever as opposed to shivering which is much milder.

HISTORY OF PRESENTING COMPLAINT (HPC)

Chronology

Clarity in the history of the onset and progression of the patient's symptoms is essential to being able to hone down to a list of potential diagnoses. The relative timing of the different symptoms can be important too. For example, a young child with coryzal symptoms and fever who a few days later develops a maculopapular rash is more likely to have measles than a child who develops a similar rash concurrently with the coryzal symptoms and fever when the diagnosis may be a non-specific viral upper respiratory tract infection. If patients have difficulty in deciding how a problem started, then a useful approach can be to ask when they last felt well.

Precipitants

It is always worth asking whether the patient has ever experienced anything similar and what the diagnosis was then. Often patients have their own idea of potential precipitants or causes that may be important, and exploring these can elicit other relevant factors. For example, a diabetic man may be concerned that he has not been able to look after his diabetes as well since starting a new job involving night shift work. As part of the discussion it transpires he now has regulation footwear as well, which has resulted in a foot ulcer. The ulcer may be a culmination of a worsening sensory neuropathy, secondary to less tight glycaemic control, in addition to increased tiredness from shift work and more hypoglycaemic episodes resulting in the patient checking his feet less often.

Risk factors

If the patient's symptoms particularly suggest a condition or group of infections, then asking about other associated features or the risk factors becomes pertinent. For example, it would be relevant to ask patients describing a productive cough and fever whether they had dyspnoea, chest pain and a reduced exercise tolerance as well as risk factors for pneumonia such as chronic obstructive pulmonary disease (COPD), working in a coal mine or an office with air conditioning, parrots as pets or a hobby racing pigeons.

Impact

The impact of patients' symptoms on their lifestyle is another area to explore. It may well be associated to the timing of a consultation or admission: either related to when symptoms become intolerable or socially embarrassing; or that the patients or their carers can no longer cope at home.

PAST MEDICAL HISTORY (PMH)

A comprehensive PMH may reveal previous medical problems or interventions that crucially affect the possible diagnoses or management. If the details are not spontaneously given it is not usually that patients wish to hide this information but merely that they do not realize the relevance. Topics to enquire about are:

- Previous infections, especially if the symptoms were similar to the current presenting complaints.
- Immunizations, especially in children and if there has been foreign travel.
- Previous operations and procedures, in particular if there is any residual prosthetic material, since this can be a source or reservoir of infection.
- Splenectomy or sickle cell disease, since these patients are more vulnerable to encapsulated bacterial infections.
- Heart valve disease or valvular surgery, as these are risk factors for endocarditis.

- Malignancy and any treatment received; if chemotherapy has been used then the dates of each course and the drugs involved determine the likelihood of neutropenic sepsis or other complications.
- Other chronic conditions that may influence the infections to which the patient is vulnerable, such as COPD or diabetes mellitus. In some chronic conditions the symptoms may reflect a flare-up or be due to an infective cause, for example a diarrhoeal episode in a patient with inflammatory bowel disease (IBD), and given that the management is markedly different, it is important to distinguish between the two.

DRUG HISTORY (DH)

The drug history should include everything the patient takes, i.e. all prescribed medications as well as over-the-counter remedies and complementary health therapies. It is not sufficient just to have a list of the prescribed drugs; this needs to include the doses and frequency at which they are taken – ideally, how the drugs are actually taken as opposed to what is directed. Discussing the drug schedule may bring out problems experienced with the timing of doses related to the patient's lifestyle and will be important for the clinician to address in order to encourage cooperation with the prescribed therapy. With elderly patients, it is helpful to ascertain whether they can manage their tablets or whether they have a dosette box.

A good mnemonic for remembering all the aspects of a drug history is:

D – Doctor prescribed

R – Reactions, i.e. allergies

U – Unprescribed, i.e. over-the-counter remedies and complementary health therapies

G – Gynaecological, e.g. oral contraceptive pill (OCP) and hormone replacement therapy (HRT); patients often tend not to mention these unless directly asked

S – Social, i.e. illicit drug habit (see Social history).

In particular with an infectious disease case, it is worth asking if the patient is taking any immuno-suppressive drugs, such as steroids or azathioprine, as these patients will be vulnerable to a broader range of organisms. Also enquiring about previous antibiotic therapy with dosages may be helpful, especially in larger patients, because if only low doses have been used (may be the limitation of oral prescribing) then a lack of response may not be as a result of a resistant organism but inadequate blood levels of the antibiotic. In very sick patients, though, the clinician would not want to repeat using a drug that had already been unsuccessful. In patients presenting with a pyrexia of unknown origin (PUO), any changes in medications may be relevant as some drugs can produce a fever, such as carbapenems.

ALLERGIES

Patients should be asked if they have ever experienced any allergic reaction to a medication and, vitally, what the effect was. After all, an episode of diarrhoea after a course of antibiotics is a side-effect not an allergic reaction. The reason for splitting hairs over this issue is that a patient should not be denied potentially life-saving therapy because of an incorrectly documented 'allergy' that in fact is not.

Many patients are allergic to penicillin. It is therefore crucial to remember that the penicillin group of drugs includes the carbapenems, such as meropenem, and that co-amoxiclav is amoxicillin with clavulinic acid. There is also a 10% crossover of allergic reactions between the penicillin group and the cephalosporins, e.g. cefuroxime and ceftriaxone. If the reaction to penicillin is severe, for example anaphylaxis rather than just a skin rash, then it would not be safe to trial using any cephalosporin.

FAMILY HISTORY (FH)

Patients should be sensitively asked if any of their close family, such as parents, siblings, children and grandparents, have suffered any serious illnesses or died. The age at death and the cause of death needs to be ascertained.

SOCIAL HISTORY (SH)

The social history may necessarily cover a broad range of aspects of a patient's life. The detail of the different elements will depend on the presenting complaints. Areas to consider are:

- Smoking – whether patients have ever smoked and if so how much they have smoked. The best way to express the amount is in 'pack years'.
- Alcohol – the consumption of alcohol on a weekly basis quoted in units and whether, in the patient's view, consumption has ever been heavy. The type of beverage may be relevant, for example more concern would be raised from large volumes of spirits or Special Brew, a high alcohol content beer.
- Travel – the places overseas the patient has visited, including stopovers on journeys. For tropical destinations, whether the patient had received the appropriate vaccinations and taken malaria prophylaxis correctly if required. The types of activities undertaken may also be relevant, such as swimming in Lake Malawi for schistosomiasis or walking in the Black Forest for Lyme disease. It is important to ask if anyone else is similarly affected and whether anyone was ill whilst abroad.
- Job – the environment of the job may influence the patient's health, for example a dusty building site, a chemical factory or forestry work. There may be other specific job-related risk factors such as animal contact or working at a sewage plant.
- Accommodation – whether the patient has adequate housing or is homeless and sleeping rough. The health of any fellow residents may be relevant, such as a child with chickenpox when the patient has never had the infection.
- Support network – in terms of psychological well-being and practical help. Areas to cover are whether the family lives locally and how available they are for helping, family dynamics relating to the patient, and other sources of help, such as neighbours, friends or social services.
- Social services – how much help is given in terms of numbers of carers and the number of times a day they visit; which services have been accessed,

A single 'pack year' is 20 cigarettes smoked per day for a year. Therefore someone who smoked 30 cigarettes a day for 30 years has a 45 pack year smoking history. The following measures are equivalents of 1 unit of alcohol: small glass of wine, half pint of beer, and one shot of spirits.

for example meals-on-wheels, home assessment by Occupational Therapy with the necessary modifications made and aids supplied.

- Mobility – whether patients require a walking frame or wheelchair. If patients are bed-bound, can they turn themselves, and who cares for pressure areas.
- Time spent in institutions – certain infections are more prevalent in institutions, such as tuberculosis in prison, hepatitis A in homes for the severely disabled.
- Illicit drug use – which drugs are taken, the size of the habit and how this is funded. Prostitution may be a concern. For intravenous drug users (IVDUs), issues related to needle sharing, hepatitis B, C and HIV status, rehabilitation programmes and previous use of methadone need to be covered. It is also important to ascertain whether the general practitioner is prepared to prescribe methadone on discharge or whether there are other possible clinics to attend for this before it is started in hospital.
- Sexual history – it may not be appropriate to discuss this on the first meeting or until a more private environment can be found. Although many students may initially find this an awkward topic to discuss, a patient with genital symptoms will be expecting to be questioned.
- Pets – what, if any, animals/birds, reptiles are kept.
- Hobbies – any hobbies that may entail risk factors for infections, such as water contact, pigeon racing or walking through forests.
- Diet – particular diets can influence health, such as veganism, or it may be important for religious reasons that the correct food is supplied in hospital, for example halal meat.

SYSTEMS REVIEW

At the end of the history it is good practice to run through a screening set of questions covering the main body systems to check there are not aspects the patient has forgotten to mention. Examples would be:

- Cardiovascular – chest pain, ankle oedema, orthopnoea
- Respiratory – cough, dyspnoea, wheeze, haemoptysis
- Abdominal – pain, change of bowel habit, blood loss
- Neurological – headaches, visual disturbances, loss of dexterity
- Musculoskeletal – arthralgia, myalgia, difficulty weight-bearing
- Skin – rashes, ulcers, bite marks.

DIFFERENTIAL DIAGNOSIS LIST

By the end of the history the information gleaned should be formulated into the most likely possible diagnoses.

Formulating a list of differential diagnoses also helps to focus the clinician's mind on which signs might be expected on examination, or those to specifically look out for.

The purpose of the examination is to elicit signs to enable the clinician to refine the list of differential diagnoses made from the history, although keeping an open mind is essential so that additional features are not missed.

The patient should be put at ease for an examination. A warm, private room with clean linen on the bed and good lighting is the ideal setting. The use of clear, easily understandable instructions is important both for the clinician to carry out a slick examination and for the patient to feel comfortable and not mauled by the end. Before starting, it is essential to ask patients if they have any pain and be respectful of this.

The use of chaperones for examinations is essential when there is to be an intimate examination. It is prudent to have a chaperone for all examinations of patients of the opposite sex, to prevent any allegations of professional misconduct. This may not always be practical in the real world, but if in doubt or you sense the patient is not comfortable with the proposed examination, offer a chaperone or consult your senior team members. Always get a chaperone for examination of the genital area.

GENERAL INSPECTION

Every examination should begin with standing at the end of the bed and inspecting the patient. This can give a gross impression of whether the patient is well or unwell. More specifically look for:

- Flushed face, dilated peripheries, sweating – reflecting a septic patient
- Mottled cool peripheries, clammy – reflecting a patient whose circulation is shut down
- Eyes kept closed – may be due to photophobia suggesting meningitis

- Restless, distressed patient – may result from pain, as with pyelonephritis when the patient cannot seem to get comfortable
- Cachexia – seen with tuberculosis and cancer patients
- Obesity – need to consider pressure areas and fungal infections in the skin folds
- Jaundice – occurs in some liver and biliary tract infections
- Anaemia – complicates malaria and hookworm infections amongst others
- Skin – rashes, cellulitic areas, abscesses, fungal infections including in the scalp.

A sick patient with a purpuric rash should ring alarm bells with the examiner for meningococcal septicaemia. A rapid assessment of the patient, immediate involvement of senior medical staff and intravenous antibiotic therapy is vital to prevent serious complications and death.

BEDSIDE ACCESSORIES

There may be many clues around the bedside as to the condition of patients and the severity of their current illness.

- Oxygen mask – suggests respiratory or cardiac compromise
- Inhalers and peak flow meter – possible exacerbation of asthma or chronic obstructive pulmonary disease (COPD)
- Drip stand with intravenous fluids or antibiotics attached – patient more unwell since intravenous therapy is required
- Cardiac monitoring equipment – more unwell patient or cardiac complications of infection as occurs with Lyme disease
- Blood glucose monitoring equipment – diabetic patient

- Specialist food brought by relatives – suggests supportive family and cultural differences
- Cards and flowers – a good indicator that the patient has a supportive network of family and friends.

- Leuconychia (white nails) occurs with chronic liver disease.
- Koilonychia (spoon-shaped nails) occurs with iron-deficiency anaemia.

HANDS

A close inspection of the hands should be the next step of the examination no matter which body system may be thought to harbour the infection.

Pulse

The rate, rhythm and character of the pulse should be noted. A tachycardia usually accompanies a fever. A bounding pulse may reflect hypercapnia in a COPD exacerbation. Pneumonia can be complicated by atrial fibrillation.

Skin

Hot, sweaty hands suggest the patient is septic. Thin skin and many bruises suggest prolonged steroid use, which can cause immunosuppression and diabetes mellitus. The signs of chronic liver disease seen in the hands include palmar erythema and Dupuytren's contracture. Nicotine staining of the fingers occurs with smoking.

Nails

- Splinter haemorrhages in the nails are usually due to trauma, especially in those who do manual labour, gardening or DIY, but they should raise the suspicion of endocarditis.
- Fungal infections of the nails leads to discoloration (yellow/green), onycholysis (lifting up of the nail from its bed) and hyperkeratosis (thickening).
- Clubbing occurs with the infections shown in Figure 28.1.

Fig. 28.1 Infection-related causes of clubbing

Respiratory	Cardiac	Abdominal
Empyema and abscesses Bronchiectasis Cystic fibrosis	Endocarditis	Chronic liver disease, e.g. due to hepatitis B or C

HEAD AND NECK

Mouth

An inspection of the interior of the mouth can reveal a number of infections. Oral candidiasis presents with white clods on the buccal mucosa and tongue. Tonsillar enlargement occurs with streptococcal pharyngitis, diphtheria and Epstein–Barr virus (EBV) infections. Oral ulceration may result from herpes simplex virus (HSV) 1, or less commonly HSV-2, and syphilis. Koplik spots on the buccal mucosa are pathognomonic for measles.

Eyes

Conjunctival erythema indicates conjunctivitis, which can occur as part of Reiter's syndrome in combination with arthritis and urethritis or gastroenteritis. The sclerae appear yellow with jaundice and are a more sensitive site to detect mild jaundice than the skin. The bilirubin needs to be more than 35 µmol/l for clinical detection. The inside of the lower eyelid is a good area to inspect for possible anaemia. Clinical detection is possible in Caucasian skin with a haemoglobin less than 9 g/dl. With *Loa loa* infections it is occasionally possible to see the worm traversing the conjunctiva.

Any visual symptoms mentioned in the history should precipitate a fundoscopy examination. Immunocompromised and diabetic patients should be routinely screened with fundoscopy for cytomegalovirus (CMV) retinitis and diabetic retinopathy respectively.

Cervical and axillary lymphadenopathy

When acute, painful and mobile lymph nodes are palpated in the neck or axillae, this suggests an oral, respiratory tract or facial infection.

Parotid enlargement

The cheeks appear fuller than normal and may be tender. The diagnosis of mumps needs to be considered.

Sinus tenderness

Tenderness on palpating over the sinuses indicates sinusitis. The positions of the sinuses are shown in Chapter 3.

Ears

Symptoms suggesting otitis media or patients presenting with an upper respiratory tract infection should have an otoscopy examination. An erythematous, swollen eardrum with a fluid level apparent indicates otitis media.

CARDIOVASCULAR

Blood pressure (BP)

The BP should be measured manually both lying and after standing for several minutes. This allows the examiner to check for a postural drop in the blood pressure, which is a more sensitive indicator of hypovolaemia, especially in younger patients who are able to compensate well.

Jugular venous pressure (JVP)

The JVP should be visible at the base of the neck with the patient resting at 45°. It can be differentiated from the arterial pulse, since the JVP has a double waveform and is compressible. If the JVP only becomes visible as the patient lies more horizontally than 45°, it indicates that the patient is hypovolaemic, which could be secondary to septic shock. The JVP can be raised with pericarditis.

Auscultation

The chest needs to be fully exposed for a cardiovascular examination, although some women may feel more comfortable leaving their brassiere loosely placed over their breasts for modesty. Initially the apex position should be felt with the examiner noting where it is in relation to intercostal spaces and whether it deviates from the mid-clavicular line towards the mid-axillary line. Aortic incompetence, for example, can result in a laterally and inferiorly displaced apex beat. The process of auscultating across the praecordium is in fact listening for the function of each of the valves in a separate area (see Fig. 28.2). It is essential to register the presence of both heart sounds and their character, as metal valves (metallic sounding) are more likely to be infected than native ones. Tissue valve replacements are indistinguishable on auscultation from native ones.

The position of the patient on the bed can be used to accentuate different heart murmurs. Asking patients to lean over to their left side increases mitral murmurs, and leaning forward makes the murmur of aortic incompetence more audible. The relationship to breathing also makes a difference: left-sided murmurs are loudest in *Expiration* and right-sided murmurs in *Inspiration*.

Any murmur should be documented with respect to the grade, character, timing within the cardiac cycle, the position where it was loudest, and the radiation, for example 4/6 pansystolic murmur, loudest at the apex and radiating to the axilla (mitral incompetence).

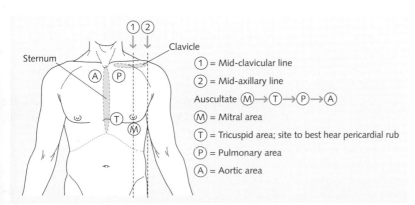

Fig. 28.2 Praecordial positions for the heart valves.

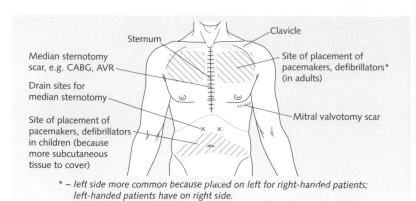

Fig. 28.3 Praecordial cardiac scars and pacemaker/defibrillator locations. CABG, coronary artery bypass graft; AVR, aortic valve repair/replacement. * Left side more common, because placed on left for right-handed patients; in left-handed patients, placement is on the right side.

Labels in figure:
Sternum
Clavicle
Median sternotomy scar, e.g. CABG, AVR
Site of placement of pacemakers, defibrillators* (in adults)
Drain sites for median sternotomy
Site of placement of pacemakers, defibrillators in children (because more subcutaneous tissue to cover)
Mitral valvotomy scar

– left side more common because placed on left for right-handed patients; left-handed patients have on right side.

Hearing a new murmur in a patient with a fever equals endocarditis until proved otherwise.

The pericardial rub of pericarditis sounds like someone crunching a crisp packet. It is audible throughout the cardiac cycle and usually best heard at the lower left sternal edge.

Extras

Whilst examining the praecordium, note should be made of any scars or pacemakers/defibrillators. The likely positions are shown in Figure 28.3. A scar from a valve replacement operation would be important to note in a suspected case of endocarditis. A fever in a patient with a recent pacemaker placement could be related to a non-sterile insertion.

RESPIRATORY

As with the cardiovascular examination, the chest needs to be fully exposed to ensure signs are not missed. Watching the patient take a deep breath in allows the examiner to identify if there is chest movement symmetry. A more sensitive method for detecting this is by placing one's hands around the patient's chest and feeling for asymmetry during inspiration. The asymmetry can arise from a unilateral pleural effusion, empyema or lobar pneumonia.

Percussion

The chest should be percussed both anteriorly and posteriorly from the apices downwards and in the mid-axillary line so as not to miss any focal dullness. A dull area indicates consolidation, whereas a stony dull area reflects fluid in the pleural space.

Auscultation

All areas of the chest should be auscultated, with the examiner paying close attention to the nature of any added sounds (see Fig. 28.4).

Vocal and tactile fremitus

Vocal and tactile fremitus are useful in differentiating between consolidated lung (dull on percussion) and fluid (stony dull). The resonance of the patient saying '99' increases over consolidated lung but reduces over an area of fluid. The resonance can be detected either by placing the ulnar border of the hand against the chest (tactile) or listening with the stethoscope (vocal). Vocal fremitus is more sensitive than tactile fremitus.

Extras

Whilst examining the chest, note should be made of any scars (see Fig. 28.5).

Fig. 28.4 Interpretations of chest signs

Sign	Interpretation
Coarse crackles	Infection, e.g. pneumonia, tuberculosis Pulmonary oedema
Fine crackles	Interstitial lung fibrosis
Wheeze	Exacerbation of asthma or COPD Pulmonary oedema
Bronchial breathing	Lung consolidation, e.g. pneumonia
Reduced breath sounds	Fluid, e.g. pleural effusion, empyema Collapsed lung, e.g. secondary to enlarged lymph nodes with TB
Absent breath sounds	Post-lobectomy or post-pneumonectomy, e.g. for TB Pneumothorax

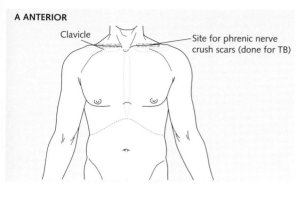

A ANTERIOR

Clavicle

Site for phrenic nerve crush scars (done for TB)

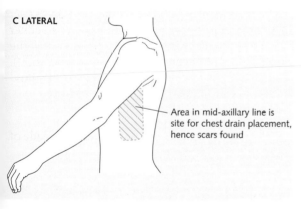

B POSTERIOR

Spine

Scapula

Scar for lobectomy or pneumonectomy

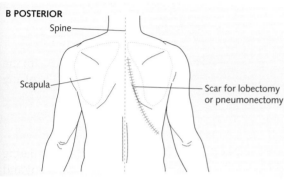

C LATERAL

Area in mid-axillary line is site for chest drain placement, hence scars found

Fig. 28.5 Chest scars (e.g. lobectomy, pneumonectomy, phrenic crush, previous chest drains): (A) anterior; (B) posterior; (C) lateral.

ABDOMINAL

The adequate exposure for an abdominal examination is always quoted as 'nipples to knees' but to help the patient remain relaxed the groin area is covered with a sheet. Inspection of the abdomen can reveal scars, signs of chronic liver disease and masses, as shown in Figures 28.6 and 28.7.

Palpation

It is crucial not to hurt the patient during the examination. Whilst superficially and deeply palpating the abdomen, examiners should keep their eyes on the patient's face the whole time to check for any indication of pain. If there is tenderness present on palpation, it is useful to check for rebound tenderness (pain on removing the hand from pressing into the abdomen) then percussion tenderness (pain on percussing the abdomen), as each of these increases the likelihood of there being peritonitis as the underlying problem.

> Asking the patient to blow out the abdomen and suck it in is a good screening test for the generalized tenderness of peritonitis. It is particularly good with children, as it does not entail touching them so their confidence in the examiner is not lost.

Once a mass is felt, it should be examined in more detail to elicit its nature. Features to check are tenderness, size, mobility and movement with respiration. There are specific manoeuvres to check for organomegaly in the abdomen. By pressing firmly into the abdomen, asking the patient to take deep breaths in and out and moving in the direction shown in Figure 28.8, it is possible to feel an enlarged liver or spleen move down from the costal margin in inspiration. The extent of any hepatomegaly or splenomegaly is expressed in finger breadths below the costal margin.

Palpation of the kidneys involves the examiner placing a hand under the patient's flank and the other on top of the abdomen and attempting to bounce the kidney onto the upper hand from below.

Ascites

There are two methods of testing for possible ascites: shifting dullness and the fluid thrill (see Fig. 28.9). Shifting dullness entails percussing the abdomen from the centre down towards the patient's left flank; when the note turns dull the patient is asked to roll onto the right side while the examiner keeps her or his hand in the same position. After waiting a moment to allow any fluid movement, the examiner re-percusses, and if the percussion note has changed to more resonant then there is shifting dullness and hence ascites.

Fig. 28.6 Abdominal scars and masses (lymphadenopathy, transplanted kidney, ileocaecal TB).

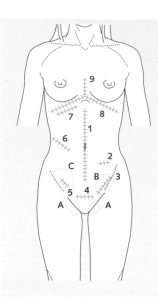

Masses
A = Inguinal lymphadenopathy

B = Kidney transplant (scar over mass)

C = Ileocaecal TB

Scars
1 = Midline, e.g. laparotomy, gastrectomy

2 = Short horizontal scar in left lower abdomen for reversal of hartmanis procedure (i.e. closure of colostomy stoma)

3 = Longer diagonal scar in either iliac fossa (with mass underneath) for kidney transplant

4 = Pfannensteil's incision for caesarean section

5 = Short diagonal scar in right iliac fossa for appendicectomy

6 = Loin scar for nephrectomy

7 = Kocher's incision, e.g. cholecystectomy

8 = Rooftop scar, e.g. liver resection

9 = Mercedes scar, e.g. liver transplantation

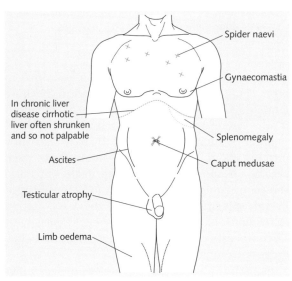

Spider naevi

Gynaecomastia

In chronic liver disease cirrhotic liver often shrunken and so not palpable

Splenomegaly

Ascites

Caput medusae

Testicular atrophy

Limb oedema

Fig. 28.7 Signs of chronic liver disease.

A splenic tip is often only palpable if patients roll slightly over towards their right. This also gives a good opportunity for the examiner to subsequently place the right hand under the patient's left flank to get a good position for the bimanual palpation of the left kidney.

Auscultation

The abdomen should be auscultated for bowel sounds and their character noted. The bowel sounds can be very active in gastroenteritis, high-pitched and tinkling with bowel obstruction, and are absent in peritonitis. Any masses should be auscultated for bruits.

LIMBS

The limbs should be inspected for swelling, erythema and increased temperature, which can be due to a deep vein thrombosis or cellulitis. In suspected cases of cellulitis, checking between the toes for the fungal infection of athlete's foot (tinea pedis) is important, as this is frequently the site of bacterial entry. Swollen ankles can occur with hypoalbuminaemia from chronic liver disease or sepsis; cardiac failure or nephrotic syndrome.

SKIN

Ulcers should be described in terms of their location, extent, depth, border and the nature of the base. The features to look for with rashes are covered in Chapter 1. Desquamation of the skin can occur with measles and scarlet fever.

DIFFERENTIAL DIAGNOSIS

The initial list of differential diagnoses made after the history should be refined after the examination. It should be possible to exclude some of the diagnoses, and others may have been suggested.

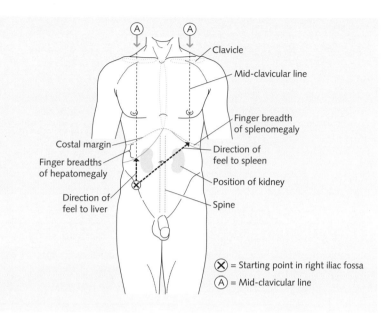

Fig. 28.8 Organomegaly palpable in abdomen.

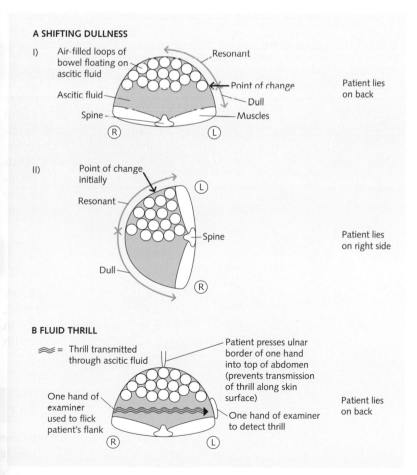

Fig. 28.9 Tests for ascites: (A) shifting dullness; (B) fluid thrill.

Common investigations

The investigations ordered for a patient should be chosen in order to confirm a diagnosis and rule out other possibilities. They are determined by the information gleaned from the history and examination.

> The clinician should be able to justify a clinical reason for each investigation ordered for a patient. 'Blanket' ordering of investigations is not appropriate, as it can then be extremely difficult to judge the importance of an unexpected abnormal result.

However, there are a number of routine tests that are usually appropriate for the majority of patients presenting with an infectious disease.

ROUTINE BLOOD TESTS

Haematology

The full blood count can elucidate numerous abnormalities, as shown in Figure 29.1.

Clotting, i.e. the prothrombin time (PT) and activated partial thromboplastin time (APTT), should be checked:

- Prior to an invasive procedure, such as a lumbar puncture, to ensure it is safe to perform
- With sick patients, as disseminated intravascular coagulation (DIC) can complicate septicaemia, e.g. meningococcal, typhoid and dengue haemorrhagic fever
- In patients with chronic liver disease as the PT is a more sensitive indicator of the synthetic function of the liver than the LFTs.

Biochemistry

- Renal function, usually abbreviated to 'U+E' which stands for 'urea and electrolytes', can be affected by infection. If the patient becomes dehydrated then the urea and creatinine will rise, with the urea rising proportionally higher. In

urinary tract infections such as pyelonephritis the kidney function may be more directly impaired, reflected in raised urea and creatinine, and potassium if severe. A raised urea (> 7 mmol/l) is one of the CURB-65 severity criteria for assessing pneumonia, and a raised creatinine is one of the King's severity criteria for assessing liver failure. Patients with profound diarrhoea can lose large quantities of sodium, potassium and chloride.

- C-reactive protein (CRP) is an acute phase protein produced by the liver. It is raised in infection and is usually more helpful than an ESR. Note that patients with severe chronic liver disease may not have the synthetic function to produce a raised CRP with infection.

- Liver function tests (LFTs) include bilirubin, the transaminases ALT (alanine transaminase) and AST (aspartate transaminase), alkaline phosphatase (ALP) and gamma-glutamyl transpeptidase (GGT). The pattern of derangement can give an indication of the source of the problem: typically a hepatitis causes the ALT and AST to be more raised than the ALP and GGT, whereas an obstruction of the biliary tree results in the ALP and GGT increasing to a greater extent than the transaminases.

- Albumin levels decrease with severe sepsis. A low albumin (<35 g/l) is one of the additional severity markers for pneumonia.

- Glucose level should be checked on all patients. A markedly raised random glucose, i.e. > 11 mmol/l, suggests diabetes mellitus and a formal fasting sample should be checked to ascertain if the infection heralds the presentation of diabetes mellitus. Hypoglycaemia can complicate infections, such as malaria, as well as chronic liver disease.

- Amylase is markedly raised in pancreatitis; lesser increases can occur with a multitude of abdominal pathologies.

- Calcium and phosphate levels are appropriate to check in cases of renal tract infections involving renal calculi, to ascertain if hypercalcaemia may be responsible for the calculi.

Fig. 29.1 Abnormalities of the full blood count

Red cells		
White cells	Anaemia	e.g. leptospirosis, malaria, typhoid, dengue fever
	Neutrophilia	Bacterial infections, e.g. pneumococcal pneumonia
	Neutropenia	Following cytotoxic chemotherapy, leaving patient vulnerable to infection
		Viral infections, e.g. influenza
	Lymphocytosis	Viral infections, e.g. croup, rotaviral diarrhoea
	Lymphopenia	e.g. HIV
	Eosinophilia	Worm infections, e.g. schistosomiasis, strongyloidiasis
Platelets	Thrombocytopenia	e.g. meningococcal septicaemia, malaria, dengue fever
Erythrocyte sedimentation rate (ESR)	Raised	Infection, but non-specific test and increases with age. Very high levels, i.e. > 100, only occur with certain infections, e.g. tuberculosis

The glycaemic control of a diabetic patient usually worsens with an infection, as a state of hyperglycaemia is induced. Infection is one of the causes of diabetic ketoacidosis (DKA). In order to control high blood sugars, diabetic patients may require a sliding scale of insulin. This has also been shown to be beneficial to intensive care patients.

Arterial blood gas (ABG)

An ABG can be a useful investigation in cases of pneumonia. The partial pressure of oxygen (P_aO_2) is one of the additional severity markers for pneumonia, with a $P_aO_2 \leq 8$ kPa being significant. The partial pressure of carbon dioxide (P_aCO_2) is important to check in patients with COPD (chronic obstructive pulmonary disease) because they rely on a hypoxic drive to breathe, and therefore oxygen therapy may result in hypercapnia. pH is one of the King's criteria for assessing the severity of liver failure.

Arterial blood gas sampling can be painful for the patient, so if repeated samples are required, for example with COPD, then capillary samples from the ear lobe can be used as an alternative, or an arterial line should be placed, e.g. in the ITU setting, so that multiple samples can be withdrawn without further venepuncture.

OTHER ROUTINE INVESTIGATIONS

Urine dipstick

This simple bedside test is very effective for assessing possible cases of urinary tract infection (UTI). A positive result for nitrites and leucocytes indicates a UTI. Some patients will also have blood and less often protein present in the urine with an infection. Diabetic patients may have glucose present. Ketones occur in the urine in starvation states and type 1 diabetes mellitus.

Electrocardiogram (ECG)

If an irregular pulse, bradycardia or tachycardia is detected on examination, then the patient should have an ECG. With an irregular pulse, the ECG can clarify whether this is due to atrial fibrillation (AF) or ectopic heart beats. Bradycardia due to heart block can complicate Lyme disease (see Ch. 14). A sinus tachycardia can occur with fevers and is usually tolerated by the patient but supraventricular and ventricular tachycardias may require intervention. Patients with pericarditis have very typical changes on the ECG with 'saddle-shaped' ST elevation globally (see Fig. 23.5).

Chest radiograph (CXR)

The CXR is essential for confirming cases of pneumonia. It will also show which lobes are affected by the pneumonia. The other changes related to

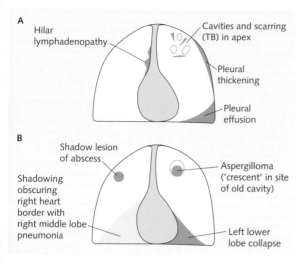

A
- Hilar lymphadenopathy
- Cavities and scarring (TB) in apex
- Pleural thickening
- Pleural effusion

B
- Shadow lesion of abscess
- Shadowing obscuring right heart border with right middle lobe pneumonia
- Aspergilloma ('crescent' in site of old cavity)
- Left lower lobe collapse

Fig. 29.2 Diagram of possible changes on CXR.

infection seen on a CXR are hilar lymphadenopathy, lobar collapse, pleural fluid, old and current tuberculosis, cavities, abscesses, septic emboli and aspergilloma, as shown in Figure 29.2.

SPECIALIZED BLOOD TESTS

Blood cultures

Any patient with a fever measuring 38 °C or more should have blood cultures taken in order to try to isolate the causative organism. Multiple sets of cultures taken at different times and from different sites increase the chances of an organism being grown. It is vital to pay meticulous attention to sterile technique when taking the cultures so as not to contaminate the specimens with skin flora (see Fig. 29.3). Further details on cultures are given below.

Blood film

A blood film is examined to:

- Investigate abnormalities of the blood cells
- Detect the presence of organisms.

A leucoerythroblastic picture, i.e. immature white and red cells in the peripheral blood, is seen in severe sepsis. Abnormal lymphocytes are a feature of Epstein–Barr virus (EBV) infection and HIV.

Both thick and thin blood films are required for diagnosing malaria. The thick film has a greater quantity of blood with several layers of cells so there is

an increased chance of seeing *Plasmodium* parasites even with a low parasitaemia. The thin film has just one layer of cells, which enables the species of *Plasmodium* to be identified. African trypanosomiasis can also be diagnosed from thin and thick blood films.

Serology

Serology involves measuring the levels of specific IgM and IgG antibodies to antigens of an organism. IgM antibodies arise acutely and IgG antibodies indicate previous exposure, although rising levels occur with a current infection. One organism may have several antigens and antibodies that can be detected, such as the hepatitis B virus with its surface, core and e antigens and respective antibodies (see Ch. 6). Antibodies can be detected using indirect immunofluorescence, enzyme-linked immunosorbent assay (ELISA; see Fig. 29.4), or complement fixation. Antigens can be detected using antisera (multiple antibodies present) or monoclonal antibodies (specific to antigen).

> It is important to remember that there may be a 'window period' between infection and seroconversion, i.e. the development of detectable antibodies. This is most marked in HIV disease when the delay between infection and seroconversion can be up to 3 months.

When an infection is endemic in an area or the organism is widespread, many of the adult population will have antibodies to the organism. In these instances, a fourfold or greater difference between the acute and convalescent titres of an antibody is suggestive of an infection. By the very nature that a convalescent titre is required, this technique does not give a rapid diagnosis.

Polymerase chain reaction (PCR)

PCR detects active replication of the organism and therefore is a more sensitive test than serology. The other major advantage is the possible speed of acquiring a result (within a few hours), unlike with serology. PCR can be performed on blood as well as other fluids such as cerebrospinal fluid (CSF) and vesicle fluid. Its use is becoming increasingly widespread for a variety of infections. Common applications are identifying *Neisseria meningitidis* from blood and CSF, hepatitis C virus (HCV) from blood and herpes simplex virus (HSV) from CSF.

Fig. 29.3 How to take sterile blood cultures.

1) Identify suitable vein (e.g. in antecubital fossa) and liberally clean area with an alcowipe, iodine or chlorhexidine solution.

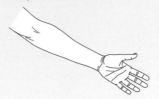

2) Without touching vein after cleaning use syringe and needle to collect 20 ml of blood from patient.

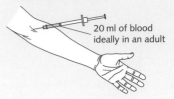

20 ml of blood ideally in an adult

3a) Remove needle used on patient and place in sharps bin. Place new sterile needle on syringe.

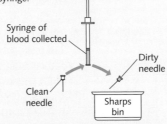

Syringe of blood collected

Dirty needle

Clean needle

Sharps bin

3b) Flick top off aerobic culture bottle without touching the surface and place an alcowipe on the surface of the bottle.

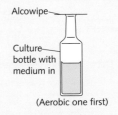

Alcowipe

Culture bottle with medium in

(Aerobic one first)

4) Inject half the volume of blood (i.e. 10 ml) into the culture bottle, (aerobic one first) needle pierces through alcowipe. Once blood injected then agitate bottle to mix blood and culture medium.

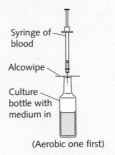

Syringe of blood

Alcowipe

Culture bottle with medium in

(Aerobic one first)

5a) Again remove needle used on aerobic bottle and place in sharps bin. Replace with new sterile needle.

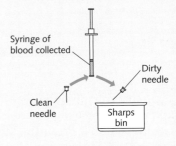

Syringe of blood collected

Dirty needle

Clean needle

Sharps bin

5b) As with aerobic bottles, flick top off anaerobic culture bottle without touching the surface and place an alcowipe on the suface of the bottle.

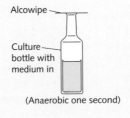

Alcowipe

Culture bottle with medium in

(Anaerobic one second)

6) Inject remainder of blood into anaerobic culture bottle, then agitate to mix blood and culture medium.

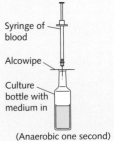

Syringe of blood

Alcowipe

Culture bottle with medium in

(Anaerobic one second)

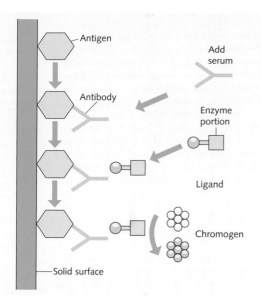

- Presence of any cells, for example red blood cells (RBC), white blood cells (WBC) and their type, casts of cells and malignant cells
- Presence of any organisms, such as bacteria, fungal hyphae, ova, parasites, cysts or viruses (if electron microscopy is used) and their identification.

With a suspected urinary tract infection the presence of > 10 WBC/mm^3 of urine confirms pyuria even if an organism is not seen or grown, as may occur with renal tuberculosis that can result in sterile pyuria. If ≥ 10^5 bacteria/mm^3 of urine are seen, this confirms a bacterial UTI. Glomerulonephritis, which can complicate HCV and Strep. pyogenes infections, gives rise to RBC casts in the urine.

Gram staining is used to classify bacteria into being positive (retain methyl violet stain to appear blue) or negative (appear red from fuchsin counterstain) as well as cocci (spheres) or bacilli (rods) from their shapes. Other stains used are shown in Figure 29.5.

Fig. 29.4 The principles of ELISA. A solid surface is labelled with antigen (the solid phase). The patient's serum is added and if the specific antibody is present, it is held by the antigen and can be detected by a labelling antibody sandwich technique with a colouring agent.
Source: Fox C, Lombard M. Crash Course: Gastroenterology, 2nd edn. Edinburgh: Mosby; 2004: Fig. 24.13.

Paul–Bunnell test

This is performed to test for EBV infection. It involves combining the patient's serum with sheep or horse erythrocytes, and if the heterophile IgM antibodies are present in the patient's serum then the erythrocytes will agglutinate.

Cultures

Cultures of the bodily fluids mentioned above can isolate the organism. Standard practice is for both aerobic and anaerobic cultures to be incubated for 48 hours. Certain organisms require particular culture media to grow and therefore, if they are suspected, specific cultures need to be set up, whereas others such as Brucella species need a prolonged incubation period. For example, Staph. aureus grows on standard agar but M. tuberculosis needs Lowenstein–Jensen or Middlebrook medium to grow; M. leprae and Chlamydia trachomatis only grow in tissue culture.

OTHER FLUIDS

There are many bodily fluids beyond blood which harbour organisms that can be visualized on microscopy and grown in culture. Examples include urine, stool, CSF, sputum, pleural fluid, bronchoalveolar lavage (BAL) washings, ascites, aspirated duodenal or gastric fluid; pus aspirated from abscesses or swabbed from ulcers; and vesicular fluid. When these specimens are sent to the laboratory the request usually states 'MC+S' which stands for 'microscopy, culture and sensitivities'.

Microscopy

When the fluid is visualized under the microscope there are two aspects to the assessment:

Fig. 29.5 Stains

Stains	Examples of use
Gram	Classification of bacteria
Ziehl–Neelsen	Mycobacteria, *Cryptosporidium parvum*
Auramine (fluorescent)	Mycobacteria
Indian ink	*Cryptococcus neoformans*
Silver stain	*Pneumocystis carinii* (or *Pneumocystis jerovecii* as it is renamed)
Giemsa stain	*Chlamydia trachomatis* and *Leishmania* species

Fig. 29.6 Diagram showing antibiotic disc testing on cultures.

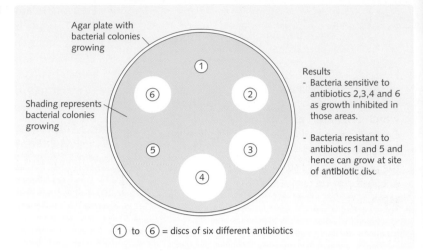

Agar plate with bacterial colonies growing

Shading represents bacterial colonies growing

Results
- Bacteria sensitive to antibiotics 2,3,4 and 6 as growth inhibited in those areas.

- Bacteria resistant to antibiotics 1 and 5 and hence can grow at site of antibiotic disc

① to ⑥ = discs of six different antibiotics

Sensitivities

Once an organism has been grown in culture then its sensitivity to a range of antibiotics can be ascertained. The simplest method for achieving this is with discs of different antibiotics placed on the culture plate (see Fig. 29.6).

Biochemistry

The levels of protein, glucose, lactate dehydrogenase (LDH) and the pH of a fluid can help to differentiate between potential causes. For example, pleural effusions are classified into transudates and exudates by their protein level being either < 30 g/l or > 30 g/l respectively. Light's criteria are a more accurate method to distinguish between transudates and exudates. A low pH and low glucose of the pleural fluid is seen with tuberculosis and empyema.

Light's criteria for an exudate are:
- Ratio of pleural fluid protein to serum protein is > 0.5
- Ratio of pleural fluid LDH to serum LDH is > 0.6
- Pleural fluid LDH is > 2/3 the upper limit for blood LDH levels.

The results from the CSF seen with different causes of meningitis are detailed in Chapter 2.

BIOPSIED TISSUE

The tissues biopsied depend on the clinical suspicion for the source of an infection. An enlarged accessible lymph node can be very useful to biopsy. Often a minor surgical procedure is required to obtain the tissue, for example a laparoscopy for peritoneal biopsies for suspected peritoneal tuberculosis, or if there is a debridement procedure then the tissue removed can be used. The tissue samples should be sent for both histology and culture.

Histology

The histological examination can identify granulomas in tissue such as lymph nodes or the liver that could be caseating, suggesting tuberculosis, or non-caseating, suggesting brucellosis. A haematological cause for a PUO may be revealed, such as lymphoma from a lymph node biopsy or leukaemia from bone marrow. HIV infection can cause typical changes that may be recognized. The stains mentioned above can be used on the tissue samples to isolate organisms, e.g. Giemsa stain on tissue samples in suspected cases of visceral leishmaniasis.

Culture

Typical examples would be tissue debrided in cases of osteomyelitis or necrotizing fasciitis that is cultured to identify the causative organism.

IMAGING

Plain radiographs

- CXR – see above.
- Abdominal radiograph (AXR) – is useful in cases of bloody diarrhoea to check for a dilated colon, which can occur rarely in *Salmonella*, *Campylobacter* and *Clostridium difficile* infections.
- Limb radiographs – are appropriate to investigate the possibility of osteomyelitis when there is deep ulceration, or joint destruction in cases of septic arthritis.

Ultrasound scans (USS)

- Abdominal USS are the most commonly requested in infectious disease cases. They are a safe and effective method for investigating abnormal liver function tests, especially relevant in those showing an obstructive picture. Hepatomegaly, hepatic abscesses and cysts, and a dilated biliary tract with or without cholelithiasis can all be identified. The other organs are also evaluated during the scan; splenomegaly, splenic abscesses, ovarian pathology and free fluid within the abdomen may be demonstrated. In cases of renal tract infections USS are used to check for structural abnormalities of the renal tract including dilatation and renal calculi.
- Chest USS may be used to evaluate the size of a pleural effusion (to assess whether or not it merits drainage) and for guided insertion of a chest drain.
- An abscess elsewhere in the body may be assessed using USS. This is done to estimate the extent of the abscess and allow guided drainage.

Echocardiography ('Echo')

Echocardiography is used to assess the heart valves in suspected cases of endocarditis (see Ch. 23). In cases of pericarditis, it is used to check for the development of a pericardial effusion and cardiac tamponade. If a pericardial effusion requires drainage then this procedure should be performed with Echo guidance.

Computerized tomography (CT) and magnetic resonance imaging (MRI)

These scans give more detailed information than either plain radiographs or USS. Typical uses would include a CT head for the investigation of neurological signs that may be due to toxoplasmosis, or for excluding any contraindications to performing a lumbar puncture, such as significant midline shift; an MRI scan for assessing possible osteomyelitis of the foot or spine, or for the investigation of a PUO when initial tests have failed to find a cause. An MRCP (magnetic resonance cholangiopancreatogram) is the non-invasive alternative to a diagnostic ERCP (endoscopic retrograde cholangiopancreatogram).

The decision between requesting a CT scan or an MRI scan needs to consider the radiation exposure involved, especially in young patients (CT scans involve a much higher radiation dose); the quality of the images for demonstrating the likely pathology (MRI has better definition for soft tissues); and the cost of the scan (MRI is much more expensive).

ENDOSCOPY

Endoscopy is useful not only for visualizing sections of the gastrointestinal tract but also for obtaining biopsies. Examples of the different types are shown in Figure 29.7.

TEST KITS

Optimal is a commercial malarial antigen test kit, looking similar to a pregnancy test kit but performed on blood, that can identify falciparum malaria in a matter of minutes.

Elispot is a test for diagnosing an active tuberculosis infection, compared with latent infection, and has just become commercially available.

Fig. 29.7 Types of endoscopy and their uses

Types of endoscopy	Example uses
Oesophagogastroduodenoscopy (OGD)	Oesophageal candidiasis (including taking biopsies to culture); gastric and duodenal aspirate samples for culture, e.g. tuberculosis, typhoid and giardiasis
Endoscopic retrograde cholangiopancreatography (ERCP)	Diagnostic: dilated biliary tree due to obstructing gallstones Therapeutic: sphincterotomy or stenting to release obstruction
Colonoscopy	Visualize pseudomembranous colitis; take biopsies to distinguish between IBD and an infective cause of bloody diarrhoea or the organism responsible for the chronic diarrhoea seen in HIV disease

IBD, inflammatory bowel disease

Writing up a medical clerking

PURPOSE

The purpose of recording a history and examination in notes is to remind yourself and convey to others what the patient's problems were at the time. Notes must be legible, timed, dated and signed in order to be used by other professionals. Do not use abbreviations unless they are so well recognized as to be easily understood.

A degree symbol is commonly used to denote a negative or absence, e.g. in the sample medical clerking in Figure 30.1, '°immunosuppression' means 'no immunosuppression', '°wheeze' means there was 'no wheeze audible on examination'.

STRUCTURE

Your history and notes will be much easier to follow if they are structured. Follow the same structure used in the history section of the sample medical clerking in Figure 30.1 on the following pages.

ILLUSTRATION

This can be very useful to document images or to convey very precisely the site of pain. Take care if you are using illustrations that, where they convey quantitative rather than qualitative data, they are clear.

FORMULATING A DIFFERENTIAL DIAGNOSIS

It is important that you convey your impression at the time of taking a history. The clinical picture may change later, but valuable clues can be gained by recording early impressions.

INVESTIGATION

If you are ordering investigations, these should be listed and dated so that it is clear when they were ordered. It is also very useful, if a list of investigations is required, that a summary of results is put alongside the list as they come through.

CONTINUITY

Clinical situations are rarely static. For subsequent entries, it is useful to state briefly the purpose or context of your review (e.g. 'called to see because complaining of chest pains).

If the clinical notes are extended because the patient has a long or complex history, a frequent update or summary is very useful to keep everyone focused on the problems. Some clinicians find it useful to keep a problem list which is updated daily. The important element throughout is clarity of thought and intent.

SAMPLE MEDICAL CLERKING

An example of a medical clerking is shown overleaf. It highlights some of the points discussed earlier in this chapter.

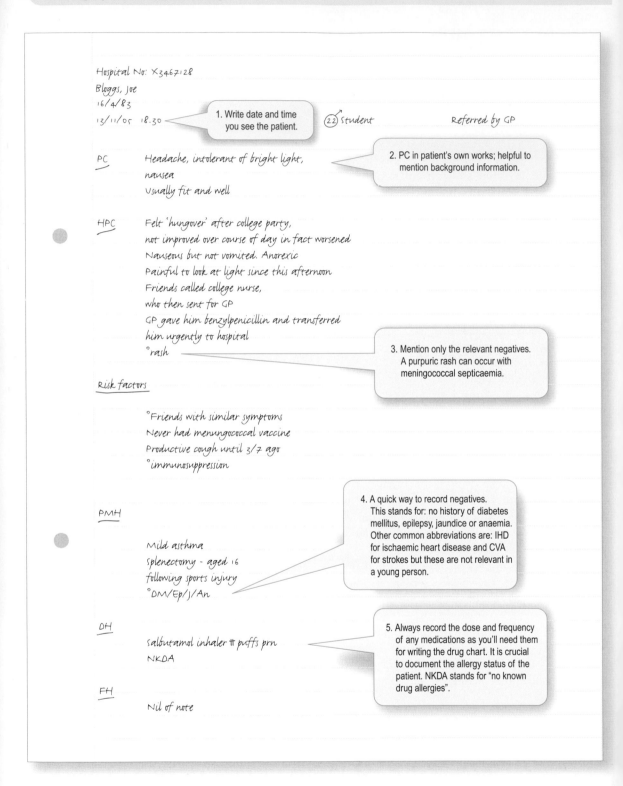

Hospital No: X3467128
Bloggs, Joe
16/4/83
13/11/05   18.30

1. Write date and time you see the patient.

(22) Student   Referred by GP

PC   Headache, intolerant of bright light,
          nausea
          Usually fit and well

2. PC in patient's own works; helpful to mention background information.

HPC   Felt 'hungover' after college party,
          not improved over course of day in fact worsened
          Nauseous but not vomited. Anorexic
          Painful to look at light since this afternoon
          Friends called college nurse,
          who then sent for GP
          GP gave him benzylpenicillin and transferred
          him urgently to hospital
          °rash

3. Mention only the relevant negatives. A purpuric rash can occur with meningococcal septicaemia.

Risk factors

          °Friends with similar symptoms
          Never had menungococcal vaccine
          Productive cough until 3/7 ago
          °immunosuppression

4. A quick way to record negatives. This stands for: no history of diabetes mellitus, epilepsy, jaundice or anaemia. Other common abbreviations are: IHD for ischaemic heart disease and CVA for strokes but these are not relevant in a young person.

PMH

          Mild asthma
          splenectomy - aged 16
          following sports injury
          °DM/Ep/J/An

DH

          salbutamol inhaler ++ puffs prn
          NKDA

5. Always record the dose and frequency of any medications as you'll need them for writing the drug chart. It is crucial to document the allergy status of the patient. NKDA stands for "no known drug allergies".

FH

          Nil of note

Fig. 30.1 Sample clerking.

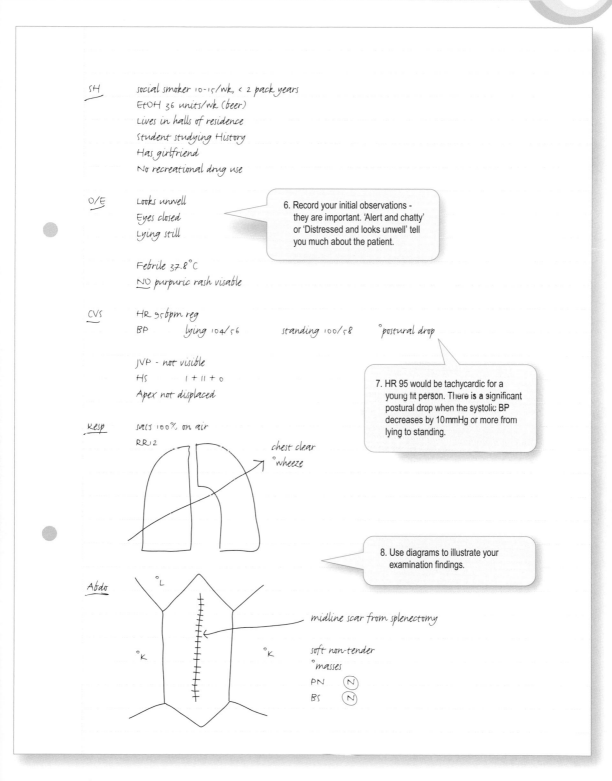

SH   social smoker 10-15/wk, < 2 pack years
      EtOH 36 units/wk (beer)
      Lives in halls of residence
      Student studying History
      Has girlfriend
      No recreational drug use

O/E   Looks unwell
      Eyes closed
      Lying still

      6. Record your initial observations -
      they are important. 'Alert and chatty'
      or 'Distressed and looks unwell' tell
      you much about the patient.

      Febrile 37.8°C
      NO purpuric rash visable

CVS   HR 95bpm reg
      BP   lying 104/56   standing 100/58   °postural drop

      JVP - not visible
      HS   I + II + 0
      Apex not displaced

      7. HR 95 would be tachycardic for a
      young fit person. There is a significant
      postural drop when the systolic BP
      decreases by 10mmHg or more from
      lying to standing.

Resp sats 100% on air
      RR 12
                              chest clear
                              °wheeze

      8. Use diagrams to illustrate your
      examination findings.

Abdo °L

      midline scar from splenectomy

      °K   °K   soft non-tender
                          °masses
                          PN   Ⓝ
                          BS   Ⓝ

Fig. 30.1 cont'd

Neuro   GCS 14/15 (E3, V5, M6)
Kernig's +ve; unable to touch
chin to chest

> 9. It is important to document the score of each of the GCS components so the deficits are recorded and hence any changes can be detected.

CNS   I   not formally tested
II - XII   N but photophobia as distressed by fundoscopy

PNS   UL   LL
         R   L   R   L
Tone   5/5   5/5   5/5   5/5
Power   N   N   N   N
Reflexes +   +   +   +
Co-ordination N N   N   N
Sensation N   N   N   N

ΔΔ   Bacterial meningitis ? meningococcal/ pneumococcal
Viral meningitis

Plan
✓ · Admit
✓ · Bloods inc   blood cultures
                       Meningococcal PCR
✓ · LP for CSF send to Biochem - protein, glucose
                         Micro - MC +S
                         Virology - viral PCR
✓ · IV access and iv fluids
✓ · Neuro observations hourly
✓ · Anti-emetic

> 10. Always include a management plan even when you are still a student. It might not be right but you need to start training yourself to think like a doctor. Tick jobs on list so that it is clear when they have been done.

   · Ceftriaxone 2g bd iv post-LP
   · Senior review

Signature

M N̶

NICKERSON
5050

> 11. Sign your notes, including printed surname and bleep number.

Fig. 30.1 cont'd

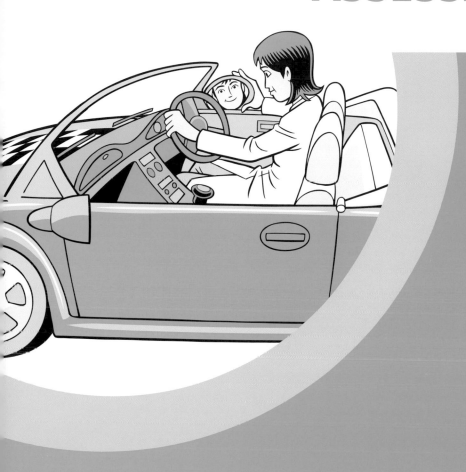

SELF-ASSESSMENT

Multiple-choice Questions (MCQs)

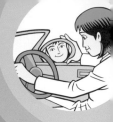

Indicate whether each answer is true or false.

1. **Intravenous drug users (IVDUs):**
   a. Rarely have more than one pathology at a time.
   b. Never exaggerate their drug habit.
   c. Most commonly have mitral valve involvement with endocarditis.
   d. Are at an increased risk of cirrhosis.
   e. Only get deep vein thromboses in the lower limbs.

2. **Pyrexia of unknown origin:**
   a. Can be diagnosed in patients on their presentation to their GP or to hospital.
   b. Cannot be caused by Munchausen's disease.
   c. Is unlikely to be caused by lymphoma.
   d. Cannot be associated with granulomas.
   e. Has an infectious cause in less than 50% of cases.

3. **The following are not given as routine childhood immunizations in the UK:**
   a. Pneumococcal (PCV).
   b. MMR (measles, mumps and rubella).
   c. Hepatitis B.
   d. *Haemophilus influenzae* type b (Hib).
   e. Polio.

4. **A maculopapular rash is not a feature of:**
   a. Measles.
   b. Mumps.
   c. Scarlet fever.
   d. Erythema infectiosum.
   e. Typhus.

5. **Meningitis due to *Neisseria meningitidis*:**
   a. Will demonstrate strings of cocci on Gram stain of the CSF (cerebrospinal fluid).
   b. Can only be diagnosed from CSF.
   c. Has a purpuric rash as an essential feature.
   d. Is rarely fatal.
   e. Is sensitive to penicillins.

6. **The following CSF results would make you suspect bacterial meningitis:**
   a. 500 lymphocytes per mm^3.
   b. Gin clear CSF.
   c. Protein 1.2 g/l.
   d. Glucose 4.2 mmol/l (blood glucose 6.1 mmol/l).
   e. Opening pressure < 10 cm H$_2$O.

7. **Tonsillar enlargement is not a feature of:**
   a. Diphtheria.
   b. Streptococcal pharyngitis.
   c. Epstein–Barr virus.
   d. *Haemophilus influenzae* type b.
   e. Viral pharyngitis.

8. **Diarrhoea:**
   a. Is bloody with *Salmonella* species.
   b. Is steatorrhoeic in nature with *Entamoeba histolytica*.
   c. May have worms visible in the stool with *Giardia lamblia* infection.
   d. Is mild with *Vibrio cholerae* infection.
   e. Associated with abdominal pain is predominant with *Bacillus cereus*.

9. **Concerning hepatitis serology:**
   a. Anti-HBe antibodies are always absent in chronic hepatitis B infection.
   b. Anti-HBc IgG is present post-vaccination against hepatitis B.
   c. HBsAg can be used to distinguish between chronic infection and post-infection states.
   d. The presence of e antigen denotes a low infectivity state.
   e. There is no PCR for hepatitis C available at present.

10. **Regarding urinary tract infections (UTIs):**
    a. A UTI is an indication to check for diabetes mellitus.
    b. A positive urinary dipstick result always indicates there is a clinical infection.
    c. All cases should routinely have a renal tract ultrasound scan.
    d. UTIs are only caused by Gram-negative organisms.
    e. There is typically a lymphocytosis.

11. **In syphilis:**
    a. A hard chancre is typical of secondary syphilis.
    b. Oral ulceration occurs in primary syphilis.
    c. The VDRL is a more accurate test for diagnosing syphilis than the FTA.
    d. Syphilis testing is a routine part of a dementia screen.
    e. TPHA becomes negative after successful treatment of syphilis.

12. **Cellulitis:**
    a. Infrequently has positive blood cultures.
    b. Is always caused by *Staph. aureus*.
    c. Does not occur in conjunction with a DVT.
    d. Only affects the epidermis.
    e. Can only be diagnosed if there is a known port of entry for the bacteria.

13. **Endocarditis:**
    a. Is most commonly caused by *Streptococcus pyogenes*.
    b. Due to *Coxiella burnetii* can be diagnosed from blood cultures.

c. Can be diagnosed with one major and two minor Duke's criteria being met.
d. Is unusual more than 1 year after a prosthetic heart valve is placed.
e. Affects the mitral valve most commonly.

14. **Regarding malaria:**
   a. Rigors only occur with falciparum malaria.
   b. Patients with haemoglobinopathies are at a higher risk of malaria.
   c. With *P. falciparum*, a parasitaemia of 3% is severe malaria.
   d. A dormant stage involving hypnozoites only occurs with *P. vivax*.
   e. Chloroquine is not useful in the treatment of malaria.

15. **Regarding HIV:**
   a. The risk of acquiring HIV is greater than the risk of acquiring hepatitis C from injecting drug use.
   b. The HIV virus does not pass into breast milk.
   c. Two negative HIV tests performed 3 months apart always confirms the patient does not have HIV.
   d. Once the CD4$^+$ cell count has dropped, it will only rise with treatment.
   e. The viral load can become undetectable whilst the patient is on treatment.

16. *Mycobacterium tuberculosis:*
   a. Is not present if three sputum smears are negative.
   b. Can be found in gastric washings.
   c. Can be grown easily from blood cultures.
   d. Gives rise to granulomas that are pathognomonic.
   e. Has a high yield from urine culture.

17. **Multidrug-resistant (MDR) tuberculosis:**
   a. Must be treated with DOT (directly observed therapy).
   b. Requires 9 months of therapy with at least four drugs.
   c. Often does not include resistance to rifampicin.
   d. Must be considered in those from Eastern Europe.
   e. Can be cured with an intermittent antibiotic regimen.

18. **The following drugs are not used in the treatment of tuberculosis:**
   a. Streptomycin.
   b. Cycloserine.
   c. Trimethoprim.
   d. Ethionamide.
   e. Capreomycin.

19. **Therapeutic drug monitoring (TDM) can be useful for:**
   a. Zidovudine.
   b. Gentamicin.
   c. Amphotericin B.
   d. Fluconazole.
   e. Ganciclovir.

20. **The following organisms do not cause pneumonia:**
   a. *Chlamydia trachomatis*.
   b. *Chlamydia pneumoniae*.

   c. Influenza B virus.
   d. *Staphylococcus aureus*.
   e. *Mycoplasma tuberculosis*.
   f. *Klebsiella* species.
   g. *Corynebacterium diphtheriae*.
   h. *Legionella pneumophila*.
   i. *Mycoplasma pneumoniae*.
   j. *Haemophilus influenzae* type b.

21. **Regarding a PUO:**
   a. A bone marrow biopsy will only identify a haematological cause.
   b. Repeating sets of blood cultures is not beneficial.
   c. A young person should routinely have a whole body CT scan to investigate a PUO.
   d. Ideally all medications should be stopped as part of the investigations.
   e. Performing every test you can think of is a good way to diagnose the cause of a PUO.

22. **The following childhood exanthemas are routinely vaccinated against in the UK:**
   a. Chickenpox.
   b. Mumps.
   c. Rubella.
   d. Scarlet fever.
   e. Erythema infectiosum.

23. **Erythema nodosum is not associated with the following infections:**
   a. Tuberculosis.
   b. Orf.
   c. Leprosy.
   d. Yersinia.
   e. Leptospirosis.

24. **The following rashes are correctly paired with the infections that are causative:**
   a. Cutaneous larva currens – non-human hookworm infection.
   b. Cutaneous larva migrans – *Strongyloides stercoralis*.
   c. Erythema chronicum migrans – *Borrelia burgdorferi*.
   d. Erythema marginatum – *Streptococcus viridans*.
   e. Eschar – *Salmonella typhi*.

25. **Regarding measles:**
   a. Koplik spots are a late sign.
   b. The diagnosis can only be made following viral isolation.
   c. Treatment with vitamin A is essential.
   d. It can be complicated by pneumonia.
   e. Patients with measles often develop encephalitis.

26. **The following are not features of Lyme disease:**
   a. Arthritis.
   b. Complete heart block.
   c. Conjunctivitis.
   d. Facial nerve palsy.
   e. Meningitis.

27. Regarding rheumatic fever:

a. An ECG is required for the Duckett Jones criteria.
b. An ASOT (antistreptolysin O titre) > 200 U/ml is sufficient to make the diagnosis.
c. The aortic valve is most commonly affected.
d. The chorea usually precedes the polyarthritis.
e. Post-infection prophylactic antibiotics are not required.

28. Regarding chickenpox:

a. All the vesicles tend to appear simultaneously.
b. Varicella pneumonia is uncommon in children.
c. Post-exposure VZIG (varicella zoster immunoglobulin) is widely used.
d. Antibiotics are never required.
e. Shingles can occur without a patient previously having chickenpox.

29. Regarding meningitis:

a. *Listeria monocytogenes* only causes meningitis in neonates.
b. *Haemophilus influenzae* type b (Hib) is a common cause of meningitis in children in the UK.
c. Fungal meningitis usually occurs in immunocompetent patients.
d. Meningitis associated with a rash must be due to meningococcus.
e. Meningoencephalitis is more likely than meningitis to be due to a virus.

30. The following are more common in encephalitis than in meningitis:

a. Reduced level of consciousness.
b. Neck stiffness.
c. Photophobia.
d. Headache.
e. Purpuric rash.

31. Regarding the management of a patient presenting with neck stiffness:

a. A lumbar puncture must be performed.
b. Antibiotic therapy should ideally be started before the lumbar puncture is performed.
c. Steroids should be given in conjunction with the first dose of antibiotics.
d. Intravenous aciclovir should be avoided in patients who are fitting.
e. Anticonvulsant therapy has no role.

32. Regarding glandular fever:

a. The blood film may show a haemolytic anaemia.
b. The liver function tests (LFTs) show an obstructive pattern of derangement.
c. Splenomegaly is not a feature.
d. Patients should be treated with ampicillin.
e. Glandular fever has no neurological complications.

33. Concerning influenza:

a. Influenza B viruses are responsible for epidemics and pandemics.

b. Oseltamivir should be routinely used in patients with influenza.
c. Asplenic patients do not require immunization against influenza.
d. There is no oral prophylaxis available.
e. *Staph. aureus* is a common cause of secondary bacterial pneumonia.

34. Regarding infection with *Corynebacterium diphtheriae*:

a. There is no exudate associated with the tonsillar enlargement.
b. Stridor is a symptom.
c. The pharynx is always involved.
d. Myocarditis is a complication.
e. Penicillin is the principal treatment.

35. Regarding epiglottitis:

a. Epiglottitis is most common in children over 5 years of age.
b. The first person to examine the patient should urgently attempt to look at the epiglottis.
c. Rifampicin is used for eradication of carriage.
d. Ampicillin is the treatment of choice.
e. Adults are never vaccinated against *Haemophilus influenzae* type b.

36. The following statements are true:

a. Otitis media is usually caused by Gram-negative bacilli.
b. Convulsions can complicate whooping cough.
c. The maxillary sinuses are most commonly affected by sinusitis.
d. A CT scan is the best method of imaging the sinuses for sinusitis.
e. Quinsy (peritonsillar abscess) can complicate diphtheria.

37. The most important investigation for a suspected pneumonia is:

a. Arterial blood gas (ABG).
b. Sputum culture.
c. Blood culture.
d. Chest radiograph (CXR).
e. Chest ultrasound scan.

38. A community-acquired pneumonia would be regarded as severe by the British Thoracic Society (BTS) definition:

a. Only if all the CURB-65 criteria were met.
b. If the patient was more than 65 years old and had a respiratory rate of 32.
c. If a 55-year-old patient had a $pCO_2 > 8$ kPa.
d. If the patient was confused and had a $pO_2 < 8$ kPa.
e. If a 70-year-old patient had a BP of 95/58 and the urea was 7.4.

39. The following are true of *Streptococcus pneumoniae*:

a. It causes community-acquired pneumonia exclusively.

b. It is the most likely cause of an LRTI in an asplenic patient.

c. It rarely causes fatal pneumonia.

d. Organisms will be sensitive to penicillin.

e. Infection may be complicated by acute glomerulonephritis.

40. **The following are true of atypical pneumonias:**

a. Legionella mostly occurs in outbreaks.

b. Patients with *Chlamydia psittaci* always clearly give a history of contact with birds.

c. They include *Klebsiella pneumoniae*.

d. A low sodium and abnormal liver function tests are diagnostic.

e. The chest radiograph may be normal initially.

41. **On examination of a patient with pneumonia the following signs are classically found:**

a. Reduced expansion of the affected side.

b. Stony dull percussion note.

c. Fine inspiratory crepitations.

d. Decreased vocal resonance.

e. Pericardial rub.

42. **The following are not complications of** *Mycoplasma pneumoniae* **infection:**

a. Erythema multiforme.

b. Meningoencephalitis.

c. Guillain–Barré syndrome.

d. Pancreatitis.

e. Haemolytic anaemia.

43. **Regarding mycobacterial disease:**

a. Immunocompetent patients are more likely to develop miliary tuberculosis.

b. Lupus vulgaris occurs exclusively at mucocutaneous junctions.

c. Addison's disease can complicate tuberculosis.

d. Scrofula is a manifestation of *M. avium-intracellulare* (MAI) complex.

e. MAI is more sensitive than *M. tuberculosis* to quadruple antituberculous therapy.

44. **Bloody diarrhoea is not caused by:**

a. *Staphylococcus aureus*.

b. *Campylobacter jejuni*.

c. *E. coli*.

d. *Salmonella enteritidis*.

e. *Entamoeba histolytica*.

45. **The following are infectious causes of chronic steatorrhoea:**

a. Coeliac disease.

b. *Clostridium difficile*.

c. *Giardia lamblia*.

d. *Cryptosporidium parvum*.

e. *Yersinia enterocolitica*.

46. **The following organisms are not paired with the food that they may contaminate:**

a. *Salmonella enteritidis* – chicken.

b. *E. coli* 0157:H7– unpasteurized cow's milk.

c. *Bacillus cereus* – rice.

d. *Clostridium botulinum* – beef.

e. *Staphylococcus aureus* – canned food.

47. **The following are true of cholera infection:**

a. Cholera is never seen in patients in the UK.

b. The decreased production of cyclic-AMP results in marked loss of water and electrolytes in the stool.

c. Dehydration is the usual cause of death.

d. Patients must be treated with antibiotic therapy.

e. There is no vaccine available.

48. **The following are true of** *E. coli:*

a. *E. coli* only causes bloody diarrhoea.

b. Child nursery outbreaks of diarrhoea due to *E. coli* are most commonly due to enteropathic *E. coli* (EPEC).

c. Enterotoxigenic *E. coli* (ETEC) has an enterotoxin which acts like the shigella toxin.

d. Ciprofloxacin improves the outcome of all types of *E. coli* infection.

e. Haemolytic-uraemic syndrome (HUS) is a benign complication seen primarily in children.

49. **Concerning diarrhoea:**

a. *Shigella* infections are associated with cramping abdominal pain and tenesmus.

b. *Entamoeba histolytica* is the great mimicker of an acute appendicitis.

c. Rotavirus typically affects children aged 5–10 years.

d. Culture of *C. difficile* is the best way to diagnose an infection.

e. The asymptomatic carriage of *Entamoeba histolytica* is eliminated by treatment with metronidazole.

50. **The complications of infective gastroenteritis do not include:**

a. Meningitis.

b. Guillain–Barré syndrome.

c. Osteomyelitis.

d. Anaemia.

e. Hyperkalaemia.

51. **Jaundice is not associated with the following infections:**

a. Hepatitis E.

b. Gastrointestinal tuberculosis.

c. Leptospirosis.

d. Hydatid disease.

e. Cytomegalovirus.

52. **When investigating a patient with jaundice, the most important test is:**

a. Transaminase (i.e. ALT and AST) levels.

b. Bilirubin level.

c. Full blood count.

d. Prothrombin time.

e. Liver ultrasound scan

53. **Regarding right upper quadrant (RUQ) pain:**

a. RUQ pain indicates there must be a problem with the liver.

b. A patient with an amoebic abscess is usually more unwell than a patient with a bacterial abscess.

c. RUQ pain associated with rigors suggests cholecystitis.

d. RUQ pain associated with dark urine and pale stools points to a hepatic cause for the jaundice rather than a prehepatic one.

e. The ALT is likely to be higher than the ALP in cholangitis.

54. The following are true of viruses causing hepatitis:

a. Cytomegalovirus (CMV) can be transmitted via blood transfusions.

b. EBV can lead to chronic hepatitis.

c. Hepatitis C is more easily transmitted sexually than by intravenous drug use.

d. Hepatitis A has an incubation period of up to 2 weeks.

e. Adults with hepatitis B are more likely than neonates to develop a chronic infection.

55. Regarding hepatitis A:

a. The virus is lost in the faeces whilst the patient is jaundiced.

b. Splenomegaly is not part of the clinical picture.

c. The diagnosis is usually made from microscopy.

d. There is no vaccine available in the UK.

e. Fulminant liver failure may be a complication.

56. Regarding hepatitis B and C:

a. Worldwide the most important transmission route for hepatitis B is sexual.

b. Acute hepatitis C infection tends to be a severe illness.

c. The risk of contracting hepatitis C from a needle-stick injury is higher than for hepatitis B.

d. There is no antiviral therapy for hepatitis B.

e. Glomerulonephritis is a complication of hepatitis B infection.

57. Regarding the hepatitis viruses:

a. Hepatitis C with genotype 1 has a poor response to treatment.

b. Alcohol intake does not affect chronic hepatitis B and C infections.

c. Coinfection with hepatitis B and D has a better outcome.

d. Fulminant liver failure due to hepatitis E has a very low mortality.

e. Patients co-infected with hepatitis C and HIV are unable to clear the hepatitis C virus when treated with pegylated interferon and ribavirin.

58. Regarding liver infections:

a. *Entamoeba histolytica* infection can be diagnosed from stool culture.

b. Hydatid cysts are exclusive to the liver.

c. Bacterial liver abscesses are usually single.

d. The differential diagnosis of fever and abnormal LFTs does not include *Coxiella burnetii*.

e. The triad of Weil's disease, namely jaundice, haemorrhage and renal impairment, is the commonest form of leptospirosis.

59. Regarding biliary tract infections:

a. Usually a single organism that is commensal to the gastrointestinal tract is responsible for biliary tract infections.

b. Acute cholecystitis tends to produce a deeper jaundice than cholangitis.

c. Gallstones tend to form secondary to a biliary tract infection.

d. Liver flukes are a risk factor for cholangiocarcinoma.

e. Liver flukes are acquired from eating raw or undercooked meat.

60. Regarding lower respiratory tract infections:

a. *Klebsiella pneumoniae* causes community-acquired pneumonia more commonly than nosocomial pneumonia.

b. Blood cultures are positive in about 50% of cases of community-acquired pneumonia.

c. Confusion, a severity marker, is defined as a score on the Abbreviated Mental Test of less than 7.

d. Lung cavitation is a feature of pneumonia due to *Staph. aureus*.

e. An empyema will resolve with a prolonged course of appropriate antibiotics.

61. Regarding lower respiratory tract infections:

a. A negative legionella urinary antigen excludes the diagnosis.

b. Endocarditis can complicate atypical pneumonia.

c. Diarrhoea and vomiting are seen only with *Mycoplasma pneumoniae*.

d. *Pseudomonas aeruginosa* is readily treatable with empirical antibiotic therapy.

e. Metronidazole must be given for all aspiration pneumonias.

62. The following rashes are paired with their complications:

a. Chickenpox – cerebellar atrophy.

b. Rheumatic fever – Huntington's chorea.

c. Rubella – sensorineural deafness.

d. Scarlet fever – necrotizing fasciitis.

e. Erythema infectiosum – haemolytic anaemia.

63. Regarding meningitis, the following statements are not true:

a. Subarachnoid haemorrhage is a differential diagnosis of meningitis.

b. *E. coli* is a rare cause of meningitis in neonates.

c. Rifampicin may be given to close contacts of a case of meningococcal meningitis as prophylaxis.

d. PCR (polymerase chain reaction) can be used to identify pneumococcus as the cause of meningitis.

e. When group B streptococcus causes meningitis, it is frequently acquired at the time of delivery.

64. Regarding urinary tract infections (UTIs):

a. Benign prostatic hypertrophy is protective against UTIs.

b. Sexual intercourse leads to sexually transmitted infections (STIs) rather than UTIs.
c. Haematuria does not occur with a UTI.
d. Confusion is a symptom of a UTI.
e. Rigors are unusual in combination with loin pain.

65. **Regarding the management of urinary tract infections (UTIs):**
    a. A long-term indwelling catheter can be left in situ if intravenous antibiotics are given.
    b. The correct treatment for a UTI secondary to inpatient cystoscopy is oral amoxicillin.
    c. Pyelonephritis requires a 3- to 5-day course of antibiotics.
    d. All renal calculi eventually pass in the urine.
    e. Drinking plenty of water is an important part of management of UTIs.

66. **The following statements about the bacterial causes of a UTI are not true:**
    a. Infections due to *Pseudomonas aeruginosa* are associated with the use of long-term indwelling catheters.
    b. *Staphylococcus saprophyticus* is acquired secondary to prosthetic devices, e.g. intravenous cannulas and catheters.
    c. *Proteus mirabilis* infections can predispose to renal calculi formation, particularly staghorn calculi.
    d. *Klebsiella* species are more commonly acquired nosocomially than from the community.
    e. Antibiotic resistance is becoming an increasing problem with *Enterococcus faecalis*.

67. **Concerning urinary tract infections (UTIs):**
    a. An infection involving the ureters and kidneys must be a complicated UTI.
    b. A negative 'KUB' (kidneys, ureters and bladder) radiograph excludes the diagnosis of renal calculi.
    c. Blood cultures are rarely positive with pyelonephritis.
    d. Not all patients with pyelonephritis need to undergo an ultrasound of the renal tract.
    e. Chronic pyelonephritis results from repeated UTIs in adults.

68. **Regarding gonorrhoea:**
    a. Gonorrhoea is only acquired sexually.
    b. The skin rash associated with gonorrhoea is maculopapular.
    c. Infection is limited to the genital area.
    d. *Neisseria gonorrhoeae* is a cause of infertility.
    e. Penicillin is the first-choice antibiotic for treatment of gonorrhoea.

69. **Regarding sexually transmitted infections (STIs):**
    a. Reiter's syndrome includes the triad of urethritis, arthritis and uveitis.
    b. Non-gonococcal urethritis (NGU) is more commonly asymptomatic in males than in females.
    c. The causative organism for urethritis is usually identified from serology.

d. Chlamydia is caused by *Chlamydia trachomatis* of serotypes L1–3.
e. Chlamydia is the most frequently diagnosed STI in GUM (Genitourinary Medicine) clinics in the UK.

70. **The following statements regarding herpes simplex virus (HSV) infections are true:**
    a. Genital herpes is always caused by HSV-2.
    b. Neonates only contract HSV if their mother has an active infection at the time of delivery.
    c. The ulcers of genital herpes are shallow and painful.
    d. Condoms are an effective method of preventing transmission of genital herpes.
    e. Oral lesions can reactivate to give rise to cold sores, unlike genital lesions.

71. **Regarding STIs:**
    a. Lymphogranuloma venereum causes painful ulcers and lymphadenopathy.
    b. *Treponema pallidum* infection gives rise to chancroid.
    c. Genital warts have to be treated with either cryotherapy or laser therapy.
    d. Once the treatment of genital warts has been completed, condom usage is no longer required to prevent transmission.
    e. Human papillomavirus infection is a risk factor for cervical carcinoma.

72. **Regarding investigations for STIs:**
    a. High vaginal swabs are typically collected to look for candida infections.
    b. Trichomonas is diagnosed by microscopy of a wet film of vaginal discharge.
    c. With syphilis serology, a negative VDRL with positive results for TPHA and FTA means the patient must have latent syphilis.
    d. A biopsy of a genital wart is required to make the diagnosis.
    e. Generalized screening of STIs in patients presenting to a GUM clinic is not useful.

73. **Regarding septic arthritis:**
    a. A joint affected by septic arthritis is always hot.
    b. The most common cause of septic arthritis is *Salmonella enteritidis*.
    c. Septic arthritis arises secondary to bacterial spread from cellulitis.
    d. Septic arthritis requires treatment with intravenous antibiotics, and an orthopaedic opinion is only necessary if there is no resolution after several days.
    e. Empirical therapy for septic arthritis is flucloxacillin.

74. **Regarding osteomyelitis:**
    a. Osteomyelitis tends to arise in children secondary to haematogenous seeding.
    b. Diabetic patients get cellulitis rather than osteomyelitis.
    c. *Pseudomonas aeruginosa* is more likely to cause acute osteomyelitis than chronic osteomyelitis.

d. Plain radiographs give an accurate picture of the current clinical state of the bone.
e. A prolonged course of oral antibiotics is required to treat acute osteomyelitis.

75. Concerning fungal infections:

a. All tinea infections result in 'ring' lesions on the skin.
b. Fungal nail infections are due to *Candida albicans*.
c. Intertriginous candidiasis is treated with oral itraconazole.
d. Skin scrapings that fluoresce yellow under Wood's light are diagnostic for pityriasis versicolor.
e. Infection causing pityriasis versicolor always results in hypopigmentation.

76. Regarding severe skin infections:

a. Severe pain associated with cellulitis has to be due to necrotizing fasciitis.
b. High fever and rigors are uncommon with necrotizing fasciitis.
c. The treatment of blistering, necrotic cellulitis is with high-dose intravenous antibiotic therapy and bed rest.
d. *Streptococcus pyogenes* produces an alpha toxin that is responsible for the clinical picture.
e. A patient with peripheral vascular disease undergoing an amputation must be given prophylactic penicillin (allergies permitting).

77. The following statements are true of skin infections:

a. Permanganate washes are of no benefit in the management of leg ulcers.
b. Erythema with scaling and occasional pustules occurs with candidiasis.
c. Erysipelas is more likely to affect the lower limbs than is cellulitis.
d. *Streptococcus pyogenes* only causes minor skin infections.
e. Plain radiographs are useful in the management of cellulitis.

78. The following are not clinical features of endocarditis:

a. Haemolytic anaemia.
b. Roth spots.
c. Glomerulonephritis.
d. Splenomegaly.
e. Clubbing.

79. Regarding endocarditis:

a. A negative transthoracic echocardiogram (TTE) rules out the diagnosis of endocarditis.
b. Endocarditis only occurs on previously damaged heart valves.
c. The 'HACEK' bacteria cause 3–5% of the cases of endocarditis in the UK.
d. The initial empirical treatment of endocarditis is a combination of penicillins with gentamicin.
e. Libman–Sacks syndrome is a complication of bacterial endocarditis.

80. Regarding pericarditis:

a. Fungal infections do not cause pericarditis.
b. The most common infective cause of pericarditis in the UK is Coxsackie viruses A and B.
c. Bacterial myocarditis often accompanies bacterial pericarditis.
d. Lying down can help to ease the pain of pericarditis.
e. When the pericardial rub becomes no longer clinically audible, this indicates the infection must have resolved.

81. Concerning pericarditis:

a. Pericarditis classically has widespread convex ST elevation on the ECG (electrocardiogram).
b. Development of subsequent T wave inversion in the anterior chest leads means that the pericarditis is secondary to a myocardial infarction.
c. Tuberculous pericarditis should be treated with steroids in addition to antibiotics.
d. In pericarditis, the JVP usually rises on inspiration and there is a drop in the systolic blood pressure of > 10 mmHg on inspiration.
e. Constrictive pericarditis is a complication of viral pericarditis.

82. The most important test in the investigation of fever in a traveller returning from the tropics is:

a. Stool culture.
b. Blood culture.
c. Chest radiograph.
d. Thick and thin blood films.
e. Full blood count.

83. Infection with *Salmonella typhi*:

a. Has diarrhoea as the main feature.
b. May show a hepatitic derangement on the liver function tests (LFTs).
c. Cannot be diagnosed from bone marrow.
d. Is best treated with co-trimoxazole.
e. Does not lead to chronic carriage.

84. Regarding viral haemorrhagic fevers:

a. Jaundice is an early feature of severe cases of yellow fever.
b. The majority of Lassa fever infections result in gastrointestinal haemorrhage.
c. Diarrhoea is an important severity marker in Ebola virus infections.
d. A patient presenting to hospital 28 days after returning from an area affected by Ebola virus should be isolated under strict conditions immediately.
e. The onset of bleeding coincides with the onset of fever and 'breakbone' arthralgia in dengue haemorrhagic fever (DHF).

85. The following are true of rickettsial infections:

a. An eschar is the only skin lesion associated with rickettsial infections.
b. A swinging temperature is classical for *Rickettsiae prowazekii* infection.

c. Culture is the best method to diagnose rickettsial infections.

d. Only oral prophylaxis is available.

e. The complications of rickettsial infections result from the widespread vasculitis.

86. **Concerning schistosomiasis:**

a. The clinical disease results from the immune reaction to the *Schistosoma* organisms themselves.

b. Urinary symptoms usually precede the 'Katayama fever'.

c. Rectal biopsy samples for eggs can be diagnostic in all species of *Schistosoma*.

d. Portal hypertension occurs secondary to *S. haematobium* infection.

e. Praziquantel is effective for eradication therapy in endemic areas.

87. **Regarding trypanosomiasis:**

a. Gastrointestinal complications are a part of the clinical picture of trypanosomiasis.

b. Lymphadenopathy is more prominent in *Trypanosoma brucei rhodesiense*.

c. *Trypanosoma brucei gambiense* is a more acute form of trypanosomiasis, progressing over a period of months.

d. Treatment is only effective if started before the central nervous system (CNS) features develop.

e. Trypanosomiasis is only endemic in Africa.

88. **The following statements regarding worm infections are true:**

a. Roundworms and whipworms are acquired percutaneously.

b. Epilepsy is the most common presentation of cerebral cysticercosis.

c. It is rare for nematodes to migrate through the lungs.

d. All filarial infections result in elephantiasis.

e. The pruritus ani that occurs with pinworm infections results from the migration of the worms to the anus at night.

89. **Concerning leishmaniasis:**

a. There are no skin changes with visceral leishmaniasis.

b. Cutaneous leishmaniasis is the most disfiguring form of the disease.

c. The skin ulcers in cutaneous leishmaniasis only heal with treatment.

d. In order to identify the *Leishmania* organisms microscopically from skin, the sample needs to involve the border of an ulcer.

e. A patient returning from South America with a cutaneous lesion on the lower limb can be treated with topical paromomycin or local cryotherapy.

90. **The following statements are true of leprosy:**

a. Tuberculoid leprosy occurs in those with poor cell-mediated immunity.

b. A symmetrical 'glove and stocking' sensory neuropathy is typical of tuberculoid leprosy.

c. Leprosy skin lesions are more common on the trunk.

d. The clinical suspicion of leprosy can only be confirmed by microscopy of skin smears.

e. All cases of leprosy should be treated with dapsone and clofazimine daily with rifampicin given monthly.

91. **Regarding HIV:**

a. HIV impairs only cellular immunity.

b. Heterosexual intercourse is the most common route of sexual acquisition of HIV in the UK.

c. The majority of patients experience a seroconversion illness.

d. Opportunistic infections do not occur when the CD4+ cell count is above 200×10^6/ml.

e. PCP (*Pneumocystis jerovecii* pneumonia) and other opportunistic infections are the only AIDS-defining conditions recognized.

92. **The following statements are true about antiretroviral treatment:**

a. Pregnant women taking antiretroviral therapy to prevent vertical transmission require two drugs in their regimen.

b. HAART (highly active antiretroviral therapy) usually consists of a combination of non-nucleotide reverse transcriptase inhibitors (NNRTI) and protease inhibitors (PI).

c. Lipodystrophy is always a complication of nucleotide reverse transcriptase inhibitor (NRTI) drugs.

d. Many of the antiretroviral therapies interact with the P450 system, resulting in multiple drug interactions.

e. Lactic acidosis is a side-effect of treatment with protease inhibitors.

93. **Regarding *Pneumocystis jerovecii* pneumonia (PCP):**

a. PCP classically causes the oxygen saturations to increase with exercise.

b. PCP can be diagnosed from microscopy of sputum or BAL (bronchoalveolar lavage) fluid with a silver stain.

c. PCP typically shows basal consolidation on the chest radiograph.

d. Pentamidine is the treatment of choice for PCP.

e. All patients with HIV should receive prophylactic antibiotics against PCP.

94. **Concerning toxoplasmosis:**

a. Patients with toxoplasmosis can present with either encephalitis or cerebral abscesses.

b. If seizures are part of the clinical picture an alternative diagnosis should be sought.

c. Typically a single lesion is seen on the MRI scan.

d. Once the course of treatment is complete, patients do not require additional antimicrobial medication.

e. Patients often require vitamin B_{12} supplements while on treatment, because of the pyrimethamine used in the first-line regimen.

95. **Regarding fungal infections:**

   a. *Cryptococcus neoformans* only causes meningitis.
   b. The immediate treatment for cryptococcal meningitis is fluconazole.
   c. Cryptococcal meningitis can only be diagnosed from Indian ink staining of the CSF (cerebrospinal fluid).
   d. Oral candidiasis gives rise to white plaques covering all surfaces of the tongue and the buccal mucosa.
   e. Oesophageal candidiasis results in ulceration as well as white plaques.

96. **The following are true of gastrointestinal infections:**

   a. Steatorrhoea occurs with *Mycobacterium avium-intracellulare* (MAI) complex infection.
   b. Abdominal pain that can mimic an acute appendicitis results from infection with *Isospora belli*.
   c. A rectal biopsy can be used to diagnose CMV (cytomegalovirus) colitis.
   d. *Cryptosporidium parvum* is diagnosed from seeing spores in the stool on microscopy.
   e. Microsporidia are treated with co-trimoxazole.

97. **Regarding CMV infections:**

   a. CMV infections are more common in HIV patients than in transplant patients.
   b. In CMV retinitis the optic disk appears pale due to the ischaemia.
   c. Pneumonia due to CMV causes a cough productive of large volumes of sputum.
   d. CMV encephalitis responds poorly to ganciclovir.
   e. Patients who have had CMV retinitis always require lifelong prophylaxis thereafter.

98. **The following statements are correct:**

   a. The seborrhoeic dermatitis seen in early HIV disease is due to *Staphylococcus aureus* infection.
   b. Kaposi's sarcoma exclusively affects the skin.
   c. *Aspergillus fumigatus* infection can lead to fatal haemoptysis.
   d. Progressive multifocal leucoencephalopathy (PML) is suggested by multiple contrast-enhancing lesions in the white matter on an MRI scan of the brain.
   e. Rifabutin is necessary as prophylaxis against MAI in HIV-positive patients.

99. **The following are not considered to be AIDS-defining illnesses:**

   a. Oral hairy leukoplakia.
   b. Progressive multifocal leucoencephalopathy.
   c. Chronic herpes simplex infections.
   d. Burkitt's lymphoma.
   e. *Cryptococcus neoformans*.

100. **Regarding tuberculosis:**

   a. Extrapulmonary tuberculosis has to follow pulmonary tuberculosis.
   b. Skin testing (i.e. Heaf and Mantoux tests) is a routine part of the investigations of a suspected case of tuberculosis.
   c. All patients with tuberculosis should be offered HIV counselling and testing.
   d. If the liver function tests rise to double the normal values following commencement on antituberculous therapy then the drugs must be stopped.
   e. An 18-month-old child of a mother with open pulmonary tuberculosis should be followed up closely but does not require treatment unless symptoms develop.

Short-answer Questions (SAQs)

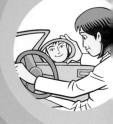

1. How would you manage the following patients:

   a. A household contact of a patient with pulmonary tuberculosis?
   b. A Ukrainian man with a chronic cough and moderate weight loss who has previously received a 3-month course of antituberculous treatment?
   c. A 26-year-old woman with one out of three sputum specimens positive for acid-fast bacilli on microscopy?

2. a. List the typical *Staph. aureus* infections.
   b. What are the potential complications of *Staph. aureus* bacteraemia?

3. What factors do you need to consider when deciding on how to treat a case of community-acquired pneumonia?

4. a. In a patient presenting with bloody diarrhoea, what aspects of the history and examination would make you suspect an infectious cause?
   b. How would you investigate the patient?

5. How do you manage a suspected case of meningitis?

6. a. What types of malaria are there that affect humans?
   b. How do you decide the severity of malaria from the blood film?

   c. How does your treatment alter depending on the type of malaria?

7. a. What is the difference between pyelonephritis and a urinary tract infection, and why is this significant?
   b. What are the potential complications of pyelonephritis?

8. What advice would you give to the following patients:

   a. A 26-year-old woman diagnosed with HIV from antenatal screening?
   b. A 24-year-old homosexual man receiving a negative HIV test result?
   c. A 30-year-old man just diagnosed with HIV after presenting with *Pneumocystis* pneumonia?

9. Outline the measures you would take in managing a patient with Gram-negative shock:

   a. General.
   b. Specific.

10. What organism(s) is (are) most likely with the following symptoms in conjunction with urethritis and what treatment is recommended?

   a. Pustular skin rash over the thighs?
   b. Vaginal pruritus?
   c. Arthritis and conjunctivitis?

Extended-matching Questions (EMQs)

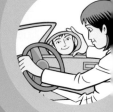

For each scenario described below, choose the *single* most likely diagnosis from the list of options. *Each option may be used once, more than once or not at all.*

1. Childhood infections

A. Measles virus
B. Mumps virus
C. Varicella-zoster virus
D. Parvovirus
E. Group A streptococcus
F. Meningococcus type b
G. *Haemophilus influenzae* type b
H. Rubella
I. Cytomegalovirus
J. Herpes simplex virus.

Instruction: *Match one of the pathogens that commonly affect children to the statements below.*

1. Although a vaccine exists for this and is in use in some countries, it is not part of the routine UK immunization programme. ☐

2. This pathogen may lead to brain damage that presents some time after the initial infection has resolved. ☐

3. Immunization of women of childbearing age has led to a large decrease in congenital infections. ☐

4. Orchitis is a recognized, and relatively common, complication. ☐

5. In addition to causing a rash, the tongue may be involved and give rise to the appearance of a 'strawberry tongue'. ☐

2. Respiratory infections

A. Cytomegalovirus
B. *Staphylococcus aureus*
C. *Pseudomonas aeruginosa*
D. *Escherichia coli*
E. *Legionella pneumophila*
F. *Streptococcus pneumoniae*
G. *Candida albicans*
H. *Mycobacterium tuberculosis*
I. *Coxiella burnetii*
J. *Mycoplasma pneumoniae.*

Instruction: *For each of the following cases of respiratory infection, select a pathogen that is most likely to account for the condition described.*

1. The patient has been ventilated on the ITU for a week following a complicated laparotomy and now has lung infiltrates and mucopurulent secretions coming up the endotracheal tube. ☐

2. A young, previously fit man presents acutely unwell with pneumonia and his chest radiograph shows numerous small abscesses ☐

3. A middle-aged man is admitted to ITU with a severe, acute pneumonia. He is the second ITU admission and the third case of pneumonia occurring in workers at the same factory in town. ☐

4. A 71-year-old woman develops a chest infection 3 days after an uncomplicated operation to remove a Duke's A colonic carcinoma. ☐

5. A 36-year-old woman has a 3-day history of fever, cough and pleuritic pain. She has coughed up a bit of blood in some purulent sputum. She has a pleural rub and her chest radiograph shows segmental consolidation in the left upper lobe. ☐

3. Helminth infections

A. *Strongyloides stercoralis*
B. *Ascaris lumbricoides*
C. *Fasciola hepatica*
D. *Enterobius vermicularis*
E. *Taenia solium*
F. *Schistosoma mansoni*
G. *Loa loa*
H. *Onchocerca volvulus*
I. *Ancylostoma duodenale*
J. *Taenia saginata.*

Instruction: *Match each of the following descriptions with the appropriate helminth from the list above.*

1. One consequence of infection is the development of hepatic fibrosis. ☐

2. This worm is associated with blindness. ☐

3. In the tropics, this worm is associated with seizures and may be the most common cause of seizures in South and Central America. ☐

4. Perianal itching is the hallmark symptom of infection. ☐

5. Biliary obstruction is a recognized complication of infection. ☐

251

4. Skin problems

A. Scarlet fever
B. Meningococcaemia
C. Syphilis
D. Dengue fever
E. Lyme disease
F. Rheumatic fever
G. Tick typhus
H. Strongyloidiasis
I. Filariasis
J. Gonococcaemia.

Instruction: *For the following skin problems, choose the disease most likely to cause the condition.*

1. Erythema chronicum migrans ☐

2. Eschar ☐

3. Pustules on the dorsum of the hand ☐

4. Migratory, serpiginous rash (larva currens) ☐

5. Erythema marginatum. ☐

5. Investigations

A. Ultrasound
B. Magnetic resonance imaging
C. Computerized tomography
D. Blood cultures
E. Paired serology (complement fixation tests)
F. ELISA
G. PCR
H. Plain radiograph
I. Paul–Bunnell test
J. Coombes' test

Instruction: *For each of the following infections, choose the best investigation to help with the diagnosis.*

1. Osteomyelitis of the femur ☐

2. Herpes simplex encephalitis ☐

3. Established HIV infection ☐

4. Miliary tuberculosis ☐

5. Acute brucellosis. ☐

6. Urinary tract infections

A. Pus cells
B. Protein and red blood cells
C. Protein and nitrites
D. *Staphylococcus saprophyticus*
E. *Escherichia coli*
F. *Pseudomonas aeruginosa*
G. *Proteus mirabilis*
H. *Candida albicans*
I. *Enterobacter cloacae*
J. *Klebsiella pneumoniae.*

Instruction: *Match each of the following statements with one of the choices above.*

1. This is commonly associated with community-acquired urinary tract infections but rarely seen in nosocomial infections. ☐

2. Renal stones are associated with this. ☐

3. This is not an uncommon finding in the blood of patients with pyelonephritis. ☐

4. Finding this in catheterized patients is more suggestive of infection than colonization of the bladder. ☐

5. Finding this in the urine can be linked to filling defects in the pelvicalyceal system on urography ☐

7. Tropical infections

A. Falciparum malaria
B. Tick typhus
C. Amoebiasis
D. Malaria
E. Lassa fever
F. Filariasis
G. Typhoid
H. Brucellosis
I. Dengue fever
J. Hepatitis E

Instruction: *Match the following clinical scenarios with the most likely diagnosis.*

1. A young woman returns from a 2-week beach holiday in Thailand and a few days later is admitted with a headache, myalgia and fever. Apart from the temperature (40°C) and a slight petechial rash on her shins, there are no other signs. ☐

2. A 19-year-old man was fully immunized before going backpacking for 3 months in south Asia and he took appropriate antimalarials as prescribed. 2 weeks following his return he is admitted with jaundice. ☐

3. A 30-year-old man from Ghana is admitted 4 weeks after arriving in the UK. He has a fever and is found to have a swollen epididymis. His malaria film is negative. ☐

4. A 54-year-old woman spent 3 months in rural Pakistan visiting relatives. About 3 weeks after returning she presents with a fever and initial malaria films are negative. ☐

5. A 25-year-old man presents a week after returning from his honeymoon in Kenya. He has had 24 hours of fever and vomiting. ☐

8. Sexually transmitted infections

A. Syphilis
B. Chancroid

C. Candidiasis
D. Trichomoniasis
E. HIV
F. Gonorrhoea
G. Genital herpes (HSV)
H. HPV (wart virus)
I. Giardiasis
J. Chlamydia

Instruction: *Match one of the sexually transmissible diseases with each of the following clinical scenarios.*

1. A 20-year-old man presents with urethritis. His urethral swab shows numerous pus cells but there is no growth on culture. ☐

2. A 30-year-old woman presents with an irritating watery discharge, and flagellated organisms are seen on a wet preparation of the discharge. ☐

3. A 20-year-old woman presents with superficial dyspareunia and has noticed vulval itchiness and a white vaginal discharge. ☐

4. A 19-year-old gay man presents with a painless ulcer on the shaft of his penis. ☐

5. A 27-year-old man with a yellow/green urethral discharge presents after his girlfriend has been admitted with pelvic inflammatory disease. ☐

9. Skin, joint and bone infections

A. *Escherichia coli*
B. *Pseudomonas aeruginosa*
C. *Proteus mirabilis*
D. Group A streptococcus
E. *Staphylococcus aureus*
F. *Staphylococcus epidermidis*
G. *Pasteurella multicida*
H. *Mycobacterium tuberculosis*

I. *Streptococcus pneumoniae*
J. *Bacteroides fragilis*.

Instruction: *For each of the following clinical problems, choose the most likely causative organism.*

1. A builder with olecranon bursitis ☐

2. Necrotizing fasciitis of the leg following a trivial injury ☐

3. Prosthetic hip infection ☐

4. An infected cat bite on the hand ☐

5. A foot infection after stepping on a nail while wearing trainers. ☐

10. Antibiotic treatment

A. Gentamicin
B. Rifampicin
C. Doxycycline
D. Penicillin G
E. Vancomycin
F. Clindamycin
G. Ceftriaxone
H. Amoxicillin
I. Flucloxacillin
J. Linezolid.

Instruction: Choose the most appropriate antibiotic for each of the following conditions.

1. Methicillin-sensitive *Staph. aureus* bacteraemia ☐

2. Listeria meningitis ☐

3. Pulmonary tuberculosis ☐

4. Primary syphilis ☐

5. Endocarditis due to *Coxiella burnetii*. ☐

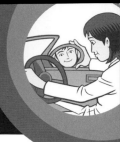

MCQ Answers

1. a. False IVDUs are more likely to have multiple coexisting problems secondary to their habit.
   b. False They may exaggerate their habit in order to receive a greater amount of methadone whilst an inpatient.
   c. False Typically the tricuspid valve is involved in endocarditis in these patients.
   d. True IVDUs are at a high risk of hepatitis C, which as a chronic infection leads to cirrhosis.
   e. False A DVT can occur in both the upper and lower limbs.

2. a. False A PUO should only be diagnosed if no cause for the fever has been found after one week's investigation in hospital.
   b. False Munchausen's disease may lead to a factitious cause for a PUO.
   c. False Lymphomas are a common malignancy to be responsible for a PUO.
   d. False There are a number of granulomatous conditions that can present as a PUO, e.g. brucellosis, tuberculosis.
   e. True Infections are common causes of PUO but still account for fewer than half of the cases.

3. a. False Pneumococcal vaccine is administered in infancy.
   b. False MMR is given at about 15 months of age.
   c. True Hepatitis B is given only to high-risk infants.
   d. False Hib is administered in infancy.
   e. False Polio is administered in infancy and boosters are given subsequently.

4. a. False
   b. True Mumps does not have a rash at all as part of the clinical features.

   c. False
   d. False
   e. False

5. a. False *Neisseria meningitidis* forms diplococci.
   b. False It can be diagnosed by PCR from blood in addition to investigations of the CSF.
   c. False A purpuric rash may occur with meningococcal meningitis but is not a requisite feature.
   d. False It is important to consider the diagnosis without the presence of the rash, since it can be rapidly fatal.
   e. True

6. a. False Acute bacterial meningitis typically has 200–2000 polymorphs per mm³.
   b. False High numbers of polymorphs give a turbid appearance to the CSF.
   c. True The protein level is high (> 0.5 g/l).
   d. False In bacterial meningitis the glucose level is significantly less than two-thirds of the blood glucose level.
   e. False The opening pressure is either normal (10–14 cmH₂O) or raised.

7. a. False
   b. False
   c. False
   d. True *Haemophilus influenzae* type b causes epiglottitis but not tonsillar enlargement.
   e. False

8. a. True
   b. False *Entamoeba histolytica* gives rise to bloody diarrhoea.
   c. False Steatorrhoea may occur with *Giardia lamblia*, and cysts are often visible in the stool on microscopy.

255

d. False   Cholera results in profuse watery diarrhoea that can rapidly lead to profound dehydration.

e. False   *Bacillus cereus* causes vomiting rather than diarrhoea.

9.
a. False   Since e antigen represents a high infectivity state, the presence of anti-HBe antibodies in a chronic infection signifies patients have a low infectivity as they have cleared the e antigen.

b. False   Vaccination against hepatitis B uses HBsAg and therefore only anti-HBs antibodies are present post-immunization.

c. True

d. False   The presence of e antigen represents a high infectivity state.

e. False   PCR is routinely used in the diagnosis of hepatitis C.

10.
a. True

b. False   Catheterized patients in particular may remain positive on dipstick testing even after successful treatment of a UTI.

c. False   An uncomplicated UTI in a woman who has not had multiple UTIs does not warrant a renal tract ultrasound.

d. False   Gram-positive bacteria can cause UTIs, although Gram-negative ones are responsible for the majority of cases.

e. False   Bacterial infections typically result in a neutrophilia on the full blood count.

11.
a. False   A chancre is present in primary syphilis.

b. False   Oral ulceration is present in the secondary phase.

c. False   There are many causes of a false positive result with the VDRL test.

d. True

e. False   TPHA remains positive even after successful treatment.

12.
a. True

b. False   Cellulitis can be caused by many organisms, with streptococci and staphylococci being the most common.

c. False   Concomitant cellulitis and a DVT is now accepted as the clinical picture in some patients.

d. False   The infection affects both the epidermis and the dermis.

e. False   The port of entry for the causative organisms may not be known.

13.
a. False   *Streptococcus pyogenes* infection can be complicated by rheumatic fever.

b. False   *Coxiella burnetii* is a cause of culture-negative endocarditis.

c. False   One major and three minor Duke's criteria are required for diagnosis.

d. False   There is an increased risk of endocarditis with a prosthetic valve both as an early (up to 60 days post-surgery) and late complication.

e. True

14.
a. False   Rigors can occur with all types of malaria.

b. False   Patients with haemoglobinopathies have some protection against severe malaria since the parasites are unable to reproduce as efficiently in the defective red blood cells.

c. True   Anything above 2% parasitaemia is considered severe.

d. False   A dormant phase can occur with any of the benign malarias.

e. False   Chloroquine is an effective treatment for benign malaria, as long as it was not used as prophylaxis.

15.
a. False   The risk of hepatitis C is greater from IVDU.

b. False   Breast-feeding is a mode of transmission for HIV.

c. False   If patients continue to practice high-risk behaviours between their two HIV tests, then they may still be in the 'window period' at the time of the second test.

d. False   The CD4+ cell count varies markedly during the course of a patient's illness, even without treatment.

e. True

16.
a. False   A patient with tuberculosis, including pulmonary, can be smear-negative for acid-fast bacilli.

b. True

c. False   *Mycobacterium tuberculosis* can usually only be cultured from blood in immuno-suppressed patients.

d. False   Caseating granulomas are highly suggestive of tuberculosis but not pathognomonic.

e. False   Urine culture has a poor yield for *M. tuberculosis*

17.
a. False   Treatment does not have to be DOT.
b. False   MDR TB requires treatment for 18–24 months usually.
c. False   MDR TB is diagnosed on the basis of resistance to rifampicin.
d. True
e. False   An interrupted drug regimen and poor compliance may predispose to MDR TB.

18.
a. False
b. False
c. True   The other drugs are all second-line antituberculous agents.
d. False
e. False

19.
a. False   The full blood count needs to be checked since zidovudine can cause myelosup-pression, but measuring the drug levels in the blood is not helpful.
b. True   Drug levels are monitored for gentamicin to avoid toxicity.
c. False   Although amphotericin B is toxic, drug levels are not measured.

d. False   Drug levels are not measured for fluconazole.

e. False   The full blood count needs to be checked since ganciclovir can cause myelosuppression, but measuring the drug levels in the blood is not helpful.

20.
a. True   *Chlamydia trachomatis* causes the sexually transmitted infection chlamydia.
b. False
c. False
d. False
e. False
f. False
g. True   *Corynebacterium diphtheriae* gives rise to diphtheria.
h. False
i. False
j. False

21.
a. False   Bone marrow biopsy tissue can also be cultured to identify an infectious cause.
b. False   Repeating blood cultures from different sites and at different times may elucidate a cause.
c. False   A whole body CT scan is a significant radiation dose and therefore the appro-priateness of the test and possible alter-natives should be carefully considered prior to ordering.
d. True
e. False   Blindly ordering batches of tests is unlike-ly to be helpful as the significance of any abnormalities can be hard to interpret.

22.
a. False   There is currently no routine immuniza-tion against chickenpox in the UK.
b. False   Mumps is not a childhood exanthema.
c. True
d. False   There is currently no routine immuniza-tion against scarlet fever in the UK.
e. False   There is currently no routine immuniza-tion against erythema infectiosum in the UK.

23. a. False   Tuberculosis is a cause of erythema nodosum.
    b. True   Orf can lead to erythema multiforme.
    c. False   Leprosy is a cause of erythema nodosum.
    d. False   Yersinia is a cause of erythema nodosum.
    e. False   Leptospirosis is a cause of erythema nodosum.

24. a. False   Cutaneous larva currens is caused by strongyloidiasis.
    b. False   Cutaneous larva migrans is caused by a non-human hookworm infection.
    c. True
    d. False   Erythema marginatum occurs with rheumatic fever.
    e. False   An eschar is seen with typhus.

25. a. False   Koplik spots usually appear before the rash.
    b. False   The diagnosis can be made clinically in the vast majority of cases.
    c. False   Vitamin A is given in developing countries to malnourished children since vitamin A deficiency is associated with an increased risk of death from measles.
    d. True
    e. False   Encephalitis is a rare complication of measles.

26. a. False   The third stage of the illness involves the joints.
    b. False   Cardiac features occur in the second stage of the illness.
    c. True
    d. False   Neurological features occur in the second stage of the illness.
    e. False   Neurological features occur in the second stage of the illness.

27. a. True   A prolonged PR interval is a minor criterion.
    b. False   The diagnosis is made from the combination of a preceding streptococcal infection, for which a raised ASOT can be used; and either two major Duckett Jones criteria or one major and more than one minor criterion.
    c. False   The mitral valve is most commonly affected.
    d. False   The chorea is usually the latest clinical feature to develop.
    e. False   Prophylactic antibiotics are very important to prevent recurrent episodes of rheumatic fever and further damage to the heart valves.

28. a. False   The vesicles tend to arise in several crops, so there are lesions at variable stages present at the same time.
    b. True
    c. False   Immunocompromised patients and pregnant women, in the peripartum period, with no previous history of chickenpox are sometimes given VZIG post-exposure.
    d. False   Secondary bacterial infection of the vesicular lesions in children commonly results from scratching of the lesions and this may require antibiotic therapy.
    e. False   A patient with shingles must have previously had chickenpox since shingles results from the reactivation of the virus which has been dormant in a sensory ganglion.

29. a. False   *Listeria monocytogenes* typically causes meningitis in neonates and immunocompromised patients.
    b. False   Hib is now a rare cause of meningitis in the UK following the introduction of the vaccine.
    c. False   Immunocompromised patients are vulnerable to fungal meningitis.
    d. False   Although a purpuric rash with meningococcal meningitis is the most important rash not to miss, patients with meningitis secondary to varicella zoster will have the vesicular rash, and immunocompromised

patients with disseminated candida may have a fungal rash.

e. True

30. a. True
b. False The triad of headache, neck stiffness and photophobia is seen both in meningitis and encephalitis.
c. False See above.
d. False See above.
e. False A purpuric rash is associated with meningococcal meningitis.

31. a. False A lumbar puncture should be performed if there are no contraindications.
b. False Ideally, antibiotics should be started post-lumbar puncture. The notable exceptions are if the patient has a purpuric rash or the patient is very sick and the lumbar puncture cannot be performed promptly.
c. True
d. False Seizures may indicate encephalitis, and intravenous aciclovir should be given empirically.
e. False Anticonvulsant therapy is used prophylactically in suspected cases of encephalitis to prevent seizures as well as for treatment.

32. a. True
b. False The LFTs show a hepatitic pattern of derangement.
c. False Splenomegaly can occur.
d. False If patients with glandular fever are treated with ampicillin they usually develop a maculopapular rash.
e. False The neurological complications of glandular fever include aseptic meningitis, encephalitis and Guillain–Barré syndrome.

33. a. False Influenza A viruses are responsible for epidemics and pandemics.
b. False There are specific NICE guidelines regarding the use of oseltamivir in influenza.

c. False Asplenic patients should be immunized against influenza as they are part of the high-risk group for infection.
d. False Oseltamivir and amantadine are both licensed for prophylactic use but amantadine is no longer recommended by NICE for this purpose.
e. True

34. a. False Diphtheria classically presents with a thick exudate over enlarged tonsils; this exudate is also known as a 'false membrane'.
b. False Stridor does not occur.
c. False *Corynebacterium diphtheriae* infection can present with the toxin-related complications arising from a contaminated skin wound.
d. True
e. False Antitoxin is the principal treatment and must be given urgently before bacterial confirmation, in order to minimize the toxin mediated effects.

35. a. False Epiglottitis typically occurs in children under the age of 5.
b. False It is essential that children are kept calm until someone able to intubate can examine them, since airway obstruction can develop rapidly.
c. True
d. False Ampicillin is no longer the treatment of choice since 15% of Hib strains are resistant.
e. False Adult patients who undergo a splenectomy or are rendered functionally asplenic require immunization against Hib.

36. a. False Otitis media is usually caused by Gram-positive cocci.
b. True
c. False Sinusitis most commonly affects the frontal sinuses.
d. False Imaging of the sinuses for sinusitis is best performed via plain radiographs or MRI.

e. False   Quinsy is a complication of streptococcal pharyngitis.

37. a. False   Whilst all the investigations listed may be performed in investigating someone with a suspected pneumonia, the diagnosis will be confirmed by the CXR.
     b. False   See above.
     c. False   See above.
     d. True
     e. False   See above.

38. a. False   The BTS define severe pneumonia as the presence of three or more of the CURB-65 criteria. Note that pCO_2 and pO_2 are not included in the criteria.
     b. False
     c. False
     d. False
     e. True

39. a. False   *Strep. pneumoniae* causes both hospital- and community-acquired pneumonia.
     b. True
     c. False   Severe pneumonia due to *Strep. pneumoniae* has a significant mortality rate.
     d. False   Resistance to penicillin in *Strep. pneumoniae* strains is increasing, with marked variation in prevalence between countries.
     e. False   *Strep. pyogenes* infection can be complicated by acute glomerulonephritis.

40. a. False   Although legionella is classically associated with outbreaks, there are in fact more cases that occur sporadically.
     b. False   Patients with pneumonia due to *Chlamydia psittaci* do not always give a clear history of avian exposure.
     c. False   *Klebsiella pneumoniae* causes typical pneumonia.
     d. False   Whilst patients with an atypical pneumonia may have a low sodium and abnormal liver function tests on

biochemical testing, these results are certainly not diagnostic.
     e. True

41. a. True
     b. False   A stony dull percussion note occurs with a pleural effusion rather than consolidation.
     c. False   Classically a pneumonia gives rise to coarse inspiratory crepitations whereas lung fibrosis produces fine crepitations.
     d. False   Decreased vocal resonance occurs with a pleural effusion rather than consolidation.
     e. False   There may be a pleural rub over an area of lung consolidation; a pericardial rub typically occurs with pericarditis.

42. a. False   The complications of *Mycoplasma pneumoniae* infection include erythema multiforme, Stevens–Johnson syndrome, meningoencephalitis, Guillain–Barré syndrome, myocarditis, pericarditis and haemolytic anaemia.
     b. False   See above.
     c. False   See above.
     d. True
     e. False   See above.

43. a. False   Immunocompromised patients are at an increased risk of miliary tuberculosis.
     b. False   Lupus vulgaris is seen on both cutaneous and mucocutaneous areas.
     c. True
     d. False   Scrofula occurs with *M. tuberculosis*.
     e. False   MAI is less sensitive to quadruple antituberculous therapy than is *M. tuberculosis*.

44. a. True   *Staphylococcus aureus* causes watery diarrhoea due to preformed toxin acting on the small bowel, whereas all the others can cause mucosal damage in the distal small bowel and colon; hence bloody diarrhoea.
     b. False
     c. False

d. False

e. False

45. a. False Whilst coeliac disease is a cause of chronic steatorrhoea, it is not an infectious one.

b. False *Clostridium difficile* causes chronic watery diarrhoea.

c. True

d. False *Cryptosporidium parvum* causes chronic watery diarrhoea.

e. False *Yersinia enterocolitica* infection results in acute watery diarrhoea.

46. a. False *Salmonella enteritidis* is found in undercooked meat, especially chicken.

b. False Although *E. coli* 0157:H7 is classically associated with undercooked beef it can also contaminate unpasteurized cow's milk.

c. False Gastroenteritis due to *Bacillus cereus* occurs from eating contaminated rice.

d. True *Clostridium botulinum* requires anaerobic conditions for growth and hence infection arises from canned and bottled foodstuffs.

e. False The toxins from *Staphylococcus aureus* can be found in processed and canned food as well as in dairy products.

47. a. False Cholera is a rare cause of diarrhoea seen in travellers returning to the UK.

b. False It is the increased production of cyclic-AMP that is responsible for the marked loss of water and electrolytes into the gut lumen.

c. True

d. False Severe cases of cholera may require antibiotic therapy but rehydration is the mainstay of treatment.

e. False There is a vaccine available but it is not efficacious.

48. a. False See below

b. True

c. False ETEC gives rise to watery diarrhoea since the toxin acts like the cholera toxin.

d. False Ciprofloxacin may worsen the outcome in verotoxigenic *E. coli* (VTEC) strain 0157, which is also associated with HUS.

e. False This has a mortality of up to 10% in children.

49. a. True

b. False The abdominal pain occurring with *Yersinia enterocolitica* infections can easily be mistaken for an acute appendicitis.

c. False Diarrhoea due to rotavirus is most commonly seen in children under the age of 5 years.

d. False Carriage of *C. difficile* occurs in many healthy individuals and so infection is best determined by detection of the toxin not culture positivity.

e. False Treatment of the asymptomatic carriage of *Entamoeba histolytica* is achieved with diloxanide furoate.

50. a. False Meningitis can occur secondary to *Salmonella* infection.

b. False Guillain–Barré syndrome may be precipitated by *Campylobacter jejuni* infection.

c. False Osteomyelitis can occur secondary to *Salmonella* infection.

d. False Heavy blood loss into the stool from an ulcerated mucosal wall can result in anaemia.

e. True Hypokalaemia can result from severe gastroenteritis due to the electrolyte losses into the stool.

51. a. False

b. True Neither ileocaecal nor peritoneal tuberculosis give rise to jaundice. All the other infections may result in jaundice as part of the clinical picture.

c. False

d. False

e. False

52. a. False
b. False
c. False
d. True   The prothrombin time reflecting the synthetic function of the liver is more valuable in assessing hepatocyte damage than the so-called liver function tests (LFTs), i.e. ALT, AST, bilirubin and alkaline phosphatase (ALP).
e. False

53. a. False   RUQ pain can also be caused by non-hepatic problems, e.g. right-sided lower lobe pneumonia or pyelonephritis.
b. False   Patients with bacterial abscesses are generally more unwell than those with amoebic abscesses.
c. True
d. False   RUQ pain associated with dark urine and pale stools points to a posthepatic cause for jaundice, such as obstructing gallstones.
e. False   In biliary tract infections there is an obstructive picture to the LFTs, i.e. ALP higher than ALT.

54. a. True
b. False   EBV does not occur as a chronic liver infection.
c. False   Hepatitis C is more readily acquired from intravenous drug use than sexually.
d. False   Hepatitis A has an incubation period of 2–6 weeks.
e. False   90% of neonates with hepatitis B develop a chronic infection.

55. a. False   The virus is excreted prior to the onset of jaundice.
b. False   Splenomegaly may be part of the clinical picture.
c. False   The diagnosis is usually made from serology.
d. False   There is a vaccine available in the UK for travellers to high-risk areas.

e. True   Liver failure is a very rare but recognized complication of hepatitis A infection.

56. a. False   Worldwide, vertical transmission from mother to child is the most important transmission route for hepatitis B.
b. False   Acute hepatitis C infection tends to be a mild illness.
c. False   The risk of contracting hepatitis C from a needle-stick injury is 10 times less than for hepatitis B but vaccination against hepatitis B virus has dramatically lowered the risk in healthcare workers.
d. False   Chronic hepatitis B can be treated with interferon alpha, lamivudine or adefovir but there is no antiviral therapy for acute hepatitis B.
e. True

57. a. True
b. False   A heavy alcohol intake can hasten the progression to cirrhosis in chronic hepatitis B and C infections.
c. False   Coinfection with hepatitis B and D worsens the outcome of the hepatitis B infection.
d. False   Fulminant liver failure due to hepatitis E in pregnant women has a significant mortality, up to 20%.
e. False   Studies have shown that patients co-infected with hepatitis C and HIV are in fact able to clear the hepatitis C virus when treated with pegylated interferon and ribavirin.

58. a. True
b. False   Hydatid cysts can occur at multiple sites including lungs, bone and the brain.
c. False   Amoebic liver abscesses are usually single.
d. False   The differential diagnosis of fever and abnormal LFTs includes *Coxiella burnetii* (Q fever).

e. False   The classical triad of Weil's disease is only seen in severe leptospirosis infections, accounting for 10–15% of cases.

59.
a. False   In many cases more than one organism is responsible for biliary tract infections.

b. False   The jaundice with acute cholecystitis tends to be milder than that occurring with cholangitis.

c. False   Biliary tract infections often occur due to bile stagnation secondary to biliary tract obstruction from gallstones.

d. True

e. False   *Clonorchis sinensis* and *Fasciola hepatica* are acquired from eating raw fish and watercress respectively.

60.
a. False   *Klebsiella pneumoniae* causes hospital-acquired pneumonia more commonly.

b. False   Blood cultures are usually positive in less than 30% of cases of community-acquired pneumonia.

c. False   Confusion is defined as an Abbreviated Mental Test score of less than or equal to 8.

d. True

e. False   An empyema requires drainage in addition to appropriate antibiotics for resolution.

61.
a. False   The legionella urinary antigen test only detects serotype 1, which accounts for 80% of cases.

b. True   Endocarditis can complicate pneumonia due to *Coxiella burnetii* (Q fever).

c. False   Diarrhoea and vomiting also occur with *Legionella pneumophila* and *Coxiella burnetii*.

d. False   *Pseudomonas aeruginosa* can be extremely difficult to eradicate and is only susceptible to a limited range of antibiotics.

e. False   Most oral anaerobes are penicillin susceptible, so there is no need to add metronidazole if the aspiration has occurred in the community.

62.
a. False   Chickenpox may cause a benign cerebellar ataxia but does not lead to permanent damage.

b. False   A feature of rheumatic fever is Sydenham's chorea rather than Huntington's chorea.

c. True

d. False   Group A streptococcus can result in both scarlet fever and necrotizing fasciitis but one infection does not lead to the other.

e. False   Erythema infectiosum can cause aplastic anaemia in those with a haemoglobinopathy.

63.
a. False   Subarachnoid haemorrhage is a differential diagnosis of headache, neck stiffness and photophobia (meningitis triad).

b. True   *E. coli* is a common cause of meningitis in neonates, although group B streptococcus is the most common.

c. False   Rifampicin can and is used as prophylaxis for meningococcal meningitis contacts.

d. False   PCR on blood can detect pneumococcus.

e. False   Meningitis due to group B streptococcus occurring within the first week of life occurs as a result of acquisition of the bacteria from the birth canal.

64.
a. False   Benign prostatic hypertrophy is a risk factor for a UTI because unvoided urine stagnates and is liable to become infected.

b. False   Sexual intercourse can lead to both STIs and UTIs.

c. False   Haematuria is more common with pyelonephritis than in a simple UTI but can be present with either.

d. True   In the elderly, confusion may be the only presenting symptom of a UTI.

e. False   Rigors and loin pain are classic symptoms of pyelonephritis.

65.
a. False   A long-term indwelling catheter should be removed in addition to giving the

patient antibiotic therapy to resolve an infection.

b. False   The correct treatment for a hospital-acquired UTI is a second-generation cephalosporin, e.g. cefuroxime, not an oral agent.

c. False   Pyelonephritis should be treated with a 7- to 10-day course of antibiotics.

d. False   Renal calculi over 5 mm diameter may not necessarily pass through the urinary tract and require removal either by lithotripsy or surgically.

e. True

66. a. False   There is a higher risk of *Pseudomonas aeruginosa* causing a urinary infection in those with long-term indwelling catheters.

b. True   *Staphylococcus saprophyticus* is most common in sexually active young women whereas *Staphylococcus epidermidis* is associated with prosthetic devices.

c. False   *Proteus mirabilis* infections can lead to the development of renal calculi.

d. False   *Klebsiella* species are more commonly acquired in hospital.

e. False   The number of resistant strains of *Enterococcus faecalis* isolated is increasing.

67. a. True   Pyelonephritis involves the ureters and kidneys and is a complicated UTI.

b. False   An intravenous urogram should be performed if no calculi are apparent on the KUB radiograph since 10% of renal calculi are radiolucent.

c. False   Blood cultures are more frequently positive with pyelonephritis than a simple UTI.

d. False   All patients with pyelonephritis should have an ultrasound of the renal tract to look for hydronephrosis.

e. False   Chronic pyelonephritis results from repeated UTIs in childhood.

68. a. False   Gonorrhoea can be transmitted vertically from mother to child.

b. False   Gonorrhoea can cause a pustular skin rash, which usually occurs in the genital area but can spread haematogenously to other sites around the body.

c. False   Severe infections may result in septicaemia and septic arthritis.

d. True   *Neisseria gonorrhoeae* can cause pelvic inflammatory disease and hence infertility.

e. False   Many gonococci now produce penicillinase so that third-generation cephalosporins and quinolones have replaced penicillin as first-line therapy.

69. a. False   The triad of Reiter's syndrome consists of urethritis, arthritis and conjunctivitis.

b. False   Females are more likely than males to be asymptomatic with NGU.

c. False   The organism responsible for a urethritis infection is diagnosed by microscopy and/or culture.

d. False   *Chlamydia trachomatis* of serotypes D to K cause chlamydia, whereas serotypes L1–3 cause lymphogranuloma venereum.

e. True

70. a. False   Genital herpes infections are more commonly caused by HSV-2, although HSV-1 may be responsible.

b. False   Mothers with asymptomatic genital herpes infection can transmit the virus to their offspring during delivery but the risk of vertical transmission is highest in those mothers with an active infection at the time of delivery.

c. True

d. False   Condoms may not prevent sexual transmission of genital herpes as there may be lesions left uncovered, so sexual abstinence is imperative until treatment is completed.

e. False   Just like oral lesions, genital lesions can reactivate after treatment and cause recurrent genital cold sores.

71.
a. False   Whilst lymphogranuloma venereum causes painful lymphadenopathy, the ulcers are painless.

b. False   Chancroid is due to *Haemophilus ducreyii*, whereas a chancre is present with primary syphilis.

c. False   Genital warts can also be treated with topical podophyllin or imiquimod.

d. False   Condom usage is necessary for up to 8 months after treatment of genital warts, to prevent further spread.

e. True

72.
a. False   High vaginal swabs are typically taken to screen for *Chlamydia trachomatis* infections.

b. True

c. False   A negative VDRL with positive results for TPHA and FTA can occur with early primary, latent, tertiary and treated syphilis.

d. False   The diagnosis of genital warts can usually be made clinically without a biopsy being necessary.

e. False   If the patient consents, then a general screen of STIs should be performed as many infections are asymptomatic.

73.
a. False   Septic arthritis due to tuberculosis produces a cold joint.

b. False   Whilst *Salmonella enteritidis* is a common cause of septic arthritis in sickle cell patients, the most common cause in the general population is *Staphylococcus aureus*.

c. False   Septic arthritis can result from both local and haematogenous spread.

d. False   Septic arthritis can destroy a joint in a matter of hours so an urgent orthopaedic opinion is crucial. A washout of the joint can be an essential addition to the intravenous antibiotic therapy required for a successful resolution of the infection.

e. True

74.
a. True

b. False   Diabetic patients are liable to get osteomyelitis secondary to cellulitis associated with ulceration, since the ulcers are slow to heal, hence allowing time for extension of the infection down to bone.

c. False   On the contrary, *Pseudomonas aeruginosa* is more likely to cause chronic osteomyelitis than acute osteomyelitis.

d. False   Radiographs may lag 1–2 weeks behind the clinical picture.

e. False   A prolonged course of intravenous antibiotics is usually required initially to treat osteomyelitis and this is usually followed by prolonged oral antibiotic therapy.

75.
a. False   Tinea capitis can result in a kerion on the scalp, tinea pedis is athlete's foot and tinea unguium affects the nails.

b. False   The differential diagnosis of fungal nail infections includes both tinea unguium and *C. albicans*

c. False   Only extensive skin involvement with candidiasis or nail infections require oral therapy; topical therapy is fine for most infections.

d. True

e. False   The change in pigmentation that occurs in pityriasis versicolor depends on the patient's natural skin colour.

76.
a. False   The differential diagnosis of cellulitis with severe pain is necrotizing fasciitis and clostridial gas gangrene.

b. False   A patient with necrotizing fasciitis usually suffers with high fever and rigors.

c. False   In both necrotizing fasciitis and clostridial gas gangrene the most important part of the management is urgent surgical debridement and possibly amputation depending on the severity. Antibiotics alone are insufficient.

d. False   *Clostridium perfringens* produces an alpha toxin (phospholipase), whereas

Streptococcus pyogenes produces exotoxins, such as streptokinase and hyaluronidase.

e. True   A patient with peripheral vascular disease undergoing an amputation is at risk of clostridial gas gangrene and therefore must be given prophylactic penicillin (allergies permitting).

77. a. False   Permanganate washes can be very useful in helping to dry out ulcers and the solution acts as an antiseptic.

b. False   Erythema with scaling and occasional pustules is seen with tinea corporis, whereas candidiasis does not scale and tends to have more pustules as well as vesicles.

c. False   Erysipelas is more likely than cellulitis to affect the face and cellulitis most commonly affects the legs.

d. False   *Streptococcus pyogenes* can cause necrotizing fasciitis as well as erysipelas and cellulitis.

e. True   Plain radiographs can be used to detect gas in the tissues indicating necrotizing fasciitis or gas gangrene; or bone involvement from osteomyelitis secondary to the cellulitis.

78. a. True   Patients with endocarditis have a normochromic normocytic anaemia, which is either secondary to splenomegaly or an anaemia of chronic disease. The other clinical features can all occur with endocarditis.

b. False

c. False

d. False

e. False

79. a. False   If the clinical suspicion remains high despite a negative TTE result, then a transoesophageal echocardiogram (TOE) should be performed.

b. False   Endocarditis is more likely to occur on damaged or prosthetic heart valves but

virulent bacteria, such as *Staph. aureus*, are able to infect normal valves.

c. False   The 'HACEK' bacteria are a very rare cause of endocarditis.

d. True

e. False   Libman–Sacks syndrome, or systemic lupus erythematosus (SLE)-related endocarditis as it is otherwise known, is one of the non-infective causes of endocarditis.

80. a. False   Fungal infections are a rare cause of pericarditis.

b. True

c. False   While viral myocarditis can accompany viral pericarditis, bacterial myocarditis is extremely rare.

d. False   Classically the pain of pericarditis is lessened by sitting forward and exacerbated by lying down.

e. False   The development of a reactive pericardial effusion leads to the loss of the pericardial rub.

81. a. False   Pericarditis classically has widespread concave ST elevation on the ECG initially and subsequently T wave inversion develops.

b. False   See above.

c. True   Trials indicate that steroid therapy in addition to antituberculous therapy reduces the risk of subsequent constrictive pericarditis.

d. False   Cardiac tamponade, a medical emergency, can complicate pericarditis and requires urgent pericardiocentesis. The clinical signs of cardiac tamponade are a JVP that rises on inspiration and a drop in the systolic blood pressure of > 10 mmHg on inspiration.

e. False   Constrictive pericarditis complicates bacterial, especially tuberculous, pericarditis.

82. a. False

b. False

c. False

d. True   Malaria should be top of any list of differential diagnoses in a traveller returning with fever from the tropics, since it can be rapidly fatal and is therefore crucially important not to miss. The diagnosis can be confirmed or excluded by examination of three sets of thick and thin blood films taken at intervals.

e. False

83.   a. False   *Salmonella enteritidis* gives rise to gastroenteritis whereas *Salmonella typhi* results in typhoid. Diarrhoea can be a part of the clinical picture more latterly in the illness but is not a prominent feature.

b. True   The hepatitic derangement of the LFTs can be very similar to that seen with the hepatitis viruses.

c. False   Cultures of bone marrow can be extremely useful in diagnosing typhoid.

d. False   Multidrug-resistant strains of *S. typhi* are common so the first-line treatment is now either a quinolone or a third-generation cephalosporin.

e. False   1–3% of infections result in chronic carriage.

84.   a. False   Jaundice is seen in the third phase of a severe case of yellow fever.

b. False   Most Lassa fever infections are asymptomatic.

c. True   The severity of the diarrhoea in an Ebola virus infection is the best clinical indicator of the severity of the disease.

d. False   The viral haemorrhagic fevers: Lassa fever, Ebola virus disease and Congo-Crimean haemorrhagic fever, have a short incubation period so that anyone presenting more than 21 days after exposure does not have the infection.

e. False   The haemorrhagic features of DHF occur from 2–7 days after the onset of fever and 'breakbone' arthralgia.

85.   a. False   An eschar may be seen with Rocky Mountain spotted fever (RMSF) and African tick typhus but is not the only skin lesion to occur. A generalized maculopapular rash can arise with epidemic typhus, RMSF and African tick typhus; this may develop into a purpuric rash. Vesicular lesions are seen with African tick typhus.

b. False   Epidemic typhus, caused by *Rickettsiae prowazekii*, typically results in a high fever that remains high.

c. False   Rickettsiae bacilli are notoriously difficult to culture so the diagnosis of typhus is made using serology.

d. False   Travellers to a high-risk area can take oral doxycycline and there is an immunization to protect against *Rickettsiae prowazekii*.

e. True

86.   a. False   The clinical picture results from fibrosis formation stimulated by the type IV hypersensitivity reaction to the presence of the eggs in the tissues rather than the *Schistosoma* organisms themselves.

b. False   The features of the 'Katayama fever' occur as the first symptoms after the incubation period. Subsequently, urinary symptoms develop in those with *S. haematobium* whereas bloody diarrhoea and abdominal pain arise in those with *S. mansoni* and *S. japonicum*.

c. True

d. False   Portal hypertension can occur secondary to infection with either *S. mansoni* or *S. japonicum*, whereas *S. haematobium* infection can lead to hydronephrosis and chronic renal failure.

e. False   Although praziquantel is effective treatment against all species of *Schistosoma*, the repeated exposures incurred in an endemic area mean that eradication is impossible.

87. a. True   Gastrointestinal complications, such as megaoesophagus, dilated stomach and megacolon, are seen in American trypanosomiasis, otherwise known as Chagas' disease.

b. False   Lymphadenopathy is more prominent in *Trypanosoma brucei gambiense* and can give rise to 'Winterbottom's sign'.

c. False   *Trypanosoma brucei rhodesiense* results in the more acute form of African trypanosomiasis.

d. False   The drugs used for treatment differ depending on whether CNS features have developed, because those used pre-CNS involvement do not penetrate the blood–brain barrier. Treatment is more effective if started before the clinical CNS features arise but can be successful subsequently.

e. False   There are three forms of trypanosomiasis: two African (*Trypanosoma brucei gambiense* and *Trypanosoma brucei rhodesiense*) and one American (*Trypanosoma cruzi*).

88. a. False   Strongyloidiasis and hookworm infections result from percutaneous transmission whereas roundworm and whipworm infections are acquired via the oral–faecal route.

b. True

c. False   Passage through the lungs occurs with strongyloidiasis, hookworm and roundworm infections.

d. False   *Loa loa* infections do not result in elephantiasis.

e. False   It is the eggs laid by the female pinworm (or threadworm) at night that are so intensely itchy rather than the worm itself.

89. a. False   The skin can become hyperpigmented on the face, hands, feet and abdomen with visceral leishmaniasis, hence the alternative name 'kala-azar', which means black sickness.

b. False   Mucocutaneous leishmaniasis is the most disfiguring form of the disease.

c. False   Some skin lesions in cutaneous leishmaniasis heal spontaneously without treatment.

d. True   The border of the ulcer is the active site of infection; hence this area needs to be sampled in order for organisms to be seen on microscopy.

e. False   A patient returning from South America is at risk of being infected with *L. braziliensis* so should be treated with systemic treatment to prevent subsequent mucocutaneous leishmaniasis.

90. a. False   Those with good cell-mediated immunity develop tuberculoid leprosy but those with poor cell-mediated immunity have lepromatous leprosy.

b. False   A symmetrical 'glove and stocking' sensory neuropathy is typical of lepromatous leprosy, whereas nerve palsies are more common in tuberculoid leprosy.

c. False   *M. leprae* prefers cooler conditions for growth; hence the extremities are more commonly involved.

d. False   Leprosy can be confirmed by microscopy of skin or nasal mucosal smears; the histological appearance of skin or nerve biopsies, and PCR.

e. True

91. a. False   HIV undermines both the humoral and cellular immune systems.

b. True

c. False   Most patients are asymptomatic at the time of seroconversion.

d. False   Although the risk of acquiring an opportunistic infection is much higher when the CD4+ cell count falls to below 200×10^6/ml, these infections can occur with a count above this level.

e. False   AIDS-defining illnesses include infectious and non-infectious diseases, e.g. tumours.

92.
a. False — All patients must receive triple therapy as a minimum to prevent the development of drug resistance.
b. False — HAART typically uses two NRTIs and either a PI or an NNRTI.
c. False — Lipodystrophy is a side-effect of therapy but does not always occur.
d. True
e. False — Lactic acidosis occurs with NRTI therapy. There are many concerns over this side-effect (and that of lipodystrophy, see above), especially with long-term treatment.

93.
a. False — Classically the patient desaturates on exercise.
b. True — The fungal hyphae of *Pneumocystis jerovecii* can be seen on microscopy with a silver stain.
c. False — The chest radiograph can be normal or shows diffuse alveolar shadowing, often sparing the lower zones.
d. False — Pentamidine is second-line treatment for PCP; the treatment of choice is co-tri-moxazole with high-dose steroids.
e. False — Patients who have previously had PCP or have a CD4+ cell count less than 200×10^6/ml should receive prophylaxis against PCP with co-trimoxazole.

94.
a. True
b. False — Seizures may be a presenting symptom and are liable to occur until treatment is completed.
c. False — Classically multiple lesions are seen on the MRI scan; if only a single lesion is present then an alternative diagnosis should be sought.
d. False — HIV-positive patients require prophylaxis with co-trimoxazole after their course of treatment to prevent reinfection.
e. False — Since pyrimethamine is a folate antagonist, patients may require folinic acid supplements while on treatment.

95.
a. False — The most common cryptococcal infection is meningitis but lower respiratory tract and disseminated infections do occur.
b. False — Cryptococcal meningitis should be treated initially with amphotericin B and flucytosine, with fluconazole used for the completion of therapy.
c. False — The cryptococcal antigen test on CSF is a rapid method for diagnosing cryptococcal meningitis.
d. False — Oral candidiasis does not affect the lateral borders of the tongue; if these have white plaques then the diagnosis is oral hairy leucoplakia.
e. True

96.
a. False — Steatorrhoea occurs with *Giardia lamblia* infection, whereas MAI infection leads to chronic diarrhoea.
b. False — Acute abdominal pain is typical of CMV colitis but pain is not a feature of *Isospora belli* infection.
c. True — A rectal biopsy demonstrating inclusion bodies is the hallmark of CMV colitis.
d. False — Spores in the stool result from Microsporidia infection whereas *Cryptosporidium parvum* gives rise to cysts.
e. False — Microsporidia are treated with albendazole.

97.
a. False — CMV infections are more common in transplant patients.
b. False — CMV retinitis causes both ischaemia and haemorrhage on the retina, classically described as looking like 'cheese and tomato ketchup' on fundoscopy; the disk is unaffected.
c. False — CMV pneumonia results in a dry cough and desaturation on exercise, like PCP.
d. True
e. False — Lifelong prophylaxis is not required if the patient starts HAART.

98.
a. False — Seborrhoeic dermatitis is associated with the yeast *Pityrosporum ovale*.

b. False   Kaposi's sarcoma affects the skin but can also involve the buccal mucosa, gastrointestinal tract, lungs and lymph nodes.

c. True   In invasive aspergillosis, if the *A. fumigatus* erodes into a pulmonary vessel then the haemoptysis can be massive.

d. False   PML gives rise to multiple lesions in the white matter that do not enhance with contrast.

e. False   Rifabutin should no longer be necessary as prophylaxis against MAI since the CD4$^+$ cell count can be improved with HAART.

99.   a. True   Although oral hairy leukoplakia occurs frequently in HIV-positive patients, is not an AIDS-defining illness. All the other conditions are AIDS-defining illnesses.

b. False

c. False

d. False

e. False

100.   a. False   Extrapulmonary tuberculosis can occur independently of pulmonary tuberculosis.

b. False   Skin testing is mostly used for contact tracing and is not usually performed in the routine investigation of suspected cases.

c. True

d. False   Antituberculous medications should not be stopped because of the development of hepatitis until the liver function tests are five times normal, although this needs to be monitored closely.

e. False   All children under the age of 2 years who are close contacts of 'smear-positive' tuberculosis should be treated.

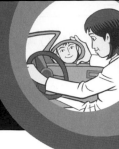
1. a. Household contacts of a case of pulmonary tuberculosis should have a Mantoux skin test and a chest radiograph to assess if they are infected or require prophylactic treatment. Any children under the age of 2 years living in the same household as a case of 'smear-positive' or open tuberculosis, should receive a course of treatment.

b. 3 months is an inadequate course of treatment for tuberculosis, and additionally the former Soviet Union is a high-risk area for multidrug-resistant tuberculosis (MDRTB). Obtaining multiple, good-quality specimens for culture is essential and then performing drug sensitivity testing if any organisms are grown is extremely important to guide therapy. Also, PCR can be used to look for the resistance gene for rifampicin. Expert advice should be sought regarding the drug regimen. The patient should be followed-up by a specialist in either respiratory medicine or infectious diseases who has experience of treating MDRTB.

c. This is a 'smear-positive' case of pulmonary tuberculosis. Treatment with quadruple therapy involving rifampicin, isoniazid, pyrazinamide and ethambutol (recommended regimen by NICE) can be started before the culture results. Baseline blood tests including full blood count, renal and liver function and an ophthalmology review should be performed before starting treatment in light of the potential side-effects of the drugs used. Given the increased incidence of HIV in tuberculosis patients, this woman should additionally be counselled and tested for HIV. She will need follow-up appointments organized to monitor progress, ensure compliance, and to check for potential drug side-effects. The Public Health Department needs to be notified of the case so that they can investigate potential contacts who need screening.

2. a. The typical *Staph. aureus* infections include:
- Skin/soft tissue: cellulitis, wound infections, device-associated infections, abscesses, impetigo, folliculitis, furunculosis, carbuncles, pyomyositis
- Bone/joints: osteomyelitis, septic arthritis
- Respiratory tract: pneumonia, abscesses
- Heart: endocarditis
- Gastrointestinal tract: food poisoning, peritonitis (especially with peritoneal dialysis)
- Urinary tract: urethritis, pyelonephritis
- Eyes: conjunctivitis
- Central nervous system: abscesses, subdural empyema, meningitis.

b. Sites of haematogenous seeding:
- Heart: endocarditis
- Bone/joints: osteomyelitis, septic arthritis
- Respiratory tract: multiple abscesses, pneumonia
- Central nervous system: meningitis, abscesses
- Urinary tract: pyelonephritis.

Other complications from *Staph. aureus* bacteraemia:
- Septic shock
- Multiorgan failure
- Death.

3. The factors affecting treatment choice decisions include:
- Likely causative organisms
- CURB-65 severity scoring (see Fig. 4.3)
- Other severity markers, i.e. clinical (comorbidities, atrial fibrillation, multilobar involvement on the chest radiograph) or laboratory (low serum albumin, hypoxia, leucopenia or leucocytosis)
- Home circumstances and support network of the patient.

4. a. Infectious bloody diarrhoea:
- History:
  - Acute onset
  - First episode
  - Travel history to tropical destination
  - Suspicious or different food eaten
  - Other people affected who ate the same food
  - Associated vomiting
  - Broad-spectrum antibiotic treatment of a hospital inpatient (*C. difficile*).
- Examination:
  - Fever
  - Dehydration.

b. Investigations:
- Stool for microscopy and culture
- Blood tests: full blood count, renal function, blood cultures
- Abdominal radiograph if indicated
- Consider flexible sigmoidoscopy

5. Essential meningitis management:
- If seen by GP, benzylpenicillin given intramuscularly prior to transfer to hospital

- Rapid assessment of how ill the patient is, particularly noting presence of purpuric rash and signs of septicaemia
- Early involvement of senior staff in sick patients, transfer to ITU if appropriate
- Lumbar puncture if no contraindications, as long as will not delay treatment in very sick patients
- Assessment of cerebrospinal fluid (CSF) results (Fig. 2.3)
- For suspected bacterial meningitis (importantly if the CSF is not clear, treatment should not wait for CSF analysis.), empirical antibiotic treatment: intravenous third-generation cephalosporin such as cefotaxime or ceftriaxone for children and adults; intravenous penicillin combined with an aminoglycoside (gentamicin) or a third-generation cephalosporin in neonates
- Steroid therapy in conjunction with antibiotic therapy
- Supportive care as required.

6. a. Types of malaria:
   - *Plasmodium falciparum* – potentially fatal malaria
   - Benign malarias: *P. ovale, P. vivax, P. malariae.*

   b. Severity of malaria:
   - *P. falciparum* seen
   - Parasitaemia > 2%
   - Presence of a schizont.

   c. Treatment:

   - *P. falciparum* – 7-day course of quinine or an artemisinin combination therapy
   - *P. ovale* and *P. vivax* – 3-day course of chloroquine (if not used as prophylaxis) followed by a 2-week course of primaquine to destroy the hypnozoites
   - *P. malariae* – 3-day course of chloroquine (if not used as prophylaxis)

   Supportive care as required, especially important in falciparum malaria.

7. a. Pyelonephritis describes infection that involves the ureters and kidneys, making it a complicated urinary tract infection (UTI), whereas an uncomplicated UTI affects the urethra and bladder. This is significant because an uncomplicated UTI can usually be effectively treated with a 3-day course of oral antibiotics, whereas a complicated UTI requires a 7- to 10-day course of antibiotics that initially is given intravenously.

   b. Complications:
   - Gram-negative septicaemia
   - Chronic renal failure
   - Hydronephrosis
   - Renal scarring.

8. The important issues to cover in each of these cases are:
   a. The risk of vertical transmission from mother to baby is markedly reduced (25–40% to < 2%) by taking triple therapy with HAART (highly active antiretroviral therapy) during pregnancy, delivery by caesarean section and not breast-feeding.
   b. There is a 'window period' that occurs with the antibody HIV test so that it may take around 6 weeks after infection for the test to become positive (and in some cases up to 3 months). Therefore a negative result should be re-checked after this time interval, and only then, if there has been no risk behaviour between the two tests, can he be confidently told he does not have HIV. It would also be important in this case to discuss risk behaviours and prevention measures, e.g. condom use.
   c. This man has AIDS and should be counselled that he is likely to have a positive HIV test. He should have a baseline CD4 count and HIV viral load measurement. He should be informed that he will need to start antiretrovirals once his acute pneumonia has settled. He should be advised to inform his sexual partner(s) that they should seek HIV testing.

9. Gram-negative septicaemia and shock is life-threatening.
   a. General measures: remember the 'ABC' of resuscitation. Affected patients will need intravenous fluids and may need pressor agents, such as noradrenaline (norepinephrine), to maintain blood pressure. Oxygen therapy is needed and a blood gas analysis will help to assess acid–base status. Frequently, central venous access is required to help with fluid management and to facilitate intravenous therapy. It may be appropriate to transfer the patient to an ITU or HDU.
   b. Antibiotic therapy should be given parenterally, ideally intravenously. The choice of drugs should be broad enough to cover organisms such as *E. coli* and *Pseudomonas aeruginosa*. A combination of a cephalosporin and an aminoglycoside would be suitable (e.g. cefuroxime and gentamicin) after cultures have been taken. Recent studies have suggested that activated protein C may improve outcomes. Some evidence exists for giving low-dose corticosteroids but this is more controversial.

10. a. Gonorrhoea caused by *Neisseria gonorrhoeae* – third-generation cephalosporin, ceftriaxone, or quinolones, e.g. ciprofloxacin.
    b. Candidiasis caused by *Candida albicans* – clotrimoxazole cream or pessary; oral fluconazole in more severe infections.
    c. Reiter's syndrome caused by *Chlamydia trachomatis* or other causes of non-gonococcal urethritis such as *Ureaplasma urealyticum*, *Bacteroides*, *Mycoplasma* – tetracyclines, e.g. doxycycline, or macrolides, e.g. erythromycin.

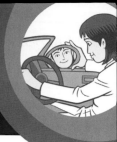
1. **Childhood infections**
   1. C
   2. A
   3. H
   4. B
   5. E

2. **Respiratory infections**
   1. C
   2. B
   3. E
   4. D
   5. F

3. **Helminth infections**
   1. F
   2. H
   3. E
   4. D
   5. C

4. **Skin problems**
   1. E
   2. G
   3. J
   4. H
   5. F

5. **Investigations**
   1. H
   2. B
   3. F
   4. C
   5. D

6. **Urinary tract infections**
   1. D
   2. G
   3. E
   4. A
   5. H

7. **Tropical infections**
   1. I
   2. J
   3. F
   4. G
   5. A

8. **Sexually transmitted infections**
   1. J
   2. D
   3. C
   4. A
   5. F

9. **Skin, joint and bone infections**
   1. E
   2. D
   3. F
   4. G
   5. B

10. **Antibiotic treatment**
   1. I
   2. H
   3. B
   4. D
   5. C

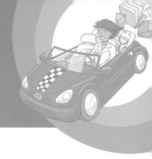

Index

Note: Page numbers in italics refer to illustrations/images.